ANNALS *of* THE NEW YORK ACADEMY OF SCIENCES

DIRECTOR AND EXECUTIVE EDITOR
Douglas Braaten

ASSISTANT EDITOR
Rebecca E. Cooney

PROJECT MANAGER
Steven E. Bohall

EDITORIAL ADMINISTRATOR
Daniel J. Becker

Artwork and design by Ash Ayman Shairzay

The New York Academy of Sciences
7 World Trade Center
250 Greenwich Street, 40th Floor
New York, NY 10007-2157

annals@nyas.org
www.nyas.org/annals

T0344669

THE NEW YORK ACADEMY OF SCIENCES BOARD OF GOVERNORS
SEPTEMBER 2010 - SEPTEMBER 2011

CHAIR
John E. Sexton

PRESIDENT
Ellis Rubinstein [ex officio]

CHAIRMAN EMERITUS
Torsten N. Wiesel

VICE-CHAIR
Kenneth L. Davis

SECRETARY
Larry Smith [ex officio]

HONORARY LIFE GOVERNORS
Karen E. Burke
Herbert J. Kayden
John F. Niblack

TREASURER
Robert Catell

GOVERNORS
Seth F. Berkley
Len Blavatnik
Nancy Cantor
Martin Chalfie
Robin L. Davisson
Mikael Dolsten
Brian Ferguson
Jay Furman
Alice P. Gast
Brian Greene

Thomas L. Harrison
Steven Hochberg
Toni Hoover
John E. Kelly III
Mehmood Khan
Abraham Lackman
Bruce S. McEwen
Russell Read
Jeffrey D. Sachs
David J. Skorton
George E. Thibault

Iris Weinshall
Anthony Welters
Frank Wilczek
Michael Zigman
Nancy Zimpher

INTERNATIONAL GOVERNORS
Manuel Camacho Solis
Gerald Chan
Rajendra K. Pachauri
Paul Stoffels

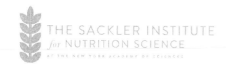

THE SACKLER INSTITUTE
for NUTRITION SCIENCE
AT THE NEW YORK ACADEMY OF SCIENCES

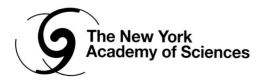

The New York
Academy of Sciences

Published by Blackwell Publishing
On behalf of the New York Academy of Sciences

Boston, Massachusetts
2011

ANNALS *of* THE NEW YORK ACADEMY OF SCIENCES

VOLUME
1229

ISSUE

Nutrition and Physical Activity in Aging, Obesity, and Cancer

ISSUE EDITORS

Young-Joon Surh, Yong Sang Song, Jae Yong Han, Tae Won Jun, and Hye-Kyung Na[a]

Seoul National University and [a]Sungshin Women's University

This volume presents manuscripts stemming from the "2nd International Conference on Nutrition and Physical Activity in Aging, Obesity, and Cancer (NAPA 2011)" held on February 16–19, 2011 in Gyeongju, South Korea. Open access to the articles online is provided by support from the Sackler Institute at the New York Academy of Sciences.

TABLE OF CONTENTS

Become a Member Today of the New York Academy of Sciences

The New York Academy of Sciences is dedicated to identifying the next frontiers in science and catalyzing key breakthroughs. As has been the case for 200 years, many of the leading scientific minds of our time rely on the Academy for key meetings and publications that serve as the crucial forum for a global community dedicated to scientific innovation.

 Select one FREE *Annals* volume and up to five volumes for only $40 each.

 Network and exchange ideas with the leaders of academia and industry.

 Broaden your knowledge across many disciplines.

 Gain access to exclusive online content.

Join Online at **www.nyas.org**

Or by phone at **800.344.6902** (516.576.2270 if outside the U.S.).

The New York Academy of Sciences believes it has a responsibility to provide an open forum for discussion of scientific questions. The positions taken by the authors and issue editors of *Annals of the New York Academy of Sciences* are their own and not necessarily those of the Academy unless specifically stated. The Academy has no intent to influence legislation by providing such forums.

Ann. N.Y. Acad. Sci. ISSN 0077-8923

Introduction to *Nutrition and Physical Activity in Aging, Obesity, and Cancer*

There is strong evidence to show that healthy aging is dependent on multiple lifestyle factors, and the importance of dietary and physical manipulation of optimal health is receiving much more attention, given society's emphasis on well-being and increased longevity. The International Conferences on Nutrition and Physical Activity (NAPA) provide a unique program that discusses both of the essential components for healthy aging, namely nutrition and physical activity. The meetings gather scientists from institutions from around the world with a wide range of competences. The topics presented are comprehensive and in depth, yet clearly focused to promote both scientific understanding and clinical application for use when combating the major degenerative diseases threatening human health.

NAPA 2011 was held on February 16–19, 2011, in Gyeongju, South Korea. Hosted in the ancient historic capital of the Silla Dynasty and surrounded by beautiful natural scenery accentuated by a fresh blanket of snow, the four-day conference was attended by more than 300 delegates from approximately 20 countries. Following the success of the first International Conference on Nutrition and Physical Activity, held in Jeju Island, South Korea on December 12–15, 2009, various scientific talks and poster presentations at the 2011 conference focused on integrating the biological complexity of intracellular signaling with obesity, aging, cancer, and other chronic conditions. A key thematic element of the conference was again the beneficial role of proper nutrition and physical activity in maintaining health and vitality.

A major strength of NAPA 2011 is that many studies, especially those represented by the host institute and organizers, explore the full potential of dietary phytochemicals that affect cell signaling, hormetic adaptation, anti-inflammation, disease prevention, and antiaging. The six main scientific sessions included presentations in the following areas (with apologies to any authors omitted because of space limitations): epigenetic mechanisms and metabolism as a key to histone deacetylase inhibition; hormetic effects of phytonutrients and exercise; mechanisms of calorie restriction–mediated epithelial carcinogenesis; epigenetic epidemiology of gastric cancer; tocotrienols and breast cancer; bioactive substances from marine organisms; aging and oxidative stress/vitamin E uptake; nutrient intake and life span in *Drosophila*; neuroprotective effects of dietary modulators; genome-wide association studies of genetic factors and physical activity; functional foods for the prevention of muscle atrophy; energy balance, metabolism, and cancer prevention; enhancing functional properties of natural compounds; transcriptome analysis and data mining of metabolic pathways in gestational diabetes; therapeutic potential of human pluripotent stem cells; genome biomarkers and clinical outcomes of physical activity; endurance exercise and DNA stability; physical activity and cancer; anti-Alzheimer's disease effects of plant materials; cardiovascular fitness and neurocognitive function; culinary plants and metabolic overload in obesity; polymeric nanomicelles for magnetic resonance imaging (MRI) and therapy; microarray analysis and functional genomics for adipocyte biology; and array-based comparative genomic hybridization (CGH) analysis of genomic aberrations in epithelial cancer.

doi: 10.1111/j.1749-6632.2011.06103.x

In addition to the main scientific sessions, there were eight selected oral presentations by young investigators chosen from submitted abstracts, plus 58 posters covering topics close to the theme of the overall conference. To provide an intimate and welcoming environment, especially for young scientists, a preconference workshop was offered. Titled "How to write a successful scientific manuscript," this half-day workshop consisted of two sessions. The first session highlighted tips for better writing, with three presentations: "How to organize the draft" (by Young-Nam Cha, Inha University, South Korea); "Making the most satisfactory revision" (by Young-Joon Surh, Seoul National University, South Korea); and "Things to consider before you begin writing" (by Lothar Hennighausen, National Institutes of Health, USA). In the second session, editors of three major journals (Douglas Braaten, *Annals of the New York Academy of Sciences*; Fabio Virgili, *Genes & Nutrition*; Myles Axton, *Nature Genetics*) shared their expertise and experience for successfully preparing a manuscript for publication, with brief introductions regarding their respective journals.

NAPA 2011 was organized to integrate multidisciplinary approaches of biomedical research with special emphasis on nutrition and exercise for the management of age-related metabolic disorders. Most of the high-quality and cutting-edge studies presented at NAPA 2011 use a wide range of methods and technologies available in modern biological scientific research. The conference benefited much from the warm hospitality and organizational skills of the hosts, the free and open interchange of scientific ideas, and the more than one dozen sponsors and supporters who were in attendance. Combined with the carefully selected location and accommodations, the conference had an efficient yet relaxed atmosphere.

This special issue of *Annals of the New York Academy of Sciences* provides a synopsis of some of the key presentations from NAPA 2011. As will be evident from the various reports herein, the bar has been raised in preparation for the third conference in the series. We sincerely hope that the NAPA conferences will maintain their tradition of high-quality, diverse science and continue to attract the attention and attendance of leading scientists around the world.

YOUNG-JOON SURH
Seoul National University, Seoul, South Korea

RODERICK H. DASHWOOD
Oregon State University, Corvallis, Oregon

HYE-KYUNG NA
Sungshin Women's University, Seoul, South Korea

LI LI JI
University of Wisconsin-Madison, Madison, Wisconsin

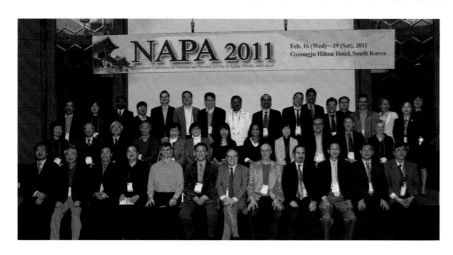

Ann. N.Y. Acad. Sci. ISSN 0077-8923

ANNALS OF THE NEW YORK ACADEMY OF SCIENCES
Issue: *Nutrition and Physical Activity in Aging, Obesity, and Cancer*

Xenohormesis mechanisms underlying chemopreventive effects of some dietary phytochemicals

Young-Joon Surh

College of Pharmacy and Cancer Research Institute, Seoul National University, Seoul, South Korea

Address for correspondence: Young-Joon Surh, College of Pharmacy, Seoul National University, 599 Kwanak-ro Kwanak-gu, Seoul 151-742, South Korea. surh@plaza.snu.ac.kr

A wide variety of phytochemicals present in our diet, including fruits, vegetables, and spices, have been shown to possess a broad range of health-beneficial properties. The cytoprotective and restorative effects of dietary phytochemicals are likely to result from the modulation of several distinct cellular signal transduction pathways. Many dietary phytochemicals that are synthesized as secondary metabolites function as toxins, that is, "phytoalexins," and hence protect plants against insects and other damaging organisms and stresses. However, at the relatively low doses consumed by humans and other mammals, these same toxic plant–derived chemicals, as mild stressors, activate adaptive cellular response signaling, conferring stress resistance and other health benefits. This phenomenon has been referred to as xenohormesis. This review highlights the xenohormesis mechanisms underlying chemopreventive effects of some dietary chemopreventive phytochemicals, with special focus on the nuclear transcription factor erythroid 2p45 (NF-E2)–related factor 2 (Nrf2) as a key player.

Keywords: hormesis; xenohormesis; phytochemicals; adaptive response; chemoprevention

All substances are poisons; there is none that is not a poison. The right dose differentiates a poison and remedy. Paracelsus (1493–1541)

Living organisms constantly cope with a broad spectrum of noxious stimuli or adverse conditions, and the adaptation to external stressors—physical, chemical, biological, and social/psychological—is an essential principle for survival. Interestingly, the response to a stressor is not necessarily linear with regards to the dose, but rather U- or J-shaped. Thus, exposure to a low level of stressful stimulus that is detrimental at higher levels can confer tolerance or resistance to a subsequent insult by the same or related stressor agent or condition. Such an adaptive stress response has been identified as an evolutionarily conserved process. The term *hormesis* defines a nonlinearity biphasic biological response where exposure to a low dose/level of an environmental toxicant or noxious condition results in a potentially beneficial effect, whereas a high dose/level has an adverse effect. In the field of biomedical disciplines, hormesis is referred to as an adaptive response or preconditioning of cells and organisms to a moderate/intermittent stress.[1,2] Hormesis represents a fundamental concept in evolutionary theory, explaining how life on earth has adapted to harsh environment. To survive environmental hazards, organisms have developed distinct cellular signaling pathways that mediate hormetic responses. These include transcription factors and their upstream kinases, which regulate the expression of genes encoding a battery of stress resistance and cytoprotective proteins (e.g., protein chaperones, heat-shock proteins, antioxidant and phase-2 detoxifying enzymes, etc.).[3]

Xenohormesis hypothesis: evolutionary adaptation to foreign stressors for survival advantage

Organisms have evolved to sense stress signaling molecules produced by other species in their environment. In this way, organisms can properly be prepared in advance for deteriorating environmental conditions. This interspecies hormesis is referred to as xenohormesis, which describes a phenomenon

doi: 10.1111/j.1749-6632.2011.06097.x

© 2011 New York Academy of Sciences.

where an organism senses chemical cues from other species about the status of environment or food supply and responds to them in a way that is beneficial.[4,5]

Mutualism between plants and animals supports a coevolutionary impetus for xenohormesis. Plants and animals share a high degree of sequence homology between their stress response signaling pathways.[6] For instance, when plants are subjected to harsh environment, such as a drought, microbial infection, attack by insects and pests, etc., they produce chemicals that help endure such stressful conditions or protect them from further environmental hazards. Since animals normally depend upon plants for their food supply, they have adapted to sense the bioactive substances produced by stressed plants in order to gauge changing external conditions.[6] In this context, those chemical substances (phytochemicals) produced from plants for self-defense in response to stress or other adverse conditions are inherently phytoalexins (plant toxins). These xenohormetic phytochemicals, which alert animals to adversity, can stimulate their stress response and eventually fortify cellular defense capacity (*vide infra*).

Cellular stress responsive gene induction by xenohormetic phytochemicals

The stress response of plants has been evolving for almost one billion years. Because most plants cannot physically move around, they must endure environmental stresses in place. This sedentary life of plants may explain the complexity of their stress response.[6] Plants produce toxins to protect themselves against fungi, insects, and animal predators. Consistent with this notion, cultivated plant foods contain on average fewer natural toxins than do their wild counterparts.[7] When plants are under stressful conditions, there might be a marked increase in their accumulation of natural pesticides (biopesticides), occasionally to the levels that can be acutely toxic to humans. As such plant toxins constitute the substantial part of chemicals present in the human diet, it has been estimated that 99.99% (by weight) of the pesticides in the American diet are chemicals that plants produce to defend themselves.[8]

Xenohormesis can explain how environmentally stressed plants produce bioactive compounds that can confer stress resistance and survival benefits to animals that consume them. Animals take advantage of exploiting the information contained in products of sophisticated stress response of plants, which has developed as a result of their stationary lifestyle.[6] Indeed, the majority of known health-beneficial effects of edible plants are attributable to the pharmacologically active substances of plants' stress response. Although the noxious properties of xenohormetic phytochemicals are detrimental to microorganisms, insects, and pests eating plants, at the subtoxic doses ingested by humans as part of their diet, the same compounds are considered to induce mild cellular stress responses.[9,10] This, in turn, activates adaptive stress response signaling pathways, leading to increased expression of genes mostly encoding cytoprotective proteins including antioxidant enzymes, phase-2 detoxifying enzymes, protein chaperones, growth factors, mitochondrial proteins, etc. For instance, the oxidative stress caused by some flavonoids with prooxidant activity can contribute to their health-promoting activity by inducing important antioxidant enzymes, pointing to a beneficial effect of a supposed toxic chemical reaction.[11]

Although there has been a paucity of solid clinical data to support the xenohormesis hypothesis in the nutritional field, accumulating evidence from recent studies suggests that xenohormetic mechanisms may underlie health-beneficial effects of some edible phytochemicals in humans. As xenohormetic phytochemicals can improve our body's functions by stimulating our cellular stress response, they can be applied in drug development and the nutritional enhancement of diet.[6] Specific examples of signal transduction molecules activated by phytochemicals that exert xenohormetic effects include Nrf-2, AMP-activated protein nkinase, histone deacetylases of the sirtuin family (e.g., SIRT-1), FOXO, and transient receptor potential vanilloid receptor.[3,10]

Nrf2 as an essential component of xenohormetic circuit

Living organisms have evolved ubiquitous mechanisms to manage a vast multitude of stressors and noxious conditions. Animals that consume plants as a primary source of their diet have apparently developed mechanisms to eliminate phytoalexins or neutralize their potentially deleterious effects. One of the most essential components of physiologically important stress response signaling pathways is the redox-sensitive transcription factor Nrf2, which is considered the cellular redox sensor. Multiple lines of evidence support that the known health-beneficial effects of low doses of phytochemicals largely depend on their ability to activate Nrf2 signaling.[9]

Under physiologic conditions, Nrf2 is normally sequestered in the cytoplasm as an inactive complex with the repressor Kelch-like ECH-associated protein 1 (Keap1). The release of Nrf2 from its repressor and subsequent nuclear translocation are most likely to be achieved by alterations in the structure of Keap1. Nrf2, once migrated to the nucleus, forms a heterodimer with another protein, such as small Maf, which in turn binds to the antioxidant response elements or more correctly electrophile response elements (EpRE), located in the promoter region of genes encoding various antioxidant and phase-2 detoxifying enzymes. Some chemopreventive and cytoprotective agents target Keap1 by oxidizing or covalently modifying one or more of its specific cysteine thiols, thereby facilitating dissociation of Nrf2 from Keap1 and nuclear translocation.[12] In addition, upstream signaling kinases, such as p38, protein kinase C, extracellular signal-regulated protein kinase, c-Jun N-terminal kinase, and phosphoinositide-3-kinase, can activate Nrf2 through phosphorylation at its specific serine residues. This may also facilitate the nuclear localization of Nrf2.

Nrf2 has evolved over millennia from primitive origins. Thus, there exist homologues of mammalian Nrf2 even in lesser-developed invertebrate species, including *Caenorhabditis elegans* and *Drosophila*. In particular, those regions essential for the regulating stability and DNA binding of Nrf2 are remarkably conserved. During evolution, organisms might have selected a distinct form of Nrf2 for optimal defense capacity to manage a broad spectrum of external insults.[13]

The primary function of Nrf2 is to protect cells and organisms from oxidative stress by upregulating the *de novo* synthesis of diverse antioxidant enzymes and cytoprotective proteins, such as heme oxygenase-1 (HO-1), NAD(P)H:quinone oxidoreductase-1, those involved in glutathione metabolism (e.g., glutamate cysteine ligase, glutathione *S*-transferase, glutathione peroxidase), and thioredoxin. Nrf2 also plays a role in facilitating the elimination of some electrophilic toxicants by in-

ducing the expression of phase-2 detoxifying enzymes. The list of stress response and cytoprotective proteins whose expression is primarily regulated by Nrf2 has been expanding.

Although Nrf2 mainly plays a major role in cellular antioxidant defense, results from recent studies have highlighted its anti-inflammatory function (Fig. 1).[14] As oxidative stress and inflammatory tissue damage are two major culprits in the pathogenesis of the majority of human malignancies, Nrf2 is recognized as a potential target for cancer chemoprevention. Some representative chemopreventive phytochemicals capable of activating Nrf2 signaling and their underlying mechanisms are described in the following section.

Activation of Nrf2 by chemopreventive and cytoprotective phytochemicals

There are numerous phytochemicals that have been reported to activate Nrf2 signaling.[15] Though their chemical structures are diverse, ranging from flavonoids (e.g., epigallocatechin gallate and quercetine) to stilbenes (e.g., resveratrol and piceatannol), diferuloylmethanes (e.g., curcumin and caffeic acid phenethylester), and organosulfur compounds (e.g., allilcin and diallyl trisulfide), there is some commonality responsible for Nrf2 activation. Two of these characteristics in common are prooxidant and electrophilic properties.[11,16]

Electrophilic and oxidant phytochemicals, which exert beneficial health effects at low doses, can alter the redox state of the target cells (Fig. 1). This can be achieved by direct generation of reactive oxygen species (ROS) or indirectly by decreasing intracellular reduced glutathione (GSH). Mild oxidative stress can activate protein kinases responsible for the activation of the Nrf2 through phosphorylation of the specific amino acids localized in this transcription factor. As a result, there will be upregulation of cytoprotective gene expression. Alternatively, ROS can oxidize critical cysteine thiol groups present in Keap1, which facilitates the dissociation of Nrf2 from a complex with its negative regulator Keap1 for nuclear translocation. Interestingly, the ability of antioxidant flavonoids to activate an EpRE-mediated response correlates well with their prooxidant properties. Thus, it has been reported that flavonoids with a higher intrinsic redox potential to generate oxidative stress and redox cycling are the most potent inducers of EpRE-mediated

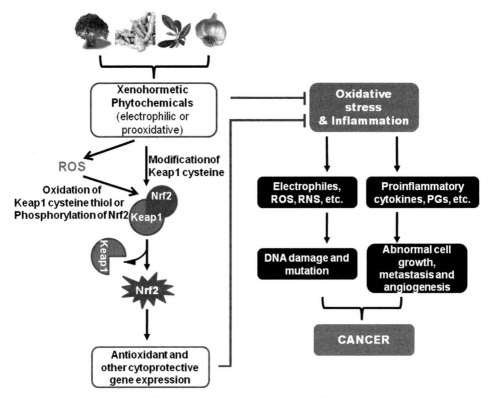

Figure 1. Activation of Nrf2-Keap1 signaling by xenohormetic phytochemicals with cancer chemopreventive potential.

cytoprotective gene expression.[11] According to this study, Nrf2-activation by flavonoids was accompanied by decreased cellular GSH, lending support to an prooxidative mechanism.

Some electrophilic phytochemicals, such as curcumin, are capable of directly modifying Keap1 cysteine thiol groups. Curcumin bears the α,β-unsaturated carbonyl moiety and hence can act as a Michael reaction acceptor capable of interacting with nucleophiles, such as protein thiols. Catalytic hydrogenation of curcumin at both double bonds conjugated with carbonyl groups produces tetrahydrocurcumin, which cannot act as a Michael reaction acceptor. Unlike curcumin, tetrahydrocurcumin failed to activate EpRE-mediated HO-1 expression in rat smooth muscle cells.[17] Oral administration of curcumin resulted in enhanced nuclear translocation and EpRE binding of Nrf2 and subsequently HO-1 expression in rat liver, but these effects were very marginal in tetrahydrocurcumin-treated animals.[18] Another example of an electrophilic phytochemical targeting Nrf2-Keap1 signaling is zerumbone, a sesquiterpene derived from tropical

ginger, which also contains an α,β-unsaturated carbonyl moiety. Zerumbone was found to suppress chemically induced papilloma formation in mouse skin.[19] Our recent study has revealed that topical application of zerumbone onto dorsal skin of hairless mice induces activation of Nrf2 and expression of HO-1.[20] Treatment of mouse epidermal JB6 cells with zerumbone caused a marked increase of Nrf2 nuclear translocation as well as the promoter activity of HO-1, and also enhanced binding of Nrf2 to the antioxidant response element. Notably, α-humulene and 8-hydroxy-α-humulene, the structural analogues of zerumbone that lack the α,β-unsaturated carbonyl group, failed to activate Nrf2 and were unable to increase HO-1 expression. Unlike zerumbone, these nonelectrophilic analogues could not suppress the phorbol ester-induced JB6 cell transformation as well.[20]

Besides the enone-type phytochemicals including curcumin and xerumbone, those with the catechol moiety are also electrophilic as they undergo oxidative conversion to a quinone. For instance, carnosic acid, a naturally occurring catechol-type polyphenolic diterpene derived from rosemary (*Rosmarinus officinalis*), has been reported to activate the Nrf/Nrf2 transcriptional pathway by binding to specific Keap1 cysteine residues.[21] Many noncatechol-type polyphenols undergo oxidative conversion to produce a catechol metabolite, which, through redox cycling, can directly modify target proteins including Keap1 via (*S*)-alkylation or provoke oxidative stress by interacting with GSH.

Other categories of electrophilic phytochemicals include isothiocyanates (e.g., sulforaphane) and some organosulfur compounds (e.g., diallyl trisulfide). Sulforaphane, abundant in broccoli sprouts, has been reported to strongly induce carcinogen detoxifying enzymes, predominantly through activation of Nrf2.[22] Sulforaphane-induced activation of Nrf2 signaling was largely attributed to its Keap1 thiol modification, especially at cysteine 151, which is supposed to facilitate release of Nrf2 from the inactive complex with Keap1. However, a later study by Egner *et al.* demonstrated that thiol modification of Keap1 cysteine 151 by sulforaphane failed to cause direct dissociation of Nrf2 from Keap1, but rather resulted in structural changes in Keap1.[23] This led to polyubiquitination and subsequent proteasomal degradation of Keap1, thereby allowing Nrf2 to escape from Cul3-dependent proteasomal degradation, providing a new insight into the mechanism underlying Nrf2 activation by sulforaphane.

Garlic oil contains several organosulfur compounds, such as diallyl sulfide, diallyl disulfide, and diallyl trisulfide. When each of these garlic-derived organosulfur compounds was treated to human hepatoma HepG2 cells, diallyl trisulfide elicited the most pronounced effects in terms of inducing nuclear translocation and transcriptional activity of Nrf2 and antioxidant gene expression.[24] Co-treatments with thiol-reducing antioxidants, such as *N*-acetylcysteine and GSH, attenuated diallyl trisulfide–induced EpRE activity and Nrf2 accumulation.

Conclusion

Xenohormesis can explain how plants challenged with environmental stressors, such as microbes, insects, animal predators, drought, and excess solar illumination, produce bioactive substances that, as chemical cues, alert animals to adversity. When consumed by animals, the same compounds stimu-

late an adaptive survival response, conferring stress resistance and health benefits.[6] One of the key molecules that plays a central role in cellular adaptive response to a wide array of external stressors is the redox-sensitive transcription factor Nrf2.

If Nrf2 plays such a pivotal role in the physiological stress response, is sustained upregulation or activation of this transcription factor beneficial? Oxidative and electrophilic stressors alter the cellular redox state, thereby rapidly activating Nrf2. However, it remains to be proven if such a situation occurs in response to chronic exposure of cells to low-dose dietary phytochemicals, which renders the target cells better able to respond to a subsequent harmful challenge.[16]

While timely transient activation of Nrf2 signaling is pivotal to boost cellular defense against acute toxicity, unnecessarily elevated Nrf2 activity may not be necessarily beneficial, and may even be detrimental to organisms. While low levels of Nrf2 activity predispose cells to chemical carcinogenesis, inappropriately overactivated Nrf2 may play a role in the progress of cancer.[25] Moreover, the overactivation of Nrf2 is associated with increased resistance to anticancer therapeutic regimens and confers survival advantage to some cancerous or transformed cells.[26] In this context, Nrf2 is a double-edged sword in regulating redox regulation in cancerous versus normal cells, and its functions may also follow the hormetic dose response.

Acknowledgments

This work was supported by the grant (No. 2008-00783) for the joint program of cooperation in Science and Technology between Korea–India supported by National Research Foundation (NRF), Republic of Korea.

Conflicts of interest

The author declares no conflicts of interest.

References

1. Calabrese, E.J. 2005. Paradigm lost, paradigm found: the re-emergence of hormesis as a fundamental dose response model in the toxicological sciences. *Env. Poll.* **138:** 379–412.
2. Mattson, M.K. 2008. Hormesis defined. *Ageing. Res. Rev.* **7:** 1–7.
3. Mattson, M.K. 2008. Dietary factors, hormesis and health. *Ageing Res. Rev.* **7:** 43–48.
4. Horwitz, K.T. & D.A. Sinclare. 2008. Xenohormesis: sensing the chemical cues of other species. *Cell* **133:** 387–391.

5. Lamming, S.W., J.G. Wood & D.A. Sinclair. 2004. Small molecules that regulate lifespan: evidence for xenohormesis. *Mol. Microbiol.* **53:** 1003–1009.

6. Hooper, P.L., P. L. Hooper, M. Tytell & L. Vigh. 2010. Xenohormesis: health benefits from an eon of plant stress response evolution. *Cell Stress Chaperones* **15:** 761–770.

7. Ames, B.N., M. Profet & L.S. Gold. 1990. Nature's chemicals and synthetic chemicals: comparative toxicology. *Proc. Natl. Acad. Sci. USA* **87:** 7782–7786.

8. Ames, B.N., M. Profet & L.S. Gold. 1990. Dietary pesticides (99.99% all natural). *Proc. Natl. Acad. Sci. USA* **87:** 7777–7781.

9. Son, T.G., S. Camandola & M.P. Mattson. 2008. Hormetic dietary phytochemicals. *Neuromol. Med.* **10:** 236–246.

10. Mattson, M.P., T.G. Son & S. Camandola. 2007. Viewpoint: mechanisms of action and therapeutic potential of neurohormetic phytochemicals. *Dose Response* **5:** 174–186.

11. Lee-Hilz, Y.Y., A.-M.J.F. Boerboom, A.H. Westphal, *et al.* 2006. Prooxidant activity of flavonoids induces EpRE-mediated gene expression. *Chem. Res. Toxicol.* **19:** 1499–1505.

12. Surh, Y.-J. 2003. Cancer chemoprevention with dietary phytochemicals. *Nat. Rev. Cancer* **3:** 768–780.

13. Maher, J. & M. Yamamoto. 2010. The rise of antioxidant signaling–The evolution and hormetic actions of Nrf2. *Toxicol. Appl. Pharmacol.* **244:** 4–15.

14. Kim, J.Y., Y.-N. Cha & Y.-J. Surh. 2010. A protective role of nuclear factor-erythroid 2-related factor Nrf2) in inflammatory disorders. *Mutat. Res.* **690:** 12–23.

15. Surh, Y.-J., J.K. Kundu & H.-K. Na. 2008. Nrf2 as a master redox switch in turning on the cellular signaling involved in the induction of cytoprotective genes by some chemopreventive phytochemicals. *Planta Med.* **74:** 1526–1539.

16. Lindsay, D.G. 2005. Nutrition, hormetic stress and health. *Nutr. Res. Rev.* **18:** 249–258.

17. Pae, H.O., G.S. Jeong, S.O. Jeong, *et al.* 2007. Roles of heme oxygenase-1 in curcumin-induced growth inhibition in rat smooth muscle cells. *Exp. Mol. Med.* **39:** 267–277.

18. Farombi, E.O., S. Shrotriya, H.-K. Na, *et al.* 2008. Curcumin attenuates dimethylnitrosamine-induced liver injury in rats through Nrf2-mediated induction of heme oxygenase-1. *Food Chem. Toxicol.* **46:** 1279–1287.

19. Murakami, A., T. Tanaka, J.Y. Lee, *et al.* 2004. Zerumbone, a sesquiterpene in subtropical ginger, suppresses skin nutition and promotion stages in ICR mice. *Int. J. Cancer.* **110:** 481–490.

20. Shin, J.-W., L. Ohnish, A. Murakami, *et al.* 2011. Zerumbone induces heme oxygenase-1 expression in mouse skin and cultured murine epidermal cells through activation of Nrf2. *Cancer Prev. Res.* **4:** 860–870.

21. Satoh, T., K. Kosaka, K. Itoh, *et al.* 2008. Carnosic acid, a catechol-type electrophilic compound, protects neurons both in vitro and in vivo through activation of the Keap1/Nrf2 pathway via *S*-alkylation of targeted cysteines on Keap1. *J. Neurochem.* **104:** 1116–1131.

22. Fahey, J.W., Y. Zhang & P. Talalay. 1997. Broccoli sprouts: an exceptionally rich source of inducers of enzymes that protectagainst chemical carcinogens. *Proc. Natl. Acad. Sci. USA* **94:** 10367–10372.

23. Eggler A.L., G. Liu, J.M. Pezzuto, *et al.* 2005. Modifying specific cysteines of the electrophile-sensing human Keap1 protein is insufficient to disrupt binding to the Nrf2 domain Neh2. *Proc. Natl. Acad. Sci. USA* **102:** 10070–10075.

24. Chen, C., D. Pung, V. Leong, *et al.* 2004. Induction of detoxifying enzymes by garlic organosulfur compounds through transcription factor Nrf2: effect of chemical structure and stress signals. *Free Radic. Biol. Med.* **37:** 1578–1590.

25. Hayes, J.D. & M. McMahon. 2006. The double-edged sword of Nrf2: subversion of redox homeostasis during the evolution of cancer. *Mol. Cell* **21:** 732–734.

26. Taguchi K., H. Motohashi & M. Yamamoto. 2011. Molecular mechanisms of the Keap1–Nrf2 pathway in stress response and cancer evolution. *Genes Cells* **16:** 123–140.

Ann. N.Y. Acad. Sci. ISSN 0077-8923

Dietary energy balance modulation of epithelial carcinogenesis: a role for IGF-1 receptor signaling and crosstalk

Tricia Moore,[1] L. Allyson Checkley,[1] and John DiGiovanni[1,2,3]

[1] Division of Pharmacology and Toxicology, The University of Texas at Austin, Austin, Texas. [2] Department of Nutritional Sciences, The University of Texas at Austin, Austin, Texas. [3] Dell Pediatric Research Institute, The University of Texas at Austin, Austin, Texas

Address for correspondence: John DiGiovanni, Ph.D., Dell Pediatric Research Institute, The University of Texas at Austin, 1400 Barbara Jordan Blvd. Austin, TX 78723. jdigiovanni@mail.utexas.edu

Obesity affects more than one third of the U.S. population and is associated with increased risk and/or disease severity for several chronic diseases, including cancer. In contrast, calorie restriction (CR) consistently inhibits cancer across species and cancer types. Differential effects on globally active circulatory proteins, particularly insulin-like growth factor-1 (IGF-1), provide a plausible mechanistic explanation for the energy balance–cancer link. Diet-induced changes in circulating IGF-1 modulate IGF-1R/EGFR activation and downstream signaling to Akt and mTOR. These dietary energy balance effects on signaling ultimately modulate the levels and/or activity of cell cycle regulatory proteins, regulating proliferation, and modulating susceptibility to tumor development. Selective targeting of mTORC1 potently inhibits tumorigenesis in several model systems producing CR mimetic effects. Targeting this and other pathways modulated by dietary energy balance may lead to the development of strategies for cancer chemoprevention and for reversing the effects of obesity on cancer development and progression.

Keywords: energy balance; tumorigenesis; IGF-1; Akt; mTOR

Introduction

Energy balance refers to the relationship between energy consumption and energy expenditure.[1] A sustained positive energy balance state (overweight or obesity) is associated with increased risk and/or mortality for multiple cancers.[2] In contrast, a chronic negative energy balance state, achieved by calorie restriction (CR), effectively inhibits tumorigenesis. With the increasing prevalence of obesity in both adults and children, it is imperative that the mechanisms underlying the effects of both positive and negative energy balance on cancer be identified.[3,4] In this regard, current research focuses on understanding and identifying biological mechanisms that are differentially regulated by CR and obesity. Additional studies have utilized pharmacological agents to target specific molecules/pathways with the purpose of identifying novel chemoprevention strategies, as well as reducing the effects of obesity on cancer development and progression.

CR, diet-induced obesity, and cancer

CR limits total energy intake (typically a 15–40% reduction in carbohydrate and/or fat calories relative to *ad libitum*–fed controls) while maintaining isonutrient conditions. This restricted regimen results in prevention of adult-onset obesity (prevalent among the *ad libitum*–fed controls), life-span extension, and suppression of multiple chronic diseases in rodents, primates, and humans. CR has consistently been shown to act as a potent inhibitor of carcinogenesis in animal models, regardless of mode of tumor induction.[5,6] Studies have been conducted using the two-stage skin carcinogenesis model, a well-established model of epithelial carcinogenesis,

doi: 10.1111/j.1749-6632.2011.06099.x

to specifically evaluate the impact of CR on tumor initiation, promotion, and progression. While CR had no apparent effect on tumor initiation or progression, CR reduced susceptibility to skin tumor promotion. Specifically, CR during tumor promotion led to a significant reduction in tumor incidence, multiplicity, and papilloma size.[7–9]

In contrast to CR, chronic, *ad libitum* consumption of a high-fat diet (45–60 kcal% fat) leads to diet-induced obesity (DIO). DIO has been positively associated with type-2 diabetes, as well as other chronic diseases, including cancer in rodents and humans. The association between DIO and cancer has been shown in multiple tissues and cell types, including breast, colon, pancreas, liver, lung, and leukocytes.[10–14] Studies have been conducted using the two-stage skin carcinogenesis model to determine the impact of a high-fat diet on epithelial carcinogenesis.[8,15,16] Administration of an *ad libitum* high-fat diet (46% vs. 11% fat) led to significant differences in body weight and more rapid development of skin tumors; however, no differences in the number of tumors were reported between these diet groups.[16] In contrast, another study using the same high-fat diet fed in an isocaloric manner reported significant differences in tumor incidence and multiplicity in the absence of significant differences in weight gain.[15] These studies, however, did not specifically evaluate the impact of DIO on susceptibility to tumor development and progression. The potential mechanisms for the effects of CR and DIO on tumorigenesis have been studied, and a brief summary of some of these mechanisms is presented in more detail in subsequent sections.

Dietary energy balance and globally active circulatory proteins

Dietary energy balance manipulation (across the spectrum of CR to DIO) induces numerous cellular, biochemical, and molecular changes, which collectively may contribute to the effects of caloric consumption on tumorigenesis. A number of studies have suggested that diet-induced changes in globally active circulatory proteins may serve as the primary mechanism whereby energy balance modulates cancer development and/or progression.[5,6,17] Specifically, CR and obesity differentially regulate levels of several serum-related hormones and growth factors (e.g., leptin, adiponectin, insulin, corticos-

terone, IGF-1), which then function to modulate intracellular signaling, hence altering cellular function and tumor development and/or progression. Figure 1 summarizes some of these circulating factors and the signaling pathways that are impacted by changes in levels of these factors. Studies have been conducted to specifically evaluate the role of each of these globally active circulatory proteins in the modulation of tumorigenesis and are summarized briefly in the sections below.

Leptin

Leptin is an adipocyte-derived hormone that regulates satiety and energy metabolism. CR consistently decreases, while obesity consistently increases circulating leptin levels.[18] Both epidemiological and animal studies suggest an association between levels of circulating leptin and cancer risk, specifically for colorectal, prostate, endometrial, and breast cancers.[19–23] *In vivo*, leptin has been shown to promote angiogenesis and tumor invasion, while *in vitro*, leptin has been shown to stimulate cellular proliferation of both preneoplastic and neoplastic cells, while having no effect on "normal" cells.[24,25] Leptin binding to its cognate receptor induces changes in intracellular signaling, which results in enhanced susceptibility to tumorigenesis. Specifically, leptin binds its transmembrane receptor (Ob-Rb), thus modulating activation of Jak-STAT and MAPK signaling pathways, which have been shown to be critical signaling pathways required for cancer development and progression. Recent studies have also suggested that the effect of leptin on tumorigenesis may be dependent on the ratio of leptin to adiponectin, as opposed to an independent effect of leptin *per se*.[21,26–28] A-ZIP/F-1 mice, which lack adipose tissue and all associated adipokines, are highly susceptible to skin tumor development using the two-stage protocol, suggesting that levels of leptin and/or adiponectin may not be as critical as the levels of circulating IGF-1.[29,30] However, it is important to point out that A-ZIP/F-1 mice have other metabolic imbalances that may cloud the overall interpretation of the role of adipokines and adipose tissue in tumor development and progression.

Adiponectin

Adiponectin is another adipokine that regulates insulin sensitivity as well as carbohydrate and lipid metabolism. Levels of adiponectin are decreased in metabolic syndromes, including type-2 diabetes,

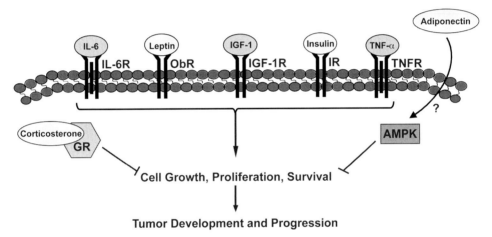

Figure 1. Summary of the effects of dietary energy balance on globally active circulatory proteins and potential cellular outcomes. Positive energy balance (overweight/obesity) increases circulating levels of leptin, insulin, IGF-1, TNF-α, and IL-6, while reducing levels of adiponectin. In contrast, negative energy balance (CR) reduces circulating levels of leptin, insulin, IGF-1, TNF-α, and IL-6, while increasing levels of adiponectin and corticosterone. These changes can then result in increased signaling through corresponding receptors or intracellular molecular targets, leading to either enhanced (positive energy balance) or reduced (negative energy balance) cell growth, proliferation, and survival. Together, these effects may modulate tumor development and progression.

dyslipidemia, and extreme obesity. This reduction can be partially reversed by weight loss, although recent reports suggest that drastic weight changes, achieved by severe CR or surgical intervention, are necessary to induce a significant increase in levels of adiponectin.[31,32] While the role of adiponectin in the modulation of tumorigenesis is not well characterized, recent data suggest an inverse correlation between levels of adiponectin and multiple cancer types, including both breast and colorectal cancers.[33–38] Mechanistic studies suggest that the inhibitory effects of adiponectin are due, at least in part, to activation of AMP-activated protein kinase (AMPK), which inhibits mTORC1 signaling.[39,40] Adiponectin also reduces Stat signaling, which may also contribute to its effects on tumor development.[34,35] Recent data suggest that these ef-

fects are closely associated with the ratio of leptin and adiponectin and that the balance between these two circulating hormones may be important.[21,26–28]

Insulin

Insulin resistance and chronic hyperinsulinemia increase risk for several cancers; however, it is unclear if these effects are due to increased insulin receptor signaling or alternatively due to indirect effects on IGF-1, estrogens, leptin, or other hormones.[41,42] Recent data suggest that crosstalk exists between the insulin receptor and multiple hormonal pathways, making it difficult to ascertain the primary role of insulin in the effects of energy balance on cancer.[43,44] Furthermore, it has been well established that increased levels of insulin lead to increased IGF-1 synthesis (hepatic) and IGF-1 bioavailability (reduced

IGF-BP-1 production), which could further contribute to the observed enhancing effect of insulin on cellular growth, proliferation, and survival *in vivo*.[42] Similar to IGF-1, CR reduces, while obesity increases, the levels of circulating insulin. Findings from the liver IGF-1–deficient (LID) mouse model, however, suggest that insulin may not be the primary mediator of the effect of energy balance on tumorigenesis. Despite high levels of insulin, a 75% reduction in levels of circulating IGF-1 has been shown to dramatically reduce susceptibility to two-stage skin carcinogenesis, colon carcinogenesis, and mammary carcinogenesis, in a manner similar to CR.[1,45]

IGF-1

IGF-1 has consistently been shown to enhance growth and proliferation in multiple cancer cell lines, and more recent epidemiological evidence supports the hypothesis that IGF-1 acts as a critical regulator of several types of human cancers.[25,46,47] Hepatic synthesis accounts for the majority of circulating IGF-1. This process is regulated by growth hormone and insulin and is influenced by nutrient intake and energy consumption. CR consistently reduces, while obesity consistently increases, levels of circulating IGF-1. Many of the anticancer effects of CR are believed to be mediated, at least in part, by reduced circulating levels of IGF-1. Specifically, restoration of IGF-1 levels in CR mice has been shown to ablate the antitumor effects of CR in multiple models.[48–50] Furthermore, as previously discussed, genetic reduction of circulating IGF-1 levels (LID mouse model) inhibits mouse skin tumorigenesis, in a manner similar to CR.[1,45] IGF-1 can act to enhance proliferation, cell growth, and cell survival through both direct and indirect effects.[51–54] IGF-1 can bind directly to the IGF-1 receptor (IGF-1R), resulting in increased activation of downstream signaling to Akt, mTOR, as well as other downstream effectors. Alternatively, IGF-1 may act indirectly through modulation of other receptors, such as the epidermal growth factor receptor (EGFR). The role of receptor crosstalk is discussed in more detail below.

Corticosterone

Early studies by Boutwell *et al.*[55] established that CR could inhibit two-stage skin carcinogenesis and that glucocorticoids might play a role in the inhibitory effect of CR on tumor development in this model. Fur-

ther studies of CR in this and other animal models have provided additional support for the connection between heightened circulating glucocorticoid levels and inhibition of tumorigenesis. It is known that severe CR (levels exceeding 30%) leads to markedly increased levels of circulating corticosterone. Several mechanisms have been proposed to account for the inhibitory effects of elevated corticosterone on tumor development, including inhibition of inflammation, induction of p27 (inhibition of proliferation), inhibition of protein kinase C, as well as reduced activation of Erk.[56–59] Further studies have evaluated the impact of adrenalectomy on CR-mediated inhibition of tumorigenesis; however, the results from these studies are less clear. Adrenalectomy abolished the inhibitory effect of CR on skin tumor promotion in mice; however, adrenalectomy of rats subjected to chemically induced mammary carcinogenesis had no impact on CR-mediated inhibition.[56,60,61] Furthermore, dietary corticosterone supplementation of rats, in the absence of CR, inhibited tumorigenesis; however, this increase in corticosterone levels also induced a dose-dependent reduction in circulating IGF-1 levels.[62] Thus, the role of circulating glucocorticoids in the effects of dietary energy balance manipulation on tumor development requires further investigation.

Inflammatory cytokines

Chronic inflammation has long been associated with cancer development and progression and, more recently, this connection has been extended to include obesity.[63,64] Obesity is associated with increased adipose tissue, especially white adipose tissue (WAT). WAT produces a number of inflammatory cytokines, including tumor necrosis factor-alpha (TNF-α), interleukin-6 (IL-6), IL-1β, monocyte chemoattractant (MCP-1), and C-reactive protein, which act both locally (tissue level) and globally (circulating in serum).[65] Increased adipose-derived cytokine production, particularly increased levels of MCP-1, enhances local macrophage infiltration, leading to further increases in the levels of secreted inflammatory cytokines, as well as heightened recruitment of other related immune cells.[65–67] These inflammatory cytokines then modulate inflammation via increased signaling through NF-κB-, STAT3-, and JNK-related pathways.[65,68] Together, the increased production of inflammatory cytokines and immune cell recruitment leads to a chronic, low-grade inflammatory response, thus increasing susceptibility to tumor development. Increasing adiposity has been shown to be positively associated with an inflammatory response in both rodents and humans.[65,69] While obesity consistently enhances inflammation through heightened proinflammatory signaling, CR has been shown to consistently inhibit an inflammatory response through reduced NF-κB, STAT3, and JNK signaling.[68,70] These findings suggest that modulation of inflammation may play a role in the effects of dietary energy balance on tumor development and progression.

Dietary energy balance and IGF-1R signaling

It is well established that the PI3K/Akt/mTOR pathway, which is commonly altered in human tumors, is a critical mediator of the effects of IGF-1 on tumorigenesis.[51,52,71–73] Binding of IGF-1 to the IGF-1R activates PI3K, which subsequently leads to activation of Akt. In turn, Akt functions to regulate cellular survival, growth, and proliferation through phosphorylation of multiple downstream effectors including Bad, Foxo1, GSK3β, TSC2 (thereby modulating mTORC1 signaling), and others.[52,74–79] Recent studies have shown that dietary energy balance, across the spectrum of CR to DIO, differentially regulates signaling through this pathway, providing a potential mechanism underlying the effects of energy balance on tumorigenesis.[80] Furthermore, these data have provided a plausible mechanism for how altered levels of IGF-1 may modulate tumor development. Finally, data generated using LID mice have provided further evidence that levels of circulating IGF-1 modulate Akt and mTOR signaling in tissues undergoing tumor development.[45]

In recent studies, CR has been shown to reduce, while DIO increases, activation of the IGF-1R in multiple epithelial tissues in mice.[80] Modulation of IGF-1R activation leads to concomitant modulation of Akt and mTORC1 activation, as well as their downstream substrates (e.g., Bad and GSK3β and p70S6K, S6 ribosomal protein, 4E-BP-1, respectively).[80,81] EGFR activation was also modulated in a similar manner by dietary energy balance manipulation and may have also contributed to the observed differences in Akt and mTORC1 signaling.[80,81] This effect of dietary energy balance on EGFR activation may be mediated, at least in part, by IGF-1R/EGFR crosstalk (see below). Diet-induced changes in Akt and mTORC1 signaling occurred under steady-state conditions in multiple epithelial tissues (i.e., skin epidermis, liver, dorsolateral prostate, and mammary fat pad) and in epidermis after treatment with TPA. Similar changes were reported in mammary tumors.[80–82] Reductions in Akt and mTORC1 activation have also been observed in TPA-treated epidermis of LID mice, which have levels of circulating IGF-1 comparable to mice on CR diets. These findings indicate that the effects of CR and DIO on Akt and mTORC1 signaling are mediated, at least in part, by diet-induced changes in levels of circulating IGF-1.[45] AMPK has also been implicated in regulation of mTORC1 signaling during dietary energy balance manipulation, a mechanism that functions independent of growth factor–mediated receptor activation. This nutrient sensing pathway becomes activated under nutrient deprivation conditions (high AMP-to-ATP ratio), leading to inhibition of mTORC1 and consequently inhibition of protein translation. While CR has been shown to activate this pathway in liver, skeletal muscle, and adipose tissue, no differences were observed between CR and DIO regimens in either the epidermis or dorsolateral prostate, suggesting a tissue-specific role for AMPK in the regulation of mTORC1 under different dietary conditions.[80,83] Figure 2 summarizes our current understanding of the effects of dietary energy balance on IGF-1/EGFR activation and subsequent downstream signaling pathways.

In addition to diet-induced changes in Akt and mTORC1 signaling, CR has also been shown to alter total levels and complex formation of cell cycle regulatory proteins. CR (40% CR) reduced the levels of cell cycle progression–related proteins (i.e., cyclins D, E, A) and increased the levels of negative cell cycle regulatory proteins (i.e., p21, p27) in rat mammary carcinomas.[58,59,62] Furthermore, 40% CR has been shown to regulate the activity of cell cycle related proteins through alterations in complex formation. Specifically, CR increased the association between cyclin-dependent kinases (cdks) and p27 or p21, while inhibiting cdk complex formation with cyclins D1 and E, thus inhibiting cell cycle progression.[58] These inhibitory effects of CR on cell cycle progression were attributed to increased levels of circulating corticosterone; however, IGF-1 levels are concomitantly reduced with CR, making it difficult to ascertain the primary mechanism that regulates the inhibitory effects of CR on cell cycle progression.

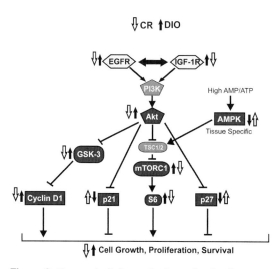

Figure 2. Proposed cellular mechanisms whereby dietary energy balance modulates tumorigenesis. DIO (black arrows) increases signaling through the IGF-1R and the EGFR in epithelial cells due to IGF-1R/EGFR crosstalk. This in turn leads to heightened activation of Akt and mTORC1. Subsequently, DIO increases protein levels of positive cell cycle regulators such as cyclin D1 while decreasing the levels of negative cell cycle regulatory proteins (p21 and p27). Overall, this leads to increased cell growth, proliferation, and survival during tumor promotion. In contrast, CR (white arrows) leads to the opposite effects on these signaling pathways and cell cycle regulators, leading to a reduction in cell growth, proliferation, and survival during tumor promotion. Note in the case of GSK-3β, DIO leads to an increase in phosphorylation, which reduces GSK-3β activity and leads to increased levels of cyclin D1. CR produces the opposite effects. Diet-induced changes in AMPK activation appear to be more tissue/cell specific, and thus its overall contribution to changes in mTORC1 and downstream signaling may not be uniform across all types of tissues. Collectively, these changes in cellular signaling modulate susceptibility to carcinogenesis.

Additional data from both skin and liver suggest that IGF-1 can mediate similar diet-induced changes in cell cycle regulatory proteins through effects on Akt and mTORC1 signaling. In this regard, moderate CR (30% CR) reduced levels of cyclin D1 in both the skin and liver, consistent with the inhibitory effect of CR on IGF-1–mediated Akt and mTORC1 activation.[80] Furthermore, DIO elicited the opposite effects, increasing levels of cyclin D1 in these same epithelial tissues. Collectively, these data suggest that several pathways, including IGF-1R/EGFR downstream signaling, may mediate changes in cell cycle regulatory protein levels and activity during dietary energy balance manipulation. The observed changes in cell cycle regulatory proteins may also provide a mechanistic explanation for the effects

of dietary energy balance manipulation on cellular proliferation. In this regard, CR consistently inhibited, while DIO consistently enhanced, cellular proliferation in both normal and tumorigenic tissue (e.g., mammary, colon, liver, bladder).[10,84–87] These diet-induced changes in cellular proliferation presumably contribute to the effect of dietary energy balance manipulation on tumorigenesis (again, see Fig. 2).

Interplay between the IGF-1R and the EGFR

As previously noted, dietary energy balance modulated activation of both the IGF-1R and the EGFR in mouse epidermis,[80] which then coordinately functions to regulate Akt and mTORC1 signaling. Under these conditions, EGFR-mediated activation of Akt and mTORC1 may be modulated, at least in part, by IGF-1R and EGFR crosstalk. Numerous studies have now established that crosstalk exists between these two receptors, and several potential mechanisms have been proposed.[88,89] Figure 3 summarizes the known mechanisms for this crosstalk, including IGF-1–induced ectodomain shedding of EGFR ligands, IGF-1–induced transcription of EGFR and EGFR ligands, and IGF-1–induced IGF-1R/EGFR heterodimerization.[90–94] Data from the LID mouse model support this notion of IGF-1–mediated IGF-1R and EGFR crosstalk. In this regard, genetically reduced levels of IGF-1 attenuated activation of not only the IGF-1R, but also the EGFR in TPA-treated skin.[45] These findings suggest that dietary energy balance may modulate Akt and mTORC1 signaling through differential effects on IGF-1R and EGFR crosstalk, as a result of diet-induced changes in circulating IGF-1 levels.

Targeting mTORC1 as a CR mimetic approach

The differential effects of CR and DIO on activation of Akt and in particular mTORC1, as well as the overall importance of these pathways on cell proliferation and cell growth, suggested that one approach to developing novel cancer prevention strategies may be to target of one or both of these pathways. Recently, rapamycin has been studied as a potential CR mimetic and chemopreventive agent. Rapamycin effectively blocks mTORC1 complex formation, thus inhibiting mTORC1-mediated cellular growth and proliferation.[95,96] Rapamycin has

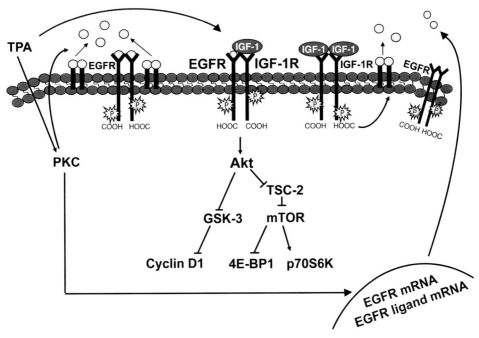

Figure 3. Proposed mechanisms of crosstalk between the IGF-1R and the EGFR. Activation of the IGF-1R by IGF-1 leads to activation of the EGFR. Several potential mechanisms have been proposed to account for this IGF-1–mediated activation of the EGFR, including IGF-1–induced ectodomain shedding of EGFR ligands, IGF-1–induced transcription of EGFR and EGFR ligands, and IGF-1R/EGFR heterodimerization.[90–94] Diet-induced changes in levels of circulating IGF-1 may modulate downstream signaling to Akt and mTORC1 through this crosstalk mechanism.

recently been shown to extend lifespan in mice, similar to CR, and is considered a lead CR mimetic compound.[97] Furthermore, rapamycin has been shown to suppress tumorigenesis in several animal models, including xenograft models; a carcinogen-induced lung cancer model; and transgenic mouse models of head and neck SCC, human breast cancer, and prostate cancer.[98–102] Additional recent studies have also evaluated the ability of rapamycin to inhibit skin tumorigenesis, using both the two-stage and UV-induced skin carcinogenesis models.[103–105] Rapamycin given topically is a potent inhibitor of skin tumor promotion by TPA during two-stage skin carcinogenesis.[103] Furthermore, rapamycin (topical or i.p.) induced regression and/or inhibited growth of existing tumors.[103,104] Using a UV skin carcinogenesis model, rapamycin (given in the diet) also delayed the appearance and reduced the multiplicity of larger tumors (>4mm).[105]

The mechanisms underlying the effects of rapamycin on tumorigenesis have been explored. Using the two-stage skin carcinogenesis model, rapamycin was shown to inhibit tumor promotion by primarily blocking mTORC1 signaling through p70S6K and inhibiting epidermal proliferation.[103] The ability of rapamycin to inhibit growth of existing tumors and to induce tumor regression correlated with reduced proliferation and increased apoptosis.[104] The antitumor effect of rapamycin was attributed to its ability to induce apoptosis in tumor cells through reduced signaling downstream of mTORC1 (as assessed by levels of p70S6K) and reduced levels of the cell cycle proteins PCNA and cyclin D1.[104] In addition to changes in cellular proliferation, rapamycin may function to reduce inflammation. Rapamycin treatment was also found to significantly reduce TPA-induced infiltration of several types of inflammatory cells (including T cells, macrophages, neutrophils, and mast cells).[103] Collectively, the current findings suggest that rapamycin may function as a potent CR mimetic compound in cancer prevention.

Conclusions

In summary, CR inhibits, while DIO enhances, tumorigenesis in multiple models. Changes in globally active circulatory proteins, particularly IGF-1, are hypothesized to be the key mediators of these dietary effects on tumorigenesis. Reduced (CR) or increased (DIO) circulating levels of IGF-1 effectively regulate activation of not only the IGF-1R, but also the EGFR (due to IGF-1R/EGFR crosstalk). CR attenuates, while DIO enhances, IGF-1R/EGFR–mediated activation of Akt and mTORC1, thus altering levels of cell cycle regulatory proteins and reducing or increasing cellular proliferation, respectively. Rapamycin effectively inhibits skin tumor promotion, mTORC1 downstream signaling, and epidermal hyperproliferation in a manner similar to CR. Future studies are needed to evaluate the potential for rapamycin to counteract the effects of obesity on cancer development and progression and to search for other CR mimetic agents to use alone or in combination to produce synergistic chemopreventive effects.

Conflicts of interest

The authors declare no conflicts of interest.

References

1. Patel, A.C. *et al.* 2004. Effects of energy balance on cancer in genetically altered mice. *J. Nutr.* **134:** 3394S–3398S.
2. Calle, E.E. *et al.* 2003. Overweight, obesity, and mortality from cancer in a prospectively studied cohort of U.S. adults. *N. Engl. J. Med.* **348:**1625–1638.
3. Hedley, A.A. *et al.* 2004. Prevalence of overweight and obesity among US children, adolescents, and adults, 1999–2002. *JAMA* **291:** 2847–2850.
4. Ogden, C.L. 2004. *Advance Data from Vital Health Statistics.* CDC.
5. Hursting, S.D. *et al.* 2010. Calories and carcinogenesis: lessons learned from 30 years of calorie restriction research. *Carcinogenesis* **31:** 83–89.
6. Hursting, S.D. *et al.* 2003. Calorie restriction, aging, and cancer prevention: mechanisms of action and applicability to humans. *Annu. Rev. Med.* **54:**131–152.
7. Birt, D.F. *et al.* 1991. Influence of diet and calorie restriction on the initiation and promotion of skin carcinogenesis in the SENCAR mouse model. *Cancer Res.* **51:** 1851–1854.
8. Birt, D.F. *et al.* 1993. Inhibition of skin tumor promotion by restriction of fat and carbohydrate calories in SENCAR mice. *Cancer Res.* **53:** 27–31.
9. Boutwell, R. 1964. Some biological aspects of skin carcinogenesis. *Prog. Exp. Tumor Res.* **4:** 207–250.
10. Lautenbach, A. *et al.* 2009. Obesity and the associated mediators leptin, estrogen and IGF-I enhance the cell proliferation and early tumorigenesis of breast cancer cells. *Nutr. Cancer* **61:** 484–491.
11. Hill-Baskin, A.E. *et al.* 2009. Diet-induced hepatocellular carcinoma in genetically predisposed mice. *Hum. Mol. Genet.* **18:** 2975–2988.
12. White, P.B. *et al.* 2010. Insulin, leptin, and tumoral adipocytes promote murine pancreatic cancer growth. *J. Gastrointest. Surg.* **14:** 1888–1893; discussion 1893–1894.
13. Yun, J.P. *et al.* 2010. Diet-induced obesity accelerates acute lymphoblastic leukemia progression in two murine models. *Cancer Prev. Res. (Phila)* **3:** 1259–1264.
14. Yakar, S. *et al.* 2006. Increased tumor growth in mice with diet-induced obesity: impact of ovarian hormones. *Endocrinology* **147:** 5826–5834.
15. Birt, D.F. *et al.* 1989. Dietary fat effects on the initiation and promotion of two-stage skin tumorigenesis in the SENCAR mouse. *Cancer Res.* **49:** 4170–4174.
16. Birt, D.F. *et al.* 1989. Acceleration of papilloma growth in mice fed high-fat diets during promotion of two-stage skin carcinogenesis. *Nutr. Cancer* **12:** 161–168.
17. Hursting, S.D. *et al.* 2007. Energy balance and carcinogenesis: underlying pathways and targets for intervention. *Curr. Cancer Drug Targets* **7:** 484–491.
18. Zhang, Y. & R. Leibel. 1998. Molecular physiology of leptin and its receptor. *Growth Genet. Hormones* **14:** 17–35.
19. Stattin, P. *et al.* 2004. Obesity and colon cancer: does leptin provide a link? *Int. J. Cancer.* **109:** 149–152.
20. Chang, S. *et al.* 2001. Leptin and prostate cancer. *Prostate* **46:** 62–67.
21. Ashizawa, N. *et al.* 2010. Serum leptin-adiponectin ratio and endometrial cancer risk in postmenopausal female subjects. *Gynecol. Oncol.* **119:** 65–69.
22. Rene Gonzalez, R. *et al.* 2009. Leptin-signaling inhibition results in efficient anti-tumor activity in estrogen receptor positive or negative breast cancer. *Breast Cancer Res.* **11:** R36.
23. Karaduman, M. *et al.* 2010. Tissue leptin levels in patients with breast cancer. *J. BUON.* **15:** 369–372.
24. Bouloumie, A. *et al.* 1998. Leptin, the product of Ob gene, promotes angiogenesis. *Circ. Res.* **83:** 1059–1066.
25. Fenton, J.I. *et al.* 2005. Leptin, insulin-like growth factor-1, and insulin-like growth factor-2 are mitogens in ApcMin/ +but not Apc+/ +colonic epithelial cell lines. *Cancer Epidemiol. Biomarkers Prev.* **14:** 1646–1652.
26. Yamaji, T. *et al.* 2010. Interaction between adiponectin and leptin influences the risk of colorectal adenoma. *Cancer Res.* **70:** 5430–5437.
27. Cleary, M.P. *et al.* 2009. Targeting the adiponectin: leptin ratio for postmenopausal breast cancer prevention. *Front Biosci. (Schol Ed)* **1:** 329–357.
28. Grossmann, M.E. *et al.* 2009. Role of the adiponectin leptin ratio in prostate cancer. *Oncol. Res.* **18:** 269–277.
29. Nunez, N.P. *et al.* 2006. Accelerated tumor formation in a fatless mouse with type 2 diabetes and inflammation. *Cancer Res.* **66:** 5469–5476.
30. Hursting, S.D. *et al.* 2007. The obesity-cancer link: lessons learned from a fatless mouse. *Cancer Res.* **67:** 2391–2393.

31. Abbasi, F. *et al.* 2004. Plasma adiponectin concentrations do not increase in association with moderate weight loss in insulin-resistant, obese women. *Metab. Clin. Exper.* **53:** 280–283.

32. Martin, B. *et al.* 2007. Sex-dependent metabolic, neuroendocrine and cognitive responses to dietary energy restriction and excess. *Endocrinology* **148:** 4318–4333.

33. Grossmann, M.E. *et al.* 2008. Effects of adiponectin on breast cancer cell growth and signaling. *Br. J. Cancer* **98:** 370–379.

34. Fenton, J.I. & J.M. Birmingham. 2010. Adipokine regulation of colon cancer: adiponectin attenuates interleukin-6-induced colon carcinoma cell proliferation via STAT-3. *Mol. Carcinog.* **49:** 700–709.

35. Kim, A.Y. *et al.* 2010. Adiponectin represses colon cancer cell proliferation via AdipoR1- and -R2-mediated AMPK activation. *Mol. Endocrinol.* **24:** 1441–1452.

36. Fujisawa, T. *et al.* 2008. Adiponectin suppresses colorectal carcinogenesis under the high-fat diet condition. *Gut* **57:** 1531–1538.

37. Otani, K. *et al.* 2010. Adiponectin suppresses tumorigenesis in Apc(Min)(/+) mice. *Cancer Lett.* **288:** 177–182.

38. Brakenhielm, E. *et al.* 2004. Adiponectin-induced antiangiogenesis and antitumor activity involve caspase-mediated endothelial cell apoptosis. *Proc. Nat. Acad. Sci. USA* **101:** 2476–2481.

39. Viollet, B. & F. Andreelli. 2011. AMP-activated protein kinase and metabolic control. *Handb. Exp. Pharmacol.* **203:** l303–1330.

40. Nawrocki, A.R. *et al.* 2006. Mice lacking adiponectin show decreased hepatic insulin sensitivity and reduced responsiveness to peroxisome proliferator-activated receptor gamma agonists. *J. Biol. Chem.* **281:** 2654–2660.

41. Calle, E.E. & R. Kaaks. 2004. Overweight, obesity and cancer: epidemiological evidence and proposed mechanisms. *Nat. Rev. Cancer* **4:** 579–591.

42. Yakar, S., D. Leroith & P. Brodt. 2005. The role of the growth hormone/insulin-like growth factor axis in tumor growth and progression: lessons from animal models. *Cytokine Growth Factor Rev.* **16:** 407–420.

43. Saxena, N.K. *et al.* 2008. Bidirectional crosstalk between leptin and insulin-like growth factor-I signaling promotes invasion and migration of breast cancer cells via transactivation of epidermal growth factor receptor. *Cancer Res.* **68:** 9712–9722.

44. Lanzino, M. *et al.* 2008. Interaction between estrogen receptor alpha and insulin/IGF signaling in breast cancer. *Curr. Cancer Drug Targets* **8:** 597–610.

45. Moore, T. *et al.* 2008. Reduced susceptibility to two-stage skin carcinogenesis in mice with low circulating IGF-1 levels. *Cancer Res.* **68:** 3680–3688.

46. LeRoith, D. *et al.* 1995. Insulin-like growth factors and cancer. *Ann. Intern. Med.* **122:** 54–59.

47. Singh, P. *et al.* 1996. Proliferation and differentiation of human colon cancer cell line (CaCo2) is associated with significant changes in the expression and secretion of insulin-like growth factor (IGF) IGF-II and IGF binding protein-4: role of IGF-II. *Endocrinology* **137:** 1764–1774.

48. Hursting, S.D. *et al.* 1993. The growth hormone: insulin-like growth factor 1 axis is a mediator of diet restriction-induced inhibition of mononuclear cell leukemia in Fischer rats. *Cancer Res.* **53:** 2750–2757.

49. Zhu, Z. *et al.* 2005. Effects of dietary energy repletion and IGF-1 infusion on the inhibition of mammary carcinogenesis by dietary energy restriction. *Mol. Carcinog.* **42:** 170–176.

50. Dunn, S. E. *et al.* 1997. Dietary restriction reduces insulin-like growth factor I levels, which modulates apoptosis, cell proliferation, and tumor progression in p53-deficient mice. *Cancer Res.* **57:** 4667–4672.

51. Taniguchi, C.M., B. Emanuelli & C.R. Kahn. 2006. Critical nodes in signalling pathways: insights into insulin action. *Nat. Rev. Mol. Cell Biol.* **7:** 85–96.

52. Hay, N. 2005. The Akt-mTOR tango and its relevance to cancer. *Cancer Cell* **8:** 179–183.

53. Resnicoff, M. *et al.* 1995. The insulin-like growth factor I receptor protects tumor cells from apoptosis in vivo. *Cancer Res.* **55:** 2463–2469.

54. Dunn, S. E. *et al.* 1998. A dominant negative mutant of the insulin-like growth factor-I receptor inhibits the adhesion, invasion, and metastasis of breast cancer. *Cancer Res.* **58:** 3353–3361.

55. Boutwell, R.K. 1964. Some biological aspects of skin carcinogenisis. *Prog. Exp. Tumor Res.* **19:** 207–250.

56. Birt, D.F. *et al.* 2004. Identification of molecular targets for dietary energy restriction prevention of skin carcinogenesis: an idea cultivated by Edward Bresnick. *J. Cell Biochem.* **91:** 258–264.

57. Birt, D. F., A. Yaktine & E. Duysen. 1999. Glucocorticoid mediation of dietary energy restriction inhibition of mouse skin carcinogenesis. *J. Nutr.* **129:** 571S–574S.

58. Jiang, W., Z. Zhu & H.J. Thompson. 2003. Effect of energy restriction on cell cycle machinery in 1-methyl-1-nitrosourea-induced mammary carcinomas in rats. *Cancer Res.* **63:** 1228–1234.

59. Zhu, Z., W. Jiang & H.J. Thompson. 1999. Effect of energy restriction on the expression of cyclin D1 and p27 during premalignant and malignant stages of chemically induced mammary carcinogenesis. *Mol. Carcinog.* **24:** 241–245.

60. Pashko, L.L. & A.G. Schwartz. 1992. Reversal of food restriction-induced inhibition of mouse skin tumor promotion by adrenalectomy. *Carcinogenesis* **13:** 1925–1928.

61. Jiang, W. *et al.* 2004. Adrenalectomy does not block the inhibition of mammary carcinogenesis by dietary energy restriction in rats. *J. Nutr.* **134:** 1152–1156.

62. Zhu, Z., W. Jiang & H.J. Thompson. 2003. Mechanisms by which energy restriction inhibits rat mammary carcinogenesis: in vivo effects of corticosterone on cell cycle machinery in mammary carcinomas. *Carcinogenesis* **24:** 1225–1231.

63. Coussens, L.M. & Z. Werb. 2002. Inflammation and cancer. *Nature* **420:** 860–867.

64. Hursting, S.D. & N.A. Berger. 2010. Energy balance, host-related factors, and cancer progression. *J. Clin. Oncol.* **28:** 4058–4065.

65. Shoelson, S.E., L. Herrero & A. Naaz. 2007. Obesity, inflammation, and insulin resistance. *Gastroenterology* **132:** 2169–2180.

66. Park, E.J. *et al.* 2010. Dietary and genetic obesity promote liver inflammation and tumorigenesis by enhancing IL-6 and TNF expression. *Cell* **140**: 197–208.

67. Wu, Y. *et al.* 2010. Insulin-like growth factor-I regulates the liver microenvironment in obese mice and promotes liver metastasis. *Cancer Res.* **70**: 57–67.

68. Grivennikov, S.I. & M. Karin. 2010. Dangerous liaisons: STAT3 and NF-kappaB collaboration and crosstalk in cancer. *Cytokine Growth Factor Rev.* **21**: 11–19.

69. Park, H.S., J.Y. Park & R. Yu. 2005. Relationship of obesity and visceral adiposity with serum concentrations of CRP, TNF-alpha and IL-6. *Diabetes Res. Clin. Pract.* **69**: 29–35.

70. Ye, J. & J.N. Keller. 2010. Regulation of energy metabolism by inflammation: a feedback response in obesity and calorie restriction. *Aging (Albany NY).* **2**: 361–368.

71. Vivanco, I. & C.L. Sawyers. 2002. The phosphatidylinositol 3-Kinase AKT pathway in human cancer. *Nat. Rev. Cancer* **2**: 489–501.

72. Luo, J., B.D. Manning & L.C. Cantley. 2003. Targeting the PI3K-Akt pathway in human cancer: rationale and promise. *Cancer Cell* **4**: 257–262.

73. Shaw, R.J. & L.C. Cantley. 2006. Ras, PI(3)K and mTOR signalling controls tumour cell growth. *Nature* **441**: 424–430.

74. Cross, D.A. *et al.* 1995. Inhibition of glycogen synthase kinase-3 by insulin mediated by protein kinase B. *Nature* **378**: 785–789.

75. Shin, I. *et al.* 2002. PKB/Akt mediates cell-cycle progression by phosphorylation of p27(Kip1) at threonine 157 and modulation of its cellular localization. *Nat. Med.* **8**: 1145–1152.

76. Diehl, J.A. *et al.* 1998. Glycogen synthase kinase-3beta regulates cyclin D1 proteolysis and subcellular localization. *Genes Dev.* **12**: 3499–3511.

77. Datta, S.R. *et al.* 1997. Akt phosphorylation of BAD couples survival signals to the cell-intrinsic death machinery. *Cell* **91**: 231–241.

78. Kops, G.J. & B.M. Burgering. 1999. Forkhead transcription factors: new insights into protein kinase B (c-akt) signaling. *J. Mol. Med.* **77**: 656–665.

79. Ruggero, D. & N. Sonenberg. 2005. The Akt of translational control. *Oncogene* **24**: 7426–7434.

80. Moore, T. *et al.* 2008. Dietary energy balance modulates signaling through the Akt/mammalian target of rapamycin pathways in multiple epithelial tissues. *Cancer Prev. Res.* **1**: 65–76.

81. Dogan, S. *et al.* 2011. Effects of intermittent and chronic calorie restriction on mammalian target of Rapamycin (mTOR) and IGF-I signaling pathways in mammary fat pad tissues and mammary tumors. *Nutr. Cancer.* **63**: 389–401.

82. Xie, L. *et al.* 2007. Effects of dietary calorie restriction or exercise on the PI3K and RAS signaling pathways in the skin of mice. *J. Biol. Chem.* **282**: 28025–28035.

83. Fulco, M. & V. Sartorelli. 2008. Comparing and contrasting the roles of AMPK and SIRT1 in metabolic tissues. *Cell Cycle* **7**: 3669–3679.

84. James, S. J. & L. Muskhelishvili. 1994. Rates of apoptosis and proliferation vary with caloric intake and may influence incidence of spontaneous hepatoma in C57BL/6 x C3H F1 mice. *Cancer Res.* **54**: 5508–5510.

85. Steinbach, G. *et al.* 1993. Effects of caloric restriction and dietary fat on epithelial cell proliferation in rat colon. *Cancer Res.* **53**: 2745–2749.

86. Zhu, Z., W. Jiang & H.J. Thompson. 1999. Effect of energy restriction on tissue size regulation during chemically induced mammary carcinogenesis. *Carcinogenesis* **20**: 1721–1726.

87. Lok, E. *et al.* 1990. Calorie restriction and cellular proliferation in various tissues of the female Swiss Webster mouse. *Cancer Lett.* **51**: 67–73.

88. Adams, T.E., N.M. McKern & C.W. Ward. 2004. Signalling by the type 1 insulin-like growth factor receptor: interplay with the epidermal growth factor receptor. *Growth Factors* **22**: 89–95.

89. Jones, H. E. *et al.* 2006. Growth factor receptor interplay and resistance in cancer. *Endocr. Relat. Cancer* **13**(Suppl 1): S45–S51.

90. Bor, M. V. *et al.* 2000. Epidermal growth factor and insulin-like growth factor I upregulate the expression of the epidermal growth factor system in rat liver. *J. Hepatol.* **32**: 645–654.

91. Nahta, R. *et al.* 2005. Insulin-like growth factor-I receptor/human epidermal growth factor receptor 2 heterodimerization contributes to trastuzumab resistance of breast cancer cells. *Cancer Res.* **65**: 11118–11128.

92. Krane, J.F. *et al.* 1991. Synergistic effects of epidermal growth factor (EGF) and insulin-like growth factor I/somatomedin C (IGF-I) on keratinocyte proliferation may be mediated by IGF-I transmodulation of the EGF receptor. *J. Invest. Dermatol.* **96**: 419–424.

93. Roudabush, F.L. *et al.* 2000. Transactivation of the EGF receptor mediates IGF-1-stimulated shc phosphorylation and ERK1/2 activation in COS-7 cells. *J. Biol. Chem.* **275**: 22583–22589.

94. El-Shewy, H.M. *et al.* 2004. Ectodomain shedding-dependent transactivation of epidermal growth factor receptors in response to insulin-like growth factor type I. *Mol. Endocrinol.* **18**: 2727–2739.

95. Garcia, J.A. & D. Danielpour. 2008. Mammalian target of rapamycin inhibition as a therapeutic strategy in the management of urologic malignancies. *Mol. Cancer Ther.* **7**: 1347–1354.

96. Kopelovich, L. *et al.* 2007. The mammalian target of rapamycin pathway as a potential target for cancer chemoprevention. *Cancer Epidemiol. Biomarkers Prev.* **16**: 1330–1340.

97. Anisimov, V.N. *et al.* 2010. Rapamycin extends maximal lifespan in cancer-prone mice. *Am. J. Pathol.* **176**: 2092–2097.

98. Granville, C.A. *et al.* 2007. Identification of a highly effective rapamycin schedule that markedly reduces the size, multiplicity, and phenotypic progression of tobacco carcinogen-induced murine lung tumors. *Clin. Cancer Res.* **13**: 2281–2289.

99. Yan, Y. *et al.* 2006. Efficacy of polyphenon E, red ginseng, and rapamycin on benzo(a)pyrene-induced lung tumorigenesis in A/J mice. *Neoplasia* **8**: 52–58.

100. Raimondi, A.R., A. Molinolo & J.S. Gutkind. 2009. Rapamycin prevents early onset of tumorigenesis in an oral-specific K-ras and p53 two-hit carcinogenesis model. *Cancer Res.* **69:** 4159–4166.

101. Liu, M. *et al.* 2005. Antitumor activity of rapamycin in a transgenic mouse model of ErbB2-dependent human breast cancer. *Cancer Res.* **65:** 5325–5336.

102. Blando, J. *et al.* 2009. PTEN deficiency is fully penetrant for prostate adenocarcinoma in C57BL/6 mice via mTOR-dependent growth. *Am. J. Pathol.* **174:** 1869–1879.

103. Checkley, A. *et al.* 2011. Rapamycin is a potent inhibitor of skin tumor promotion by 12-O-tetradecanoylphorbol-13-acetate. *Cancer Prev. Res.* in press.

104. Amornphimoltham, P. *et al.* 2008. Inhibition of mammalian target of rapamycin by rapamycin causes the regression of carcinogen-induced skin tumor lesions. *Clin. Cancer Res.* **14:** 8094–8101.

105. de Gruijl, F.R. *et al.* 2010. Early and late effects of the immunosuppressants rapamycin and mycophenolate mofetil on UV carcinogenesis. *Int. J. Cancer* **127:** 796–804.

Ann. N.Y. Acad. Sci. ISSN 0077-8923

ANNALS OF THE NEW YORK ACADEMY OF SCIENCES

Issue: *Nutrition and Physical Activity in Aging, Obesity, and Cancer*

Tocotrienols: inflammation and cancer

Kalanithi Nesaretnam and Puvaneswari Meganathan

Malaysian Palm Oil Board, Selangor, Malaysia

Address for correspondence: Kalanithi Nesaretnam, Product Development and Advisory Services Division, Malaysian Palm Oil Board, No. 6 Persiaran Institusi, Bandar Baru Bangi, 43000 Kajang, Selangor, Malaysia. sarnesar@mpob.gov.my

Inflammation is an organism's response to environmental assaults. It can be classified as acute inflammation that leads to therapeutic recovery or chronic inflammation, which may lead to the development of cancer and other ailments. Genetic changes that occur within cancer cells themselves are responsible for many aspects of cancer development but are dependent on ancillary processes for tumor promotion and progression. Inflammation has long been associated with the development of cancer. The distinct characteristics of cancer cells to proliferate, metastasize, evade apoptotic signals, and develop chemoresistance have been linked to the inflammatory response. Due to the involvement of multiple genes and various pathways, current drugs that target single genes have not been effective in providing a therapeutic cure. On the other hand, natural products target multiple genes and therefore have better success compared to drugs. Tocotrienols, the potent isoforms of vitamin E, are such a natural product. This review will discuss the relationship between cancer and inflammation with particular focus on the roles played by NF-κB, STAT3, and COX-2.

Keywords tocotrienols; inflammation; cancer; NF-κB; COX-2; STAT3; anti-inflammation

Introduction

Inflammation that results from irritation is characterized by redness (rubor), swelling (tumor), heat (calor), and pain (dolor). It has been identified as a cause for many chronic diseases, including cancer.[1] In the United States, about 1,529,560 new cases of cancer were estimated in the year 2010, and more than 1,500 people die of cancer each day as the disease accounts for one out of four deaths.[2]

Most things in life have been regarded as a "double-edged sword." Therefore, as proinflammatory genes have been found to be the mediators of cancer, the cure for cancer lies in suppressing these proinflammatory genes.[3] There have been numerous *in vitro* and *in vivo* studies conducted in order to find a suitable anti-inflammatory drug to treat inflammation. Synthetic drugs such as nonsteroidal anti-inflammatory drugs (NSAIDs) are, however, unable to offer prevention or enhance therapeutic responsiveness in patients. Earlier research also has shown that these drugs tend to induce gastric lesion in patients. As a result, clinical use of these drugs

has been limited, and attention has turned toward natural compounds.[4]

Vitamin E was discovered in 1938 and comprises tocopherols and tocotrienols, which are divided into four different analogs of α, β, δ, and γ in each category. Although tocopherols have been extensively studied, tocotrienols have been the current interest due to their greater potency and biological effects. The richest source of tocotrienols are palm, rice bran, and annatto oils.[5,6]

Nesaretnam *et al.*[7] were the first to prove that palm oil stripped of vitamin E did not protect against mammary tumorigenesis in rats, thereby proving that tocotrienols are the active compounds present in palm oil. This unique anticancer property of tocotrienols is attributed to the presence of the unsaturated phytyl chain that gives it better penetration into the lipid bilayer to produce greater physiological effects (Fig. 1).[8]

This review focuses on and summarizes the therapeutic link between tocotrienols and the proinflammatory genes as well as their gene products.

doi: 10.1111/j.1749-6632.2011.06088.x

Ann. N.Y. Acad. Sci. 1229 (2011) 18–22 © 2011 New York Academy of Sciences.

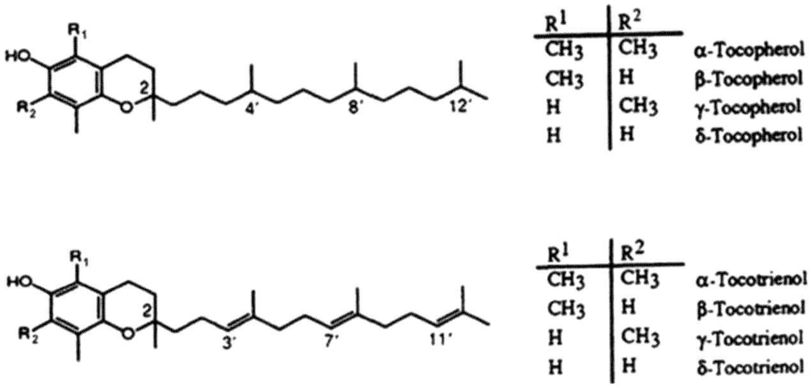

Figure 1. Chemical structure of tocopherols and tocotrienols.

NF-κB and tocotrienols

Nuclear factor κB (NF-κB) is a transcription factor discovered in 1986.[9] Since then, it has been closely linked to inflammation. NF-κB is activated in response to various environmental stimuli, viral and bacterial toxin, inflammatory cytokines, tobacco, and stress. These are the causes for 95% of all cancers.[1] Scientific evidence proves that NF-κB regulates the activity of many proinflammatory genes such as TNF-α, IL-1, and their downstream gene products, namely IL-6, IL-8, MMP-9 VEGF, and 5-LOX. In general, these genes promote and foster inflammation by controlling cellular transformation, proliferation, survival, invasion, angiogenesis, and metastasis.[1]

In the resting stage, NF-κB is sequestered in the cytoplasm by its interaction with the inhibitory IκB proteins. Once activated, the IκB proteins are degraded, leading to the activation and translocation of NF-κB into the nucleus to initiate the transcription of the target genes. The constitutive activation of NF-κB is observed in leukemia, lymphoma, breast, colon, liver, pancreas, prostate, and ovarian cancers. Moreover, this constitutive activation is associated with recurrence of cancer, poor survival, tumor progression, aggressiveness, and chemoresistance.[1]

Hence, NF-κB has been a molecular target for many chemopreventive drugs and therapies. The unique abilities of tocotrienols as antiproliferative and proapoptotic agents, as well as their ability to induce cell cycle arrest, activate p53, and inhibit angiogenesis, have been well established. Ahn et al.[10] have demonstrated that gamma-tocotrienol

displayed complete abolishment of TNF-α-induced NF-κB activation. Furthermore, it also suppressed NF-κB activation induced by phorbol myristate acetate (PMA), okadaic acid, cigarette smoke condensate, lipopolysaccharide (LPS), and epidermal growth factor (EGF). These results suggest that gamma-tocotrienol may act at a common site to all these activators. The anti-inflammatory effect of gamma-tocotrienol was found not to be cell type specific as it suppressed NF-κB activation in different cell lines, namely human lung adenocarcinoma H1299, human embryonic kidney A293, human breast cancer MCF-7, multiple myeloma U266, and human squamous cell carcinoma SCC-4 cells.[10] Although the mechanism behind the constitutive activation of NF-κB is not fully understood, IKK has been hypothesized to play a major role. The IKK kinase complex regulates the inhibitory IκB molecules that hold NF-κB dimers together in the cytoplasm. Phosphorylation of IκB by IKK complex will lead to the degradation of IkB complex that allows NF-κB to be activated and translocated into the nucleus.[11] Interestingly, gamma-tocotrienol also suppressed TNF-induced IKK in this study.[10]

Wu et al. also found similar anti-inflammatory effects in a study with palm tocotrienol rich fraction (TRF). TRF significantly inhibited lipopolysaccharide-induced NF-κB activation in human monocytic (THP-1) cells. The induced proinflammatory cytokines nitric oxide synthase (iNOS) and cyclooxygenase-2 (COX-2) were also suppressed by palm TRF.[12]

Pancreatic cancer is currently the most lethal cancer, and the standard treatments available are gemcitabine and erlotinib. These drugs have raised concern, as about 10% of patients have reported adverse effects and drug resistance. Kunnumakkara *et al.* have found that gamma-tocotrienol inhibited constitutively active NF-κB and downregulated its downstream gene products such as cyclin D1, c-myc, COX-2, Bcl-2, VEGF, and surviving in human pancreatic cell lines, namely Panc-1, MiA PaCa-2, and BxPc-3.[13] Hussien *et al.* also observed similar results in d-delta tocotrienol-mediated suppression of pancreatic tumor cells *in vitro*.[14]

Furthermore, gamma-tocotrienol downregulated the expression of Id-1 and the prosurvival proteins NF-κB and EGFR in breast cancer cell lines. Constitutive expression of Id1 has been associated with aggressive and invasive breast cancer. The inhibition of Id1 by gamma-tocotrienol has provided a novel platform for chemopreventive therapies. In addition, gamma-tocotrienol also increased the chemosensitization of cancer cells to the drug Docetaxel.[15] These findings suggest that tocotrienol is a potential anti-inflammatory agent that targets NF-κB and its gene products that mediates carcinogenesis.

STAT3 and tocotrienols

Signal transducers and activators (STAT) are made up of six different transcription factors that are linked to tumorigenesis. STAT3 has been associated with inflammation, proliferation, chemoresistance, and angiogenesis. STAT3 translocates to the nucleus upon activation by various ligands, such as IL-6 and EGF. Constitutive activation of STAT3 is a commonly observed phenomenon in multiple myeloma, chronic lymphocytic leukemia, gastric cancer, lung cancer, and laryngeal carcinoma.[16,1] Moreover, it is related to shorter disease-free survival. 44% of patients diagnosed with acute myelogenous leukemia reported shorter disease-free survival due to constitutive STAT3 activation.[17]

Gamma-tocotrienol, which is regarded as one of the most potent forms of tocotrienols, inhibited both induced and constitutive activation of STAT3 in multiple myeloma and prostate cancer cell lines. Gamma-tocotrienol also induced the expression of tyrosine phosphatase SHP-1 in both cell lines and an animal model, indicating the possible role of SHP-1 in suppressing the activity of STAT3. Additionally, gamma-tocotrienol inhibited proliferation of cancer cells by downregulating cyclin D1 and reduced

the expression of VEGF that eventually suppressed angiogenesis.[16]

ErbB is a member of the EGF family of receptors. It binds to the ligand, dimerizes and activates mitogenic signaling pathways such as the PI3K/Akt and STAT pathway. The aberrant receptor signaling is a potential target for cancer treatment, and treatment with gefitinib and erlotinib is the current approach. However, these drugs have limitations due to diversification and amplification among the receptor complexes.[18,19] Therefore, combination treatment with gamma-tocotrienol and erlotinib or gefitinib in murine mammary tumor cells (+SA) was investigated. In this study, the combination of 3 μM of gamma-tocotrienol and 0.25 μM erlotinib or 0.5 μM gefitinib inhibited cell growth and reduced cyclin expression.

The researchers suggested that this combination significantly prevents ErB receptor heterodimerization, which leads to the inhibition of mitogenic signaling. This therapeutic responsiveness may provide new avenues and lead to tangible benefits in breast cancer patients.[20]

COX-2 and tocotrienols

Cyclooxygenase (COX) is a member of the prostaglandin synthase family of enzymes that are implicated in the growth and progression of cancer. COX is made up of two main types of enzymes, namely COX-1 and COX-2. COX-1 enzyme is constitutively expressed in normal circumstances, whereas COX-2, which is an inducible enzyme, has a major role in inflammatory response.[21] The conversion of arachidonic acid to prostaglandin (PGE_2), a major metabolite in inflammation, is catalyzed by this enzyme. Overexpression of COX-2 is associated with pathophysiological diseases such as cancer, multiple sclerosis, and Alzheimer's disease. A rise in COX-2 levels is a common finding in the development of tumors.[12]

NSAIDs such as glucocorticoids and immunosuppressants target both COX-1 and COX-2 enzymes. This has led to severe gastrointestinal and renal toxicities due to the inhibition of COX-1, which is the housekeeping enzyme.[22] Thus, these drugs have limited use in chemoprevention. Research has showed that selective inhibition of COX-2 enzyme may provide a better therapeutic effect and is a suitable target for the development of anti-inflammatory drugs.[22]

Shirode *et al.* studied the effect of combination treatment of gamma-tocotrienol with celecoxib. Although celecoxib, a selective COX-2 inhibitor, displays anticancer effects, its clinical use is limited for toxicity reasons. On the other hand, gamma-tocotrienol is a potent isoform of tocotrienol. However, there have been concerns regarding its bioavailability and bioabsorption. Therefore, Shirode *et al.* treated +SA cells with a combination of 2.5 μM of celecoxib and 0.25 μM of gamma-tocotrienol. A synergistic antiproliferative effect was observed with a significant reduction in COX-2 levels. Eventually, PGE_2 expression was also downregulated due to a decrease in its precursor compound. Subsequently, Akt and NF-κB activation was also reduced. These results prove the existence of a close link between NF-κB, COX-2, and PGE_2.[23]

Meanwhile, palm TRF decreased the expression of COX-2 in LPS-induced THP-1 cell lines. Only 1 μg/mL was required to observe this effect. Apart from COX-2, the expressions of TNF-α, IL-4, and IL-8 were also significantly reduced by palm TRF. The molecular mechanism of TRF's anti-inflammatory action was found to be its ability to downregulate iNOS and COX-2.[12]

Delta tocotrienol, on the other hand, inhibited hypoxia-induced COX-2 protein expression, while hypoxia-induced COX-2 mRNA levels were unaffected. Similar results were also established by Shibata *et al.* in human colorectal adenocarcinoma cells (DLD-1) and human hepatoma cells (HepG2) cell lines. The reason for this effect was attributed to the presence of a posttranslational inhibitory mechanism.[24]

Our lab studied the anti-inflammatory effects of TRF and other individual fractions of vitamin E in lipopolysaccharide-stimulated RAW264.7 macrophages. A total of 10 ng/mL of LPS stimulated the release of PGE_2 and induced the expression of COX-2 enzymes in RAW264.7 macrophages. Significant reduction was observed in PGE_2 levels following treatment with TRF and the individual isomers α-, δ-, and γ-tocotrienols. Real-time PCR was utilized to analyze the effect on COX enzymes. COX-1 levels remained unaffected as it is a constitutively expressed housekeeping enzyme. Meanwhile, the downregulation of COX-2 expression was in the order of δ-T3 > α-T3> γ-T3>, TRF, and α-tocopherol. The reduction in the gene level was suggested as the ability of tocotrienols to inhibit gene translation that eventually suppressed PGE_2 levels, as observed earlier.[25]

In addition, tocotrienols also displayed potent anti-inflammatory activity by inhibiting IL-6 and TNF-α. These are the major proinflammatory cytokines released by activated macrophages. IL-6 has been immensely studied due to its correlation with poor prognosis and resistance to therapy.[26] Interestingly, δ-tocotrienol demonstrated a 51% reduction in IL-6 levels in LPS-stimulated RAW264.7 macrophages.[25]

Conclusion

NF-κB and its gene products have been closely linked to cancer development and progression. As synthetic drugs have adverse effects, natural chemopreventive agents have thus been vastly investigated because of their availability and reduced toxicity. Tocotrienols were initially recognized for their role as an antioxidant. However, the emerging results on their anticancer, anti-angiogenic, antiproliferative, and immune enhancement activity broaden the horizon for the usage of tocotrienols in the field of cancer research. The currently available *in vitro* and *in vivo* studies have provided valuable information that proves tocotrienols' potential beyond their antioxidant capacity. However, due to the close association between the proinflammatory cytokines and cancer, there is an urgent need to look into the molecular mechanisms on how tocotrienols may affect these inflammatory markers. The combination study of tocotrienols with low-dose celocoxib has indeed enhanced the therapeutic effect. This has provided evidence for the synergistic activity of tocotrienols with other drugs. Based on the promising results obtained from preclinical studies, more clinical trials and molecular analyses should be conducted to provide us with the essential information to utilize the anti-inflammatory effect of tocotrienols in the diagnosis, prognosis, and treatment of cancer patients.

Conflicts of interest

The authors declare no conflicts of interest.

References

1. Aggarwal, B.B. & P. Gehlot. 2009. Inflammation and cancer: how friendly is the relationship for cancer patients? *Curr. Opin. Pharmacol.* **9:** 351–369.

2. American Cancer Society (2011). *Cancer Facts & Figures 2010.* http://www.cancer.org/research/cancerfactsfigures/cancerfactsfigures/cancer-facts-and-figures-2010. Accessed 27 Mar 2011.

3. Aggarwal, B.B., S. Shishodia, S.K. Sandur, M.K. Pandey & G. Sethi. 2006. Inflammation and cancer: how hot is the link? *Biochem. Pharmacol.* **72:** 1605–1621.

4. Shafiq, N., S. Malhotra, P. Pandhi & R. Nada. 2005. Comparative gastrointestinal toxicity of selective cyclooxygenase (COX-2) inhibitors. *Indian J. Exp. Biol.* **43:** 614–619.

5. Nesaretnam, K. 2008. Multitargeted therapy of cancer by tocotrienols. *Cancer Lett.* **269:** 388–395.

6. Sen, C.K., S. Khanna & S. Roy. 2006. Tocotrienols: vitamin E beyond tocopherols. *Life Sci.* **78:** 2088–2098.

7. Nesaretnam K., N. Guthrie, A.F. Chambers & K.K. Carroll. 1992. Effect of tocotrienols on the growth of a human breast cancer cell line in culture. *Lipids* **30:** 1139–1145.

8. Nesaretnam, K., P.A. Gomez, K.R. Selvaduray & G. Abdul Razak. 2007. Tocotrienol levels in adipose tissue of benign and malignant breast lumps in patients in Malaysia. *Asia Pac. J. Clin. Nutr.* **16:** 498–504.

9. Sen, R. & D. Baltimore. 1986. Inducibility of kappa immunoglobulin enhancer-binding protein Nf-kappa B by a posttranslational mechanism. *Cell* **47:** 921–928.

10. Ahn, K.S., G. Sethi, K. Krishnan & B.B. Aggarwal. 2007. Gamma-tocotrienol inhibits nuclear factor-kappaB signaling pathway through inhibition of receptor-interacting protein and TAK1 leading to suppression of antiapoptotic gene products and potentiation of apoptosis. *J. Biol. Chem.* **282:** 809–820.

11. Tak, P.P & G.S. Firestein. 2001. NF-kB: a key role in inflammatory diseases. *J. Clin. Invest.* **107:** 7–11.

12. Wu, S.J., P.L. Liu & L.T. Ng. 2008. Tocotrienol-rich fraction of palm oil exhibits anti-inflammatory property by suppressing the expression of inflammatory mediators in human monocytic cells. *Mol. Nutr. Food Res.* **52:** 921–929.

13. Kunnumakkara, A.B., B. Sung & J. Ravindran. 2010. Gamma-tocotrienol inhibits pancreatic tumors and sensitizes them to gemcitabine treatment by modulating the inflammatory microenvironment. *Cancer Res.* **70:** 8695–8705.

14. Hussein, D. & H. Mo. 2009. d-Delta-tocotrienol-mediated suppression of the proliferation of human PANC-1, MIA PaCa-2, and BxPC-3 pancreatic carcinoma cells. *Pancreas* **38:** e124–e136.

15. Yap WN., N. Zaiden, Y.L. Tan, *et al.* 2010. Id1, inhibitor of differentiation, is a key protein mediating anti-tumor re-

sponses of gamma-tocotrienol in breast cancer cells. *Cancer Lett.* **291:** 187–199.

16. Kannappan, R., V.R. Yadav & B.B. Aggarwal. 2010. Gamma-tocotrienol but not gamma-tocopherol blocks STAT3 cell signaling pathway through induction of protein-tyrosine phosphatase SHP-1 and sensitizes tumor cells to chemotherapeutic agents. *J. Biol. Chem.* **285:** 33520–33528.

17. Benekli, M., X. Zheng., K.A. Donahue, *et al.* 2002. Constitutive activity of signal transducer and activator of transcription 3 protein in acute myeloid leukemia blasts is associated with short disease-free survival. *Blood* **99:** 252–257.

18. Normanno, N., C. Bianco, A. De Luca, *et al.* 2003. Target-based agents against ErbB receptors and their ligands: a novel approach to cancer treatment. *Endocr. Relat. Cancer* **10:** 1–21.

19. Olayioye, M.A., R.M. Neve, H.A. Lane & N.E. Hynes. 2000. The ErbB signaling network: receptor heterodimerization in development and cancer. *EMBO J.* **19:** 3159–3167.

20. Bachawal, S.V., V.B. Wali & P.W. Sylvester. 2010. Combined γ-tocotrienol and erlotinib/gefitinib treatment suppresses STAT and Akt signaling in murine mammary tumor cells. *Anticancer Res.* **30:** 429–438.

21. Mukherjee, D., S.E. Nissen & E.J. Topol. 2001. Risk of cardiovascular events associated with selective COX-2 inhibitors. *JAMA* **286:** 954–959.

22. Tomisato, W., S. Tsutsumi, T. Hoshino, *et al.* 2004. Role of direct cytotoxicity effects of NSAIDs in the induction of gastric lesions. *Biochem. Pharmacol.* **67:** 575–585.

23. Shirode, A.B. & P.W. Sylvester. 2010. Synergistic anticancer effects of combined gamma-tocotrienol and celecoxib treatment are associated with suppression in Akt and NFkB signaling. *Biomed. Pharmacother.* **64:** 327–332.

24. Shibata A, K. Nakagawa P. Sookwong, *et al.* 2008. Tocotrienol inhibits secretion of angiogenic factors from human colorectal adenocarcinoma cells by suppressing hypoxia-inducible factor-1alpha. *J. Nutr.* **138:** 2136–2142.

25. Mun-Li, Y., S.R. Abdul Hafid, C. Hwee-Ming, & K. Nesaretnam. 2009. Toocotrienols suppress proinflammatory markers and cyclooxygenase-2 expression in RAW264.7 macrophages. *Lipids* **44:** 787–797.

26. Ndlovu, M.N., C.V. Lint, K.V. Wesemael, *et al.* 2009. Hyperactivated NF-kB and AP-1 transcription factors promote highly accessible chromatin and constitutive transcription across the Interleukin-6 gene promoter in metastatic breast cancer cells. *Mol. Cell. Biol.* **29**(20): 5488–5504.

Ann. N.Y. Acad. Sci. ISSN 0077-8923

ANNALS OF THE NEW YORK ACADEMY OF SCIENCES

Issue: *Nutrition and Physical Activity in Aging, Obesity, and Cancer*

Neurogenic contributions made by dietary regulation to hippocampal neurogenesis

Hee Ra Park and Jaewon Lee

Department of Pharmacy, College of Pharmacy and Research Institute for Drug Development, Longevity Life Science and Technology Institutes, Pusan National University, Geumjeong-gu, Busan, Republic of Korea

Address for correspondence: Jaewon Lee, Department of Pharmacy, College of Pharmacy and Research Institute for Drug Development, Longevity Life Science and Technology Institutes, Pusan National University, Geumjeong-gu, Busan 609-735, Republic of Korea. neuron@pusan.ac.kr

Adult neural stem cells in the dentate gyrus of the hippocampus are negatively and positively regulated by a broad range of environmental stimuli that include aging, stress, social interaction, physical activity, and dietary modulation. Interestingly, dietary regulation has a distinct outcome, such that reduced dietary intake enhances neurogenesis, whereas excess calorie intake by a high-fat diet has a negative effect. As a type of metabolic stress, dietary restriction (DR) is also known to extend life span and increase resistance to age-related neurodegenerative diseases. However, the potential application of DR as a "neurogenic enhancer" in humans remains problematic because of the severity of restriction and the protracted duration of the treatment required. Therefore, the authors consider that an understanding of the neurogenic mechanisms of DR would provide a basis for the identification of the pharmacological and nutraceutical interventions that mimic the beneficial effects of DR without limiting caloric intake. The current review describes the regulatory effect of DR on hippocampal neurogenesis and presents a possible neurogenic mechanism.

Keywords: BDNF; curcumin; dietary restriction; hippocampal neurogenesis; neural stem cell

Introduction

Dietary restriction (DR) can increase life span in a wide variety of species, reduce neuronal damage, and improve behavioral outcome in experimental animal models relevant to the pathogenesis of several age-related neurological disorders.[1,2] Several studies have described the molecular mechanism responsible for the beneficial effects of DR on aging and age-related neurodegenerative diseases. In particular, it has been shown that DR changes metabolic processes under lower glucose conditions, and thus produces mild stress in cells to adapt to the stressed condition by orchestrating cellular and molecular changes—within physiological limits.[3,4] It has been reported that altered gene expressions by DR are related to energy metabolism, stress, inflammation, and neural plasticity.[5,6] Subsequent studies demonstrated that DR enhances neurogenesis, indicating that the metabolic environment can modulate an important brain function.[7] Our current research is aimed at developing neurogenic modulators based on the molecular mechanisms of DR and stem cell regulation. In this review, we present an overview of the regulation of adult hippocampal neurogenesis by DR and the developments of neurogenic phytochemicals.

Environmental stimuli can enhance hippocampal neurogenesis in the adult brain

Findings over the past two decades that demonstrated persistent neurogenesis in the adult brain have overturned the long-held dogma that neurons are formed exclusively before birth. The existence of neural stem cells (NSCs) in the adult brain has provoked a reevaluation of cellular plasticity in the mature brain and raised hopes that novel approaches to brain repair can be devised. The generation of

doi: 10.1111/j.1749-6632.2011.06089.x

newborn cells is maintained throughout adulthood in the mammalian brain via the proliferation and differentiation of adult NSCs.[8] Proliferating, differentiating, and migrating NSCs are eventually integrated into neural networks.[8] Adult NSCs exist in the dentate gyrus of the hippocampus and in the subventricular zone of the lateral ventricle, in which NSCs differentiate into new granular neurons and olfactory neurons, respectively.[8] Since the hippocampus is important for the storage and formation of memory, newly generating neurons in the hippocampus are considered to contribute the new memories and maintain the stability of old memories by connecting with existing neurons.[9] Adult hippocampal neurogenesis can be altered by the neuronal network activity modulating effects of neurotransmitters, growth factors, and neurotrophic factors.[10] In addition, various environmental stimuli, such as environmental enrichment and exercise, increase hippocampal neurogenesis. Interestingly, studies performed at our laboratory and those of others have reported that DR, as a metabolic stress, enhances adult hippocampal neurogenesis.[11] Voluntary running is known to enhance hippocampal neurogenesis by increasing the numbers of newly generated cells in the dentate gyrus.[12] However, DR significantly promotes the survival of newly generated neurons without affecting numbers of proliferating cells in the hippocampus. Similarly, enriched environments, such as social activity, also promote the survival of cells generated by hippocampal neurogenesis rather than elevating proliferation.[13] These findings indicate that mild stressors derived from physical, social, or metabolic alterations are beneficial in terms of the activation of NSCs and the formation of new neural circuits in the adult hippocampus.

Neurogenic mechanisms of DR

The neurotrophic factor, brain-derived neurotrophic factor (BDNF), binds to TrkB plasma membrane receptors, which leads to the autophosphorylation of its tyrosine residues in the intracellular kinase domain.[14] Tyrosine phosphorylation activates various signaling pathways, such as the phosphatidylinositol 3-kinase (PI3K)/Akt, MAPK, and PLC-γ pathways. The BDNF signaling pathway involving TrkB has been implicated in the control of cell proliferation and survival in the adult hippocampus.[15] Furthermore, hippocampal BDNF

levels were increased by both DR and an enriched environment, and it was concluded that BDNF is required for the enhancement of hippocampal neurogenesis by DR and environment enrichment in heterozygous BDNF knockout (BDNF$^{+/-}$) mice.[16] In addition, DR upregulates another neurotrophic factor, neurotrophin-3 (NT-3), in the hippocampus, and this facilitates hippocampal plasticity and neurogenesis by neuronal differentiation rather than proliferation.[17] Hippocampal NT-3 is often downregulated in response to brain damage caused by seizures, while other neurotrophic factors are dramatically upregulated in brain injury;[18] thus, DR-mediated stress response is a novel stimulus paradigm distinct from that of brain injury. Several cytokines are elevated in brain cells in response to stress, and it has been reported that interferon-gamma (IFN-γ) is upregulated in the hippocampus of rats fed on a DR regimen.[19] Interestingly, IFN-γ is known to promote neuronal differentiation and the neurite outgrowth of murine adult stem cells, and we have found that IFN-γ promotes the differentiation of NSCs via the JNK pathway.[20,21] Taken together, these results suggest that altered gene regulation by DR could explain the neurogenic mechanism underlying DR via the promotion of the differentiation of NSCs in the adult hippocampus.

Effects of DR mimetics on neurogenesis

Although it seems clear that reducing dietary intakes beneficially enhances hippocampal neurogenesis and cognitive function, practicing DR in humans is problematic for social and practical reasons in this food-rich society. In fact, previous studies have reported that a high-fat diet disrupts cognition, exacerbates neurodegenerative diseases, and impairs hippocampal synaptic plasticity and cognitive abilities, such as learning and memory.[22] In addition, elevated fasting glucose levels and hyperlipidemia induced by a high-sugar diet decrease hippocampal neurogenesis and cognitive function.[23] Therefore, efforts to search for DR mimetics are expanding in the hope of finding some treatment that does not require DR. Several DR mimetics, including 2-deoxy-D-glucose (2DG), metformin, and resveratrol, have been shown to have beneficial effects in neurodegenerative disease models by mimicking the DR-based mechanism.[24–26] 2DG is a nonmetabolizable analog of glucose that inhibits glycolysis. Furthermore, 2DG efficiently blocks neuronal loss in neurodegenerative diseases models, such as in model of Alzheimer's disease, Parkinson's disease, and stroke.[2,25,27] However, the neurogenic property of 2DG has not been tested, although we have reported that 2DG can protect NSCs against oxidative stress. In fact, 2DG appears to both have a toxic effect and reduce NSC proliferation by limiting available energy, thus activating AMP-activated protein kinase (AMPK).[28] Interestingly, AICAR, an adenosine analog used to activate AMPK, induces the astroglial differentiation of NSCs independently of AMPK. However, metformin, a DR mimetic, failed to show astrogenic activity, although it activated AMPK.[29] Resveratrol is another potent DR mimetic that stimulates Sir2, extending lifespan in yeast and nematodes.[30,31] Furthermore, the beneficial effects of resveratrol in diabetes and in age-related neurodegenerative diseases have been well documented,[32,33] and it has been recently reported that resveratrol improves cognitive function in mice by increasing hippocampal IGF-I and hippocampal neurogenesis.[34] Although only a few studies have been conducted on the neurogenic potencies of DR mimetics, novel neurogenic supplements are likely to be discovered by simulating the neurogenic molecular mechanism of DR.

Potent neurogenic phytochemicals that enhance hippocampal neurogenesis

Dietary modulation by DR, diet content, and dietary sources are important for the control of hippocampal neurogenesis and subsequent hippocampus-mediated cognitive ability. Several dietary phytochemicals, or flavonoids, are known to have beneficial effects in the central nervous system by protecting neurons against injury or diseases, although they are not classified as DR mimetics. For example, curcumin is the natural phenolic component of yellow curry spice, and it has been traditionally used in India to treat diseases associated with oxidative stress and inflammation.[35] Although curcumin research has focused primarily on cancer chemoprevention, it has been suggested that its neuroprotective properties may be useful for the treatment of neurodegenerative diseases and age-associated cognitive deficit.[36,37] Recently, it was reported that curcumin has neurogenic properties and that it stimulates embryonic NSC proliferation and adult hippocampal neurogenesis.[38] Interest-

ingly, curcumin has biphasic effects on cultured NSCs, whereby low concentrations stimulate cell proliferation and high concentrations are cytotoxic. This is consistent with the finding that high concentrations of curcumin induce oxidative stress and trigger apoptosis in cancer cells.[39] Our previous data suggest that the NSC-specific mitogenic action of low-concentration curcumin is mediated by the activation of extracellular signal-regulated kinases (ERK) and p38 MAP kinases.[38] Taken together, the concentration-dependent neurogenic property of curcumin resembles the hormesis hypothesis of DR, which is dependent on available energy. In one study, the administration of curcumin significantly increased the numbers of newly generated cells in the dentate gyrus of the hippocampus by stimulating their proliferation rather than their survival rate.[40] Enhanced neurogenesis by promoting NSC proliferation is typically observed in exercise paradigms.[12] Physical activity often elevates reactive oxygen species (ROS) production, and polyphenols including curcumin can activate the Nrf2-antioxidant response element pathway.[47] Therefore, altered redox balance in the hippocampus is supposed to trigger NSC proliferation. In addition, elevated hippocampal BDNF levels are considered to be important for enhancing neurogenesis by physical exercise or curcumin.[40,42] Hippocampal BDNF also seems to be correlated with spatial learning and memory, since flavonoid-enriched foods have been reported to increase hippocampal neurogenesis under chronically stressed condition by maintaining hippocampal BDNF levels and pCREB expression.[43] However, other dietary interventions have been found to have adverse effects on hippocampal neurogenesis. Capsaicin (*trans*-8-methyl-*N*-vanillyl-6-nonenamide) is the major pungent ingredient in red pepper, and it stimulates pain and primary afferent nerves through transient receptor vanilloid channels.[44] Capsaicin has also been reported to reduce the number of newly generated cells in the dentate gyrus of the hippocampus by attenuating the ERK signaling pathway.[45] These findings suggest that the ERK signaling pathway and BDNF signaling could constitute a neurogenic molecular mechanism that will both facilitate the discovery and development of novel drugs that induce adult hippocampal neurogenesis and be useful for the treatment of neurodegenerative diseases and disorders.

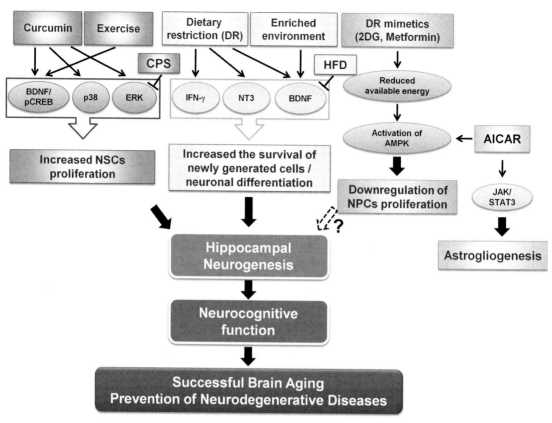

Figure 1. Neurogenic actions of environmental stimuli and dietary modulation including those of DR and its mimetics. DR and an enriched environment increase the survival rate of newly generated cells by upregulating neurotrophic factors or IFN-γ, which can promote neuronal differentiation. However, exercise and curcumin trigger the mitogenic property of NSCs by elevating BDNF levels and activating the MAP kinase signaling pathway. Inhibitions of neurogenic factors by a high-fat diet (HFD) or capsaicin (CPS) impair hippocampal neurogenesis. DR mimetics that putatively limit available energy are unlikely to be able to promote the ATP-consuming process of NPCs proliferation. Note that astrogliogenesis promoted by AICAR is independent of metformin-induced AMPK activation. Enhanced neurogenesis achieved by either increasing the survival rate and neuronal differentiation or stimulating NPC proliferation can expand the hippocampal capacity of endogenous NSCs and probably improve neurocognitive function in neurodegenerative disorders and during aging.

Conclusion

All mammals possess stem cells in many organs, notably in blood, skin, and gut, and these stem cells are considered to contribute to rapid cell replacement throughout life. The existence of NSCs in the adult mammalian brain that are capable of dividing and forming new nerve cells continues to drive the developments of novel approaches to brain repair. In particular, the enhancement of hippocampal neurogenesis is associated with the amelioration of the cognitive deficits associated with aging and Alzheimer's disease.[46] Therefore, much recent focus has been placed on the discovery and development of novel compounds that are capable of specifically

promoting adult NSCs.[47–49] The factors that control the formation of new nerve cells in the human brain are largely unknown, and identifying such factors is likely to lead to new ways of preventing or treating brain disorders. This review introduces the neurogenic properties and molecular mechanisms of DR and provides a basis for a possible preventative strategy whereby endogenous NSCs are recruited by dietary and/or pharmaceutical modulation to address neuronal loss and damage. DR and an enriched environment increase the survival rates of newly generated cells and enhance neurogenesis by upregulating neurotrophic factors. However, exercise and curcumin activate the mitogenic property of NSCs and promote NPC proliferation by BDNF and MAP kinase activation. The action mechanism of DR mimetics is primarily due to energy limitation and the activation of AMPK, and probably the stimulation of astrogliogenesis rather than neurogenesis (Fig. 1). Collectively, understanding the neurogenic mechanisms of DR, DR mimetics, and other small molecules could provide a neurorestorative strategy that stimulates endogenous NSCs and thereby prevents age-related cognitive deficits in aging and age-related neurodegenerative diseases.

Acknowledgments

This research was supported by the National Research Foundation of Korea (NRF) grant funded by the Korea government (MEST) (grant no. 20090093229).

Conflicts of interest

The authors have no conflicts of interest to declare.

References

1. Duan, W. *et al.* 2001. Dietary restriction stimulates BDNF production in the brain and thereby protects neurons against excitotoxic injury. *J. Mol. Neurosci.* **16:** 1–12.
2. Duan, W. & M.P. Mattson. 1999. Dietary restriction and 2-deoxyglucose administration improve behavioral outcome and reduce degeneration of dopaminergic neurons in models of Parkinson's disease. *J. Neurosci. Res.* **57:** 195–206.
3. Prolla, T.A. & M.P. Mattson. 2001. Molecular mechanisms of brain aging and neurodegenerative disorders: lessons from dietary restriction. *Trends Neurosci.* **24:** S21–S31.
4. Yu, Z.F. & M.P. Mattson. 1999. Dietary restriction and 2-deoxyglucose administration reduce focal ischemic brain damage and improve behavioral outcome: evidence for a preconditioning mechanism. *J. Neurosci. Res.* **57:** 830–839.
5. Swindell, W.R. 2009. Genes and gene expression modules associated with caloric restriction and aging in the laboratory mouse. *BMC Genomics* **10:** 585–612.
6. Xu, X. *et al.* 2007. Gene expression atlas of the mouse central nervous system: impact and interactions of age, energy intake and gender. *Genome Biol.* **8:** R234–234-17.
7. Fontan-Lozano, A. *et al.* 2008. Molecular bases of caloric restriction regulation of neuronal synaptic plasticity. *Mol. Neurobiol.* **38:** 167–177.
8. Zhao, C., W. Deng & F.H. Gage. 2008. Mechanisms and functional implications of adult neurogenesis. *Cell* **132:** 645–660.
9. Deng, W., J.B. Aimone & F.H. Gage. 2010. New neurons and new memories: how does adult hippocampal neurogenesis affect learning and memory? *Nat. Rev. Neurosci.* **11:** 339–350.
10. Li, G. & S.J. Pleasure. 2010. Ongoing interplay between the neural network and neurogenesis in the adult hippocampus. *Curr. Opin. Neurobiol.* **20:** 126–233.
11. Lee, J. *et al.* 2000. Dietary restriction increases the number of newly generated neural cells, and induces BDNF expression, in the dentate gyrus of rats. *J. Mol. Neurosci.* **15:** 99–108.
12. van Praag, H., G. Kempermann & F.H. Gage. 1999. Running increases cell proliferation and neurogenesis in the adult mouse dentate gyrus. *Nat. Neurosci.* **2:** 266–270.
13. Kempermann, G., H.G. Kuhn & F.H. Gage. 1997. More hippocampal neurons in adult mice living in an enriched environment. *Nature* **386:** 493–495.
14. Blum, R. & A. Konnerth. 2005. Neurotrophin-mediated rapid signaling in the central nervous system: mechanisms and functions. *Physiology* **20:** 70–78.
15. Gustafsson, E., O. Lindvall & Z. Kokaia. 2003. Intraventricular infusion of TrkB-Fc fusion protein promotes ischemia-induced neurogenesis in adult rat dentate gyrus. *Stroke* **34:** 2710–2705.
16. Lee, J., W. Duan & M.P. Mattson. 2002. Evidence that brain-derived neurotrophic factor is required for basal neurogenesis and mediates, in part, the enhancement of neurogenesis by dietary restriction in the hippocampus of adult mice. *J. Neurochem.* **82:** 1367–1375.
17. Lee, J., K.B. Seroogy & M.P. Mattson. 2002. Dietary restriction enhances neurotrophin expression and neurogenesis in the hippocampus of adult mice. *J. Neurochem.* **80:** 539–547.
18. Rocamora, N., J.M. Palacios & G. Mengod. 1992. Limbic seizures induce a differential regulation of the expression of nerve growth factor, brain-derived neurotrophic factor and neurotrophin-3, in the rat hippocampus. *Brain Res. Mol. Brain Res.* **13:** 27–33.
19. Lee, J. *et al.* 2006. Interferon-gamma is up-regulated in the hippocampus in response to intermittent fasting and protects hippocampal neurons against excitotoxicity. *J. Neurosci. Res.* **83:** 1552–1557.
20. Kim, S.J. *et al.* 2007. Interferon-gamma promotes differentiation of neural progenitor cells via the JNK pathway. *Neurochem. Res.* **32:** 1399–1406.
21. Wong, G., Y. Goldshmit & A.M. Turnley. 2004. Interferon-gamma but not TNF alpha promotes neuronal differentiation and neurite outgrowth of murine adult neural stem cells. *Exp. Neurol.* **187:** 171–177.
22. Greenwood, C.E. & G. Winocur. 1990. Learning and memory impairment in rats fed a high saturated fat diet. *Behav. Neural. Biol.* **53:** 74–87.
23. Stranahan, A.M. *et al.* 2008. Diet-induced insulin resistance impairs hippocampal synaptic plasticity and cognition in middle-aged rats. *Hippocampus* **18:** 1085–1088.
24. El-Mir, M.Y. *et al.* 2008. Neuroprotective role of antidiabetic drug metformin against apoptotic cell death in primary cortical neurons. *J. Mol. Neurosci.* **34:** 77–87.
25. Guo, Z.H. & M.P. Mattson. 2000. In vivo 2-deoxyglucose administration preserves glucose and glutamate transport and mitochondrial function in cortical synaptic terminals after exposure to amyloid beta-peptide and iron: evidence for a stress response. *Exp. Neurol.* **166:** 173–179.
26. Rocha-Gonzalez, H.I., M. Ambriz-Tututi & V. Granados-Soto. 2008. Resveratrol: a natural compound with pharmacological potential in neurodegenerative diseases. *CNS Neurosci. Ther.* **14:** 234–247.
27. Lee, J. *et al.* 1999. 2-Deoxy-D-glucose protects hippocampal neurons against excitotoxic and oxidative injury: evidence for the involvement of stress proteins. *J. Neurosci. Res.* **57:** 48–61.

28. Park, M. *et al.* 2009. 2-Deoxy-d-glucose protects neural progenitor cells against oxidative stress through the activation of AMP-activated protein kinase. *Neurosci. Lett.* **449:** 201–206.

29. Zang, Y. *et al.* 2008. AICAR induces astroglial differentiation of neural stem cells via activating the JAK/STAT3 pathway independently of AMP-activated protein kinase. *J. Biol. Chem.* **283:** 6201–6208.

30. Howitz, K.T. *et al.* 2003. Small molecule activators of sirtuins extend Saccharomyces cerevisiae lifespan. *Nature* **425:** 191–196.

31. Viswanathan, M. *et al.* 2005. A role for SIR-2.1 regulation of ER stress response genes in determining C. elegans life span. *Dev. Cell* **9:** 605–615.

32. Marambaud, P., H. Zhao & P. Davies. 2005. Resveratrol promotes clearance of Alzheimer's disease amyloid-beta peptides. *J. Biol. Chem.* **280:** 37377–37382.

33. Szkudelski, T. & K. Szkudelska. 2011. Anti-diabetic effects of resveratrol. *Ann. N. Y. Acad. Sci.* **1215:** 34–39.

34. Harada, N. *et al.* 2011. Resveratrol improves cognitive function in mice by increasing production of insulin-like growth factor-I in the hippocampus. *J. Nutr. Biochem.* doi:10.1016/j.jnutbio.2010.09.016

35. Huang, M.T. *et al.* 1991. Inhibitory effects of curcumin on in vitro lipoxygenase and cyclooxygenase activities in mouse epidermis. *Cancer Res.* **51:** 813–819.

36. Chuang, S.E. *et al.* 2000. Curcumin-containing diet inhibits diethylnitrosamine-induced murine hepatocarcinogenesis. *Carcinogenesis* **21:** 331–335.

37. Frautschy, S.A. *et al.* 2001. Phenolic anti-inflammatory antioxidant reversal of Abeta-induced cognitive deficits and neuropathology. *Neurobiol. Aging* **22:** 993–1005.

38. Kim, S.J. *et al.* 2008. Curcumin stimulates proliferation of embryonic neural progenitor cells and neurogenesis in the adult hippocampus. *J. Biol. Chem.* **283:** 14497–14505.

39. Divya, C.S. & M.R. Pillai. 2006. Antitumor action of curcumin in human papillomavirus associated cells involves downregulation of viral oncogenes, prevention of NFkB and AP-1 translocation, and modulation of apoptosis. *Mol. Carcinog.* **45:** 320–332.

40. Xu, Y. *et al.* 2007. Curcumin reverses impaired hippocampal neurogenesis and increases serotonin receptor 1A mRNA and brain-derived neurotrophic factor expression in chronically stressed rats. *Brain Res.* **1162:** 9–18.

41. Kang, E.S. *et al.* 2007. Up-regulation of aldose reductase expression mediated by phosphatidylinositol 3-kinase/Akt and Nrf2 is involved in the protective effect of curcumin against oxidative damage. *Free Radic. Biol. Med.* **43:** 535–545.

42. Cotman, C.W. & N.C. Berchtold. 2002. Exercise: a behavioral intervention to enhance brain health and plasticity. *Trends Neurosci.* **25:** 295–301.

43. An, L. *et al.* 2008. The total flavonoids extracted from Xiaobuxin-Tang up-regulate the decreased hippocampal neurogenesis and neurotrophic molecules expression in chronically stressed rats. *Prog. Neuropsychopharmacol. Biol. Psychiatr.* **32:** 1484–1490.

44. Millar, J. *et al.* 1993. The effects of iontophoretic clonidine on neurones in the rat superficial dorsal horn. *Pain* **53:** 137–145.

45. Kong, K.H. *et al.* 2010. Capsaicin impairs proliferation of neural progenitor cells and hippocampal neurogenesis in young mice. *J. Toxicol. Environ. Health A* **73:** 1490–1501.

46. Lazarov, O. *et al.* 2010. When neurogenesis encounters aging and disease. *Trends Neurosci.* **33:** 569–579.

47. MacMillan, K.S. *et al.* 2011. Development of proneurogenic, neuroprotective small molecules. *J. Am. Chem. Soc.* **133:** 1428–1437.

48. Pieper, A.A. *et al.* 2010. Discovery of a proneurogenic, neuroprotective chemical. *Cell* **142:** 39–51.

49. Spencer, J.P., D. Vauzour & C. Rendeiro. 2009. Flavonoids and cognition: the molecular mechanisms underlying their behavioural effects. *Arch Biochem. Biophys.* **492:** 1–9.

Ann. N.Y. Acad. Sci. ISSN 0077-8923

ANNALS OF THE NEW YORK ACADEMY OF SCIENCES
Issue: *Nutrition and Physical Activity in Aging, Obesity, and Cancer*

Growth hormone–STAT5 regulation of growth, hepatocellular carcinoma, and liver metabolism

Myunggi Baik,[2] Ji Hoon Yu,[1] and Lothar Hennighausen[1,2]

[1]Laboratory of Genetics and Physiology, National Institutes of Health, Bethesda, Maryland. [2]Deptartment of Molecular Biotechnology, WCU-RNNM, Chonnam National University, Gwangju, Republic of Korea

Address for correspondence: Lothar Hennighausen, Laboratory of Genetics and Physiology, National Institutes of Health, Bethesda, MD, 20892. lotharh@mail.nih.gov

The liver is a primary target of growth hormone (GH). GH signals are mediated by the transcription factor signal transducer and activator of transcription 5 (STAT5). Here, we focus on recent discoveries about the role of GH–STAT5 signaling in hepatic physiology and pathophysiology. We discuss roles of the GH–STAT5 axis in body growth, lipid metabolism, and the cell cycle pertaining to hepatosteatosis, fibrosis, and hepatocellular carcinoma. Finally, we discuss recent discoveries about the role of GH–STAT5 in sex-specific gene expression and bile acid, steroid, and drug metabolism.

Keywords: growth hormone; STAT5; liver function

Introduction

In the liver, growth hormone (GH) binds its cognate receptor (GHR), which results in the activation of JAK2, which in turn phosphorylates the signal transducer and activator of transcription 5 (STAT5) (Fig. 1A). Phosphorylated STAT5 translocates to the nucleus, where it binds to GAS motifs to regulate target genes. In the liver, GH–STAT5 signaling regulates expression of target genes associated with several physiological processes, including body growth, cell cycle, lipid, bile acid (BA), steroid, and drug metabolism (Fig. 1; Table 1). Disruption of STAT5 signaling is associated with liver disease, including fatty liver, fibrosis, and hepatocellular carcinoma (HCC). Here, we review the current status of GH–STAT5 signaling on these topics.

STAT5, growth, lipid metabolism, cell cycle, and HCC

STAT5 and body growth

GH–STAT5 signaling regulates postnatal body growth by inducing *Igf-1* gene expression.[1] Kofoed *et al.* described a patient with a homozygous mutation in the *Stat5b* gene, which resulted in IGF-1 deficiency and growth hormone insensitivity with impairment of body growth.[2] The *Igf-1* gene is a direct target of STAT5, and our studies revealed that IGF-1 concentrations were reduced in STAT5-deficient mice.[3,4] Two distinct GH-inducible STAT5B binding motifs have been identified in human *Igf-1* and rat *Igf-1* loci.[5] Other studies have suggested the potential existence of multiple STAT5B-binding sites in the *Igf-1* gene.[6] Recently, it has been demonstrated that upon GH stimulation, STAT5B is recruited to a least seven distinct chromosomal domains throughout the *Igf-1* locus, some of them with the potential of long-range enhancers.[7]

The six-exon *Igf-1* gene in rats contains two promoters with distinct tissue-limited profiles of expression.[8] GH-mediated signaling caused acute alterations in hepatic chromatin architecture at the *Igf-1* locus.[9] At promoter 1, GH caused RNA Pol II to be released from a previously recruited paused preinitiation complex. In contrast, at promoter 2, hormone treatment facilitates recruitment followed by the activation of RNA Pol II to initiate transcription. It appears that both *Igf-1* promoters reside in open chromatin, despite minimal transcription in the absence of GH, as inferred from relatively high levels of core histone acetylation and enhanced histone H3K4 trimethylation. It has been suggested

doi: 10.1111/j.1749-6632.2011.06100.x

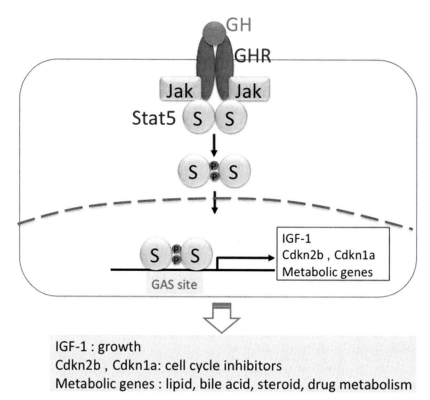

IGF-1 : growth
Cdkn2b , Cdkn1a: cell cycle inhibitors
Metabolic genes : lipid, bile acid, steroid, drug metabolism

Figure 1. GH–STAT5 signaling pathway. GH binds its receptor and then activates Jak2, which in turn activates STAT5 by phosphorylation. Phosphorylated STAT5 goes to the nucleus, where it binds to gamma interferon–activated sequence (GAS) site of target gene's promoters. It activates transcription of the *Igf-1* gene.[3,4] It activates cell cycle inhibitors *Cdkn2b* (cyclin-dependent kinase inhibitor 2B; p15[INK4B]) and *Cdkn1a* (p21[CIP1]).[13] It also activates metabolic genes associated with lipid, bile acid, and steroid/drug metabolism, signal transducer and activator of transcription 5.

that this landscape of open chromatin may reflect the impact of previous long-term exposure to GH.

STAT5 and lipid metabolism

Several studies have suggested that GH–STAT5 signaling plays an important role in controlling hepatic lipid metabolism. Mice with a liver-specific STAT5 ablation developed hepatosteatosis, glucose intolerance, insulin resistance, late-onset obesity, and impaired liver regeneration.[3] Notably, expression of genes associated with adipogenesis (PPARγ) and fatty acid uptake (CD36) was upregulated in STAT5A/B-deficient mice.[3] These changes may partially explain hepatosteatosis induced by loss of STAT5. Liver-specific deletion of the growth hormone receptor also displayed marked hepatic steatosis, insulin resistance, glucose intolerance, and increased triglyceride synthesis and decreased efflux.[10] Recent studies with STAT5-deficient mice suggest that elevated CD36, PPARγ, and PGC1α/β, along

with increased fatty acid synthesis, lipoprotein lipase, and very low-density lipoprotein receptor, are responsible for hepatic steatosis in these mice.[11] Further studies with hepatocyte-specific STAT5-null mice will contribute to an understanding of the underlying molecular mechanisms.

STAT5, cell cycle, and HCC

Loss of STAT5 in hepatocytes caused steatosis, liver fibrosis, and promoted chemically induced liver cancer,[12] which was associated with altered expression of cell cycle regulators.[13] Loss of STAT5 from mouse embryonic fibroblasts (MEFs) leads to enhanced proliferation and was linked to reduced levels of the cell cycle inhibitors *Cdkn2b* (cyclin-dependent kinase inhibitor 2B; p15[INK4B]) and *Cdkn1a* (p21[CIP1]). Growth hormone, through STAT5 binding to promoter-bound GAS motifs, enhanced expression of the *Cdkn2b* and *Cdkn1a* genes. In mouse liver, STAT5, like in MEFs, activated

Table 1. Genes regulated by STAT5 and sex in the liver

Gene	STAT5 deletion effect in males	STAT5 regulation	References
Growth			
IGF-1, IGFALS, IGFBP3, EGFR	↓	STAT5A/B	3,4
Lipid metabolism			
PPARγ, CD36	↑	STAT5A/B	3
Cell cycle inhibitor			
Cdkn1a, Cdkn2b	↓	STAT5A	13
Cell cycle regulator			
Cyclin D1	↑	STAT5A/B	3,4,13
JAK-STAT pathway associated genes			
Socs2, Cish	↓	STAT5A/B	3,4
Socs3, STAT1, STAT3	↑	STAT5A/B	3,4
Male-specific genes			
Cyp4a12, Gstπ, Slp, Elovl3, Mup3, Cyp7b1, Slco1a1(Oatp1), Hsd3b5, Moxdl1	↓	STAT5B	22–34
B cell leukemia/lymphoma 6 (Bcl6)	–	STAT5A/B	40,44
Female-specific genes			
Cyp2a4, Cyp39a1, Sult1e1, Nnmt	↑	STAT5B	22, 35–37
Cyp2b9, Cyp2b13	↑	–	22,38,39
Cyp2b10	↓	STAT5B	17

Arrows indicate changes in gene expression (up, down, no change).

expression of the *Cdkn2b* gene. This study demonstrated that cytokines, through STAT5, induce the expression of key cell cycle inhibitors. STAT5 might promote cell cycle arrest in chronically injured liver hepatocyte and HCC as a critical tumor suppressor. STAT5 also regulates tumor suppressor and antiproliferating activities in other cell types. In T cells, oncogenic tyrosine kinase NPM1-ALK induces epigenetic silencing of STAT5A gene, and STAT5A protein can act as a key tumor suppressor by reciprocally inhibiting expression of NPM1-ALK.[14] It has been suggested that loss of STAT5A is crucial for NPM1-ALK-mediated oncogenesis as this permits uninterrupted transcription of NPM1-ALK. In human diploid fibroblasts, constitutive activation of STAT5A also induced a cell cycle arrest with the characteristics of cellular senescence including the nuclear accumulation of the p53 tumor suppressor protein and accumulated DNA damage foci and activated ATM and ATR.[15] SOCS1 can link the DNA

damage signals characteristic of STAT5A-expressing cells to p53, serving as a mediator for p53 phosphorylation by ATM and ATR.[15,16] These results suggest that STAT5 can regulate senescence by activating the tumor suppressors SOCS1 and p53.[16]

STAT5, sex-specific gene expression, bile acid, drug, and steroid metabolism

STAT5 and sex-specific gene expression

The liver is a sexually dimorphic organ, with sex-dependent differential expression of more than 1,000 genes in rats and mice.[17,18] In several species, including mice and rats, pulsatile secretion of GH in males is distinct from that in females, and sexual dimorphic expression patterns of genes in liver tissue have been observed.[19] In males, testosterone acts on the hypothalamic–pituitary axis to drive pronounced pulsatile GH secretion. The androgenic hormones testosterone and dihydroxytestosterone convey their signals through the androgen receptor

(AR).[20] Recent studies have revealed that expression of the AR gene in skeletal muscle is directly controlled by GH through STAT5A/B.[21] This finding opens studies to explore links between AR, GH, and sex-specific gene expression.

Many of the sex-specific genes in liver are regulated by the GH–STAT5 pathway (Table 1).[19] In liver, STAT5B is ~20-fold more abundant than STAT5A, suggesting that the vast majority of GH signaling is mediated through STAT5B. STAT5B-deficient male mice are characterized by reduced body growth and a loss of sex-specific expression of genes encoding cytochrome *P-450* (*Cyp*) enzymes.[1] Many studies showed that male-specific genes including *Cyp4a12*,[22–24] *Gstπ*,[22,25] *Slp*,[22,26] *Elovl3*,[22,27] *Mup3*,[22,28] *Mup1/2/6/8*,[22] *Cyp7b1*,[22,29] *Slco1a1*,[22,30,31] *Hsd3b5*,[22,32,33] and *Moxdl1*[22,34] were downregulated in the male liver of hepatocyte STAT5A/B-deficient mice. In contrast, female-specific liver genes including *Cyp2a4*,[22,35] *Cyp39a1*,[22] *Sult1e1*,[22,36] *Nnmt*,[22,37] *Cyp2b9*,[22,38] and *Cyp2b13*[22,39] were upregulated (derepressed). Microarray analysis showed that 90% of male-predominant genes were suppressed and 60% of female-predominant genes were induced in liver tissue of STAT5B-null male mice.[17] Another study also identified several gene sets displaying sexual dimorphic expression.[18] Gene expression profiling on global STAT5A- and STAT5B-null mice confirmed STAT5B as the transcription factor conveying sexual dimorphism, but a distinct role for STAT5A has been established as well. The expression of 15% of female-predominant genes was dependent on the presence of STAT5A. These studies highlight sex-specific roles of the two STAT5 isoforms, with STAT5A preferentially regulating gene expression in the female liver while STAT5B plays the predominant role in the male.

The regulation of sex-specific genes through both transcriptional activators and repressors has been investigated. STAT5B synergistically enhanced the transcriptional activity of HNF4-α toward two other male-specific liver target genes, *Cyp2d9* and *Cyp8b1*.[40] These results highlight the ability of STAT5B to act in concert with HNF4-α to regulate male-specific liver *Cyp* genes. They also proposed that HNF-6 and HNF-3β are female-predominant, positive regulators of *Cyp2c12* (female specific) and negative regulators of *Cyp2a2* (male specific). The transcriptional repressor *Bcl6* is a male-specific rat liver gene product.[41] The DNA recognition motif of *Bcl6*[42] resembles the STAT5 consensus site TTC-NNNGAA.[43] This raises the possibility that *Bcl6* and STAT proteins may regulate overlapping sets of genes. *Bcl6* was bound to a subset of STAT5-binding sites in male liver chromatin, including a *Socs2* STAT5-binding site where *Bcl6* binding increased substantially between plasma GH pulses when STAT5 binding was low.[44] Thus, *Bcl6* and STAT5 binding was inversely coordinated by the endogenous pulses of pituitary GH release. They suggest that this male-specific transcriptional repressor modulates hepatic GH signaling to select STAT5 target genes.

Chromatin structure affected sex-dependent gene expression. The sex-related expression of the *Cyp2c12* gene resulted from the inaccessibility of STAT5 to the GH-responsive element by chromatin condensation in male rat livers.[45] Sex-specific differential binding affinity of STAT5 to target genes was observed in rats. Phylogenetic footprinting was used to predict functional transcription factor binding sites STAT5 in the GH-responsive genes *Igf-1*, *SOCS2*, and *HNF-6*.[46] In female rat liver, where nuclear STAT5 activity is generally low, STAT5 binding to *Igf-1* and *SOCS2* was limited to high-affinity sites, while male-specific gene expression was associated with male-specific STAT5 binding to multiple low-affinity STAT5 sites.

STAT5 and bile acid/drug metabolism

Many sex-specific genes belong to the *Cyps*, sulfotransferases (Sults), or glutathione transferase (Gst) family that play important roles in BA, steroid, and drug metabolism. Several studies report that GH–STAT5 signaling regulates expression of genes associated with BA metabolism including BA synthesis, BA uptake, BA detoxification, and excretion (Fig. 2). Conversion of cholesterol to 7α-hydroxycholesterol by Cyp7a1 cholesterol 7a-hydroxylase is the initial and rate-limiting step in BA synthesis.[47] In addition, *Cyp7b1* oxycholesterol 7α-hydroxyase catalyzes the alternative pathway of cholesterol metabolism. Expression of *Cyp7b1* (oxysterol 7α-hydroxylase) was downregulated in the liver of STAT5-deleted mice.[22,29] Expression of Hsd3b5 (3βHSD; 3β-hydroxysteroid dehydrogenase type 5), which is involved in the oxidation of the 3β-OH and isomerization of the C5-C6 double bond, was also downregulated in the liver of

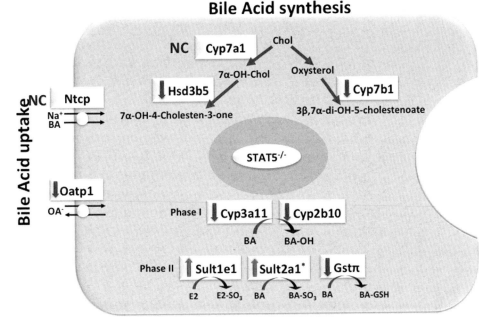

Figure 2. Changes in hepatic gene expression of BA metabolism in STAT5-deficient mice. STAT5 liver–specific knockout mice (STAT5$^{-/-}$) exhibited changes in gene expression of BA metabolism including synthesis,[22,29,32,33] uptake,[22,30,31] and detoxification.[17,22,25] Sult2a1 gene was induced in GH-releasing hormone receptor-deficient little (lit/lit) mouse.[50] Ntcp, Na$^+$/taurocholate cotransporter; Oatp1, organic anion transporter 1; BA, bile acid; Gstπ, glutathione S-transferase pi class; Chol, cholesterol; E2, estradiol; OA$^-$, organic anions; BA-OH, hydroxylated BA; BA-SO3, sulfated BA; GSH, glutathione. Arrows indicate changes in gene expression (up, down). NC, no change.

STAT5-deleted mice.[22,32,33] Secondary BAs, lithocholic acid and deoxycholic acid, are synthesized in the gut lumen from the primary BAs by microbial enzymes and are reabsorbed into the enterohepatic circulation. *Cyp3a10/6β*-hydroxylase is a male-specific P450 that catalyzes 6β-hydroxylation of lithocholic acid.[47,48] STAT5a/b positively mediated GH-dependent regulation of *Cyp3a10* promoter activity.[49]

GH–STAT5 signaling regulates gene expression associated with BA transport. *Slco1a1* (the organic anion transporter *Oatp1*) is an uptake transport of a variety of organic endo- and exogenous compounds, such as BAs, steroid and thyroid hormones and their conjugates, and numerous drugs and toxins.[30,31] Expression of BA transporter *Slco1a1* was downregulated in STAT5-deleted male mice.[22,30,31] To investigate the physiologic and pharmacologic roles of Oatps of the 1a and 1b subfamilies, mice were generated lacking all established and predicted mouse Oatp1a/1b transporters (referred to

as *Slco1a/1b$^{-/-}$* mice).[30] *Slco1a/1b$^{-/-}$* exhibited markedly increased plasma levels of bilirubin conjugated to glucuronide and increased plasma levels of unconjugated BAs, indicating that Oatp1a/1b transporters normally mediate extensive hepatic reuptake of glucuronidated bilirubin. *Slco1a/1b$^{-/-}$* mice also showed marked decrease in hepatic uptake and consequently increased systemic exposure following intravenous or oral administration of the OATP substrate drugs methotrexate and fexofenadine. These data indicate that Oatp1a/1b transporters play an essential role in hepatic reuptake of conjugated bilirubin and uptake of unconjugated BAs and drugs.

The GH–STAT5 pathway also regulates gene expression associated with BA detoxification. Hydroxylation of BAs is mediated by the phase I-detoxifying *Cyp* enzymes *Cyp3a11* and *Cyp2b10*.[17] The expression of *Cyp3a11* and *Cyp2b10* genes was downregulated in STAT5B-deficient male mice.[17] Sult2a1 catalyzes the formation of BAs sulfates

(BA-sulfates). Sulfation of BAs increases their solubility, decreases their intestinal absorption, and enhances their fecal and urinary excretion. Sult2a1 is female-predominant Sult in mouse liver. Expression of Sult2a1 is suppressed by androgens and male-pattern GH secretion, while it is induced by estrogens and female-pattern GH secretion.[50] Hepatic expression of Sult2a1 was increased in GH-releasing hormone receptor-deficient little (*lit/lit*) mouse in males.[50] In mice, STAT5 deletion in the liver resulted in decreased glutathione S-transferase pi class (Gstπ), which is one of phase II detoxification enzymes, catalyzing the conjugation of glutathione to BA.[22,25]

Recent studies pointed to the importance of GH-STAT5 signaling for maintaining BA homeostasis. Deletion of the STAT5A/B locus in hepatocyte and cholangiocytes in the multidrug resistance gene 2 knockout (*Mdr2$^{-/-}$*), resulted in an early and severe liver fibrosis phenotype, accompanied by deregulated expression of important regulators of BA homeostasis,[51] suggesting that loss of STAT5 sensitizes hepatocytes to BA-induced damage.

Overall, loss of liver-specific STAT5 resulted in decreases in *Cyp7b1* and *Hsd3b5* gene expression for BA synthesis and a decrease in Oapt1 gene expression for BA uptake. In addition, deletion of the STAT5 gene resulted in a decrease in phase I detoxifying *Cyp3a11* and *Cyp2b10* gene expression, whereas phase II detoxifying Sult1e1 gene expression was increased in these mice. Thus, these studies imply that the GH–STAT5 pathway has an important function in regulating BA metabolism including synthesis, transport, and detoxification. Whether these changes are either directly or indirectly regulated by GH–STAT5 signaling remains to be determined. Elucidating the direct or indirect molecular mechanisms involved in these processes should lead to a better understanding of the role of GH–STAT5 in BA metabolism, cholesterol homeostasis, and liver diseases such as cholestasis and gallstones.

STAT5 and steroid hormone metabolism

Liver is a target organ for steroid hormone metabolism. Several studies have suggested that GH–STAT5 regulates genes linked to steroid metabolism (Fig. 3). One of these genes, *HSD3b5*, catalyzes the formation of the relatively inactive androstanediol from the active dihydrotestos-

terone.[33] *HSD3B5* gene expression was downregulated in the liver of STAT5-deleted male mice.[22,32,33] In contrast, another gene involved in testosterone metabolism, testosterone 16α-hydroxylase (*Cyp2b9*), which hydroxylates testosterone at the 16α position, was upregulated in STAT5-deleted male mice.[22] Cyp7b1 (oxysterol 7α-hydroxylase), responsible for the hydroxylation of dehydroepiandrosterone, androstenediol, androstanetriol, and 25-hydroxycholesterol, was downregulated in STAT5-deleted male mice.[22,29]

Genes associated with estrogen metabolism are also regulated by GH–STAT5. Sult1e1 is the major Sult isoform responsible for the inactivation of β-estradiol via sulfation at physiological concentrations.[52] Expression of sult1e1 gene was upregulated in STAT5-deficient male mice.[22,36] Changes in Sult1e1 activity may alter E2 levels and E2-regulated processes in tissues and cells, including those of the liver where it is expressed at significant levels. Sult1e1 was also shown to have high affinity (nM range) for diethylstilbestrol and tamoxifen as well as for E2 and estrone.[53,54] Testosterone or estradiol 15alpha-hydroxylase *Cyp2a4* gene is female specific, and this gene is upregulated in STAT5-deleted male mice.[22,35,38]

Thus, hepatic GH–STAT5 signaling regulates, at least in part, genes involved in hepatic testosterone/estrogen and drug metabolism. Changes in the metabolism of steroid hormones may have a role in alterations in liver function or the development of liver disease. Further studies regarding direct or indirect molecular mechanisms that regulate steroid/drug metabolism by GH–STAT5 pathway will enhance our understanding of functional significance of GH–STAT5 pathway on steroid metabolism in the liver. Overall, many studies have established that GH–STAT5 signaling is key in dictating sex differences in the expression of a large number of liver gene products, including many *Cyps* and other DMEs. Additional investigations are needed to elucidate mechanisms that control expression of these genes by GH–STAT5 and to understand functional roles of GH–STAT5 regulating BA, steroid, and drug metabolism and its clinical implications. Studies with hepatocyte-specific STAT5-deleted mice will allow further understanding of the functional role of sex-specific genes for controlling drug, steroid, and BA metabolism and of related liver diseases.

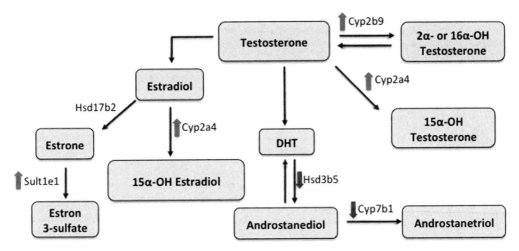

Figure 3. Changes in hepatic gene expression of testosterone and estrogen metabolism in STAT5-deficient mice. STAT5 liver–specific knockout mice downregulated expression of *Hsd3b5*[22,32] and *Cyp7b1* genes,[22,29] whereas it upregulated expression of *Cyp2b9*,[22,38] *Cyp2a4*,[22,35] and *Sult1e1* genes[22,36] in the liver. DHT, dihydrotestosterone; OH, hydroxylated. Arrows indicate changes in gene expression (up, down).

Acknowledgments

This work was funded in part through the Intramural program of the NIH and through a grant from WCU Project (R33-10059) through the NRF and by a grant from the Next-Generation BioGreen 21 Program (No. PJ008191032011), Rural Development Administration, Republic of Korea.

Conflicts of interest

The authors declare no conflicts of interest.

References

1. Udy, G.B., R.P. Towers, R.G. Snell, *et al.* 1997. Requirement of STAT5b for sexual dimorphism of body growth rates and liver gene expression. *Proc. Natl. Acad. Sci. USA* **94:** 7239–7244.
2. Kofoed, E.M., V. Hwa, B. Little, *et al.* 2003. Growth hormone insensitivity associated with a STAT5b mutation. *N. Engl. J. Med.* **349:** 1139–1147.
3. Cui, Y., G. Riedlinger, K. Miyoshi, *et al.* 2004. Inactivation of STAT5 in mouse mammary epithelium during pregnancy reveals distinct functions in cell proliferation, survival, and differentiation. *Mol. Cell. Biol.* **24:** 8037–8047.
4. Engblom, D., J.W. Kornfeld, L. Schwake, *et al.* 2007. Direct glucocorticoid receptor-STAT5 interaction in hepatocytes controls body size and maturation-related gene expression. *Genes Dev.* **21:** 1157–1162.
5. Chia, D.J., M. Ono, J. Woelfle, *et al.* 2006. Characterization of distinct STAT5b binding sites that mediate growth hormone-stimulated IGF-I gene transcription. *J. Biol. Chem.* **281:** 3190–3197.
6. Eleswarapu, S., X. Ge, Y. Wang, *et al.* 2009. Growth hormone-activated STAT5 may indirectly stimulate IGF-I gene transcription through HNF-3{gamma}. *Mol. Endocrinol.* **23:** 2026–2037.
7. Chia, D.J., B. Varco-Merth & P. Rotwein. 2010. Dispersed Chromosomal STAT5b-binding elements mediate growth hormone-activated insulin-like growth factor-I gene transcription. *J. Biol. Chem.* **285:** 17636–17647.
8. Hall, L.J., Y. Kajimoto, D. Bichell, *et al.* 1992. Functional analysis of the rat insulin-like growth factor I gene and identification of an IGF-I gene promoter. *DNA Cell. Biol.* **11:** 301–313.
9. Chia, D.J., J.J. Young, A.R. Mertens, *et al.* 2010. Distinct alterations in chromatin organization of the two IGF-I promoters precede growth hormone-induced activation of IGF-I gene transcription. *Mol. Endocrinol.* **24:** 779–789.
10. Fan, Y., R.K. Menon, P. Cohen, *et al.* 2009. Liver-specific deletion of the growth hormone receptor reveals essential role of growth hormone signaling in hepatic lipid metabolism. *J. Biol. Chem.* **284:** 19937–19944.
11. Barclay, J.L., C.N. Nelson, M. Ishikawa, *et al.* 2011. GH-dependent STAT5 signaling plays an important role in hepatic lipid metabolism. *Endocrinology* **152:** 181–192.
12. Hosui, A., A. Kimura, D. Yamaji, *et al.* 2009. Loss of STAT5 causes liver fibrosis and cancer development through increased TGF-{beta} and STAT3 activation. *J. Exp. Med.* **206:** 819–831.
13. Yu, J.H., B.M. Zhu, M. Wickre, *et al.* 2010. The transcription factors signal transducer and activator of transcription 5A (STAT5A) and STAT5B negatively regulate cell proliferation through the activation of cyclin-dependent kinase inhibitor 2b (Cdkn2b) and Cdkn1a expression. *Hepatology* **52:** 1808–1818.
14. Zhang, Q., H.Y. Wang, X. Liu, *et al.* 2007. STAT5A is epigenetically silenced by the tyrosine kinase NPM1-ALK and acts as a tumor suppressor by reciprocally inhibiting NPM1-ALK expression. *Nat. Med.* **13:** 1341–1348.

15. Mallette, F.A., M.F. Gaumont-Leclerc & G. Ferbeyre. 2007. The DNA damage signaling pathway is a critical mediator of oncogene-induced senescence. *Genes Dev.* **21:** 43–48.

16. Calabrese, V., F.A. Mallette, X. Deschênes-Simard, *et al.* 2009. SOCS1 links cytokine signaling to p53 and senescence. *Mol. Cell.* **36:** 754–767.

17. Clodfelter, K.H., M.G. Holloway, P. Hodor, *et al.* 2006. Sex-dependent liver gene expression is extensive and largely dependent upon signal transducer and activator of transcription 5b (STAT5b): STAT5b-dependent activation of male genes and repression of female genes revealed by microarray analysis. *Mol. Endocrinol.* **20:** 1333–1351.

18. Clodfelter, K.H., G.D. Miles, V. Wauthier, *et al.* 2007. Role of STAT5a in regulation of sex-specific gene expression in female but not male mouse liver revealed by microarray analysis. *Physiol. Genomics* **31:** 63–74.

19. Waxman, D.J. & C. O'Connor. 2006. Growth hormone regulation of sex-dependent liver gene expression. *Mol. Endocrinol.* **20:** 2613–2629.

20. Herbst, K.L. & S. Bhasin. 2004. Testosterone action on skeletal muscle. *Curr. Opin. Clin. Nutr. Metab. Care* **7:** 271–277.

21. Klover, P., W. Chen, B.M. Zhu, *et al.* 2009. Skeletal muscle growth and fiber composition in mice are regulated through the transcription factors STAT5a/b: linking growth hormone to the androgen receptor. *FASEB J.* **23:** 3140–3148.

22. Holloway, M.G., Y. Cui, E.V. Laz, *et al.* 2007. Loss of sexually dimorphic liver gene expression upon hepatocyte-specific deletion of STAT5a-STAT5b locus. *Endocrinology* **148:** 1977–1986.

23. Okita, R.T. & J.R. Okita. 2001. Cytochrome P450 4A fatty acid omega hydroxylases. *Curr. Drug Metab.* **2:** 265–281.

24. Hardwick, J.P. 2008. Cytochrome P450 omega hydroxylase (CYP4) function in fatty acid metabolism and metabolic diseases. *Biochem. Pharmacol.* **75:** 2263–2275.

25. Hayes, J.D., J.U. Flanagan & I.R. Jowsey. 2005. Glutathione transferases. *Annu. Rev. Pharmacol. Toxicol.* **45:** 51–88.

26. Krebs, C.J., S. Khan, J.W. MacDonald, *et al.* 2009. Regulator of sex-limitation KRAB zinc finger proteins modulate sex-dependent and -independent liver metabolism. *Physiol. Genomics* **38:** 16–28.

27. Brolinson, A., S. Fourcade, A. Jakobsson, *et al.* 2008. Steroid hormones control circadian Elovl3 expression in mouse liver. *Endocrinology* **149:** 3158–3166.

28. Chamero, P., T.F. Marton, D.W. Logan, *et al.* 2007. Identification of protein pheromones that promote aggressive behaviour. *Nature* **450:** 899–902.

29. Schwarz, M., E.G. Lund & D.W. Rusell. 1998. Two 7 alpha-hydroxylase enzymes in bile acid biosynthesis. *Curr. Opin. Lipidol.* **9:** 113–118.

30. van de Steeg, E., E. Wagenaar, C.M. van der Kruijssen, *et al.* 2010. Organic anion transporting polypeptide 1a/1b-knockout mice provide insights into hepatic handling of bilirubin, bile acids, and drugs. *J. Clin. Invest.* **120:** 2942–2952.

31. Kalliokoski, A. & M. Niemi. 2009. Impact of OATP transporters on pharmacokinetics. *Br. J. Pharmacol.* **158:** 693–705.

32. Mason, J.I., D.S. Keeney, I.M. Bird, *et al.* 1997. The regulation of 3 beta-hydroxysteroid dehydrogenase expression. *Steroids* **62:** 164–168.

33. Abbaszade, I.G., T.R. Clarke, C.H. Park, *et al.* 1995. The mouse 3 beta-hydroxysteroid dehydrogenase multigene family includes two functionally distinct groups of proteins. *Mol. Endocrinol.* **9:** 1214–1222.

34. Xin, X., R.E. Mains & B.A. Eipper. 2004. Monooxygenase X, a member of the copper-dependent monooxygenase family localized to the endoplasmic reticulum. *J. Biol. Chem.* **279:** 48159–48167.

35. Lavery, D.J., L. Lopez-Molina, R. Margueron, *et al.* 1999. Circadian expression of the steroid 15 alpha-hydroxylase (Cyp2a4) and coumarin 7-hydroxylase (Cyp2a5) genes in mouse liver is regulated by the PAR leucine zipper transcription factor DBP. *Mol.Cell. Biol.* **19:** 6488–6499.

36. Li, L., D. He, T.W. Wilborn, *et al.* 2009. Increased SULT1E1 activity in HepG2 hepatocytes decreases growth hormone stimulation of STAT5b phosphorylation. *Steroids* **74:** 20–29.

37. Weinshilboum, R. 1989. Methyltransferase pharmacogenetics. *Pharmacol. Ther.* **43:** 77–90.

38. Sakuma, T., K. Kitajima, M. Nishiyama, *et al.* 2004. Suppression of female-specific murine Cyp2b9 gene expression by growth or glucocorticoid hormones. *Biochem. Biophy. Res. Commun.* **323:** 776–781.

39. Lakso, M., R. Masaki, M. Noshiro, *et al.* 1991. Structures and characterization of sex-specific mouse cytochrome P-450 genes as members within a large family. Duplication boundary and evolution. *Eur. J. Biochem.* **195:** 477–486.

40. Wiwi, C.A. & D.J. Waxman. 2005. Role of hepatocyte nuclear factors in transcriptional regulation of male-specific CYP2A2. *J. Biol.Chem.* **280:** 3259–3268.

41. Wauthier, V. & D.J. Waxman. 2008. Sex-specific early growth hormone response genes in rat liver. *Mol. Endocrinol.* **22:** 1962–1974.

42. Seyfert, V.L., D. Allman, Y. He, *et al.* 1996. Transcriptional repression by the proto-oncogene BCL-6. *Oncogene* **12:** 2331–2342.

43. Ehret, G.B., P. Reichenbach, U. Schindler, *et al.* 2001. DNA binding specificity of different STAT proteins. Comparison of in vitro specificity with natural target sites. *J. Biol. Chem.* **276:** 6675–6688.

44. Meyer, R.D., E.V. Laz, T. Su, *et al.* 2009. Male-specific hepatic Bcl6: growth hormone-induced block of transcription elongation in females and binding to target genes inversely coordinated with STAT5. *Mol. Endocrinol.* **23:** 1914–1926.

45. Endo, M., Y. Takahashi, Y. Sasaki, *et al.* 2005. Novel gender-related regulation of CYP2C12 gene expression in rats. *Mol. Endocrinol.* **19:** 1181–1190.

46. Laz, E.V., A. Sugathan & D.J. Waxman. 2009. Dynamic in vivo binding of STAT5 to growth hormone-regulated genes in intact rat liver. Sex-specific binding at low- but not high-affinity STAT5 sites. *Mol. Endocrinol.* **23:** 1242–1254.

47. Teixeira, J. & G. Gil. 1991. Cloning, expression, and regulation of lithocholic acid 6b-hydroxylase. *J. Biol. Chem.* **266:** 21030–21036.

48. Chang, T. K. H., J. Teixeira, *et al.* 1993. The lithocholic acid 6b-hydroxylase cytochrome P-450, CYP 3A10, is an active catalyst of steroid-hormone 6b-hydroxylation. *Biochem. J.* **291:** 429–434.

49. Subramanian, A., J. Wang & G. Gil. 1998. STAT 5 and NF-Y are involved in expression and growth hormone-mediated sexually dimorphic regulation of cytochrome P450 3A10/lithocholic acid 6beta-hydroxylase. *Nucleic Acids Res.* **26:** 2173–2178.

50. Alnouti, Y. & C.D. Klaassen. 2011. Mechanisms of gender-specific regulation of mouse sulfotransferases (Sults). *Xenobiotica* **41:** 187–197.

51. Blaas, L., J.W. Kornfeld, D. Schramek, *et al.* 2010. Disruption of the growth hormone–signal transducer and activator of transcription 5-insulinlike growth factor 1 axis severely aggravates liver fibrosis in a mouse model of cholestasis. *Hepatology* **51:** 1319–1326.

52. Falany, J.L., H. Greer, T. Kovacs, *et al.* 2002. Elevation of hepatic sulphotransferase activities in mice with resistance to cystic fibrosis. *Biochem. J.* **364:** 115–120.

53. Falany, C.N. 1997. Enzymology of human cytosolic SULTs. *FASEB J.* **11:** 206–216.

54. Falany, C.N., V. Krasnykh & J.L. Falany. 1995. Bacterial expression and characterization of a cDNA for human liver estrogen sulfotransferase. *J. Steroid Biochem. Molec. Biol.* **52:** 529–539.

Ann. N.Y. Acad. Sci. ISSN 0077-8923

Practical issues in genome-wide association studies for physical activity

Jaehee Kim,[1] Sohee Oh,[2] Haesook Min,[3] Yeonjung Kim,[3] and Taesung Park[1,2]

[1]Interdisciplinary Program in Bioinformatics, Seoul National University, Kwan-ak St. 599, Kwan-ak Gu, Seoul, South Korea. [2]Department of Statistics, Seoul National University, South Korea. [3]Division of Epidemiology and Health Index, Center for Genome Science, KNIH, KCDC, South Korea

Address for correspondence: T. Park, Department of Statistics, Seoul National University, Kwan-ak St. 599, Kwan-ak Gu, Seoul 151-741, South, Korea. tspark@stats.snu.ac.kr

Genome-wide association studies (GWAS) have successfully identified many genetic variants that are associated with many complex traits. For example, GWAS can be useful for understanding the genetic basis of physical activity (PA). To date, however, there have been only a few GWAS regarding PA. In this article, we overview some practical issues for more efficient GWAS for PA: phenotype definition of PA, the analysis method, population stratification, replication, and sample size. We discuss these issues within a large-scale GWA data set from the Korea Association REsource (KARE) project, including 8,842 samples and 352,228 single nucleotide polymorphism (SNP) markers. Information on PA was obtained from questionnaires, and GWA analysis was performed to find genetic associations between PA and SNP markers in the Korean population.

Keywords: Physical activity; GWAS; KARE

Introduction

According to the World Health Organization (WHO), physical activity (PA) is any bodily movement produced by skeletal muscles that requires energy expenditure. It includes exercise as well as other activities that involve bodily movement and are done as part of playing, working, active transportation, house chores and recreational activities. Notably, exercise is a subcategory of PA. PA is an important component of the total daily energy expenditure.[1]

Recent genetic association studies aim to identify genetic variables associated with a trait and to understand genetic basis of the trait. Although genetic studies on PA have not been extensive, it was suggested that genetic factors may contribute to exercise participation.[2] For example, Stubbe *et al.* described that the variance in adult exercise behavior explained by genetic factors ranged between 48% and 71% depending on the study population.[2] In a comprehensive twin study on PA, data from seven large twin studies were pooled to create a cohort of 37,051 twin pairs: 13,676 monozygotic (MZ) pairs,

17,340 same-sex dizygotic (DZ) pairs, and 6,035 opposite-sex DZ pairs.[2,3] Information on exercise participation was derived from questionnaires from which each individual was classified as exercisers and nonexercisers. The mean prevalence of exercise participation was 44% in men and 35% in women. The intrapair resemblance in exercise participation was significantly higher in MZ twins than that in DZ twins. Furthermore, correlations among same-sex DZ twins tended to be greater than that in opposite-sex DZ pairs.

Genetic association studies can be categorized into candidate gene association studies and genome-wide association studies (GWAS). Candidate gene association studies are used to discover different polymorphic sites within the targeted candidate gene regions. On the other hand, GWAS search the entire genome for associations rather than focusing on small candidate areas. By virtue of innovative advances in high-throughput genotyping technology, GWAS have revealed links between DNA sequence variation and diverse health-index phenotypes.[4] A major advantage of the GWAS is that GWAS cover the entire genome uniformly and thereby are not

doi: 10.1111/j.1749-6632.2011.06102.x

restricted by *a priori* hypotheses as in candidate gene studies.[5]

The first GWA study on leisure-time exercise reported the results from two cohort studies: 1,644 unrelated individuals from The Netherlands Twin Register and 978 subjects living in Omaha, Nebraska.[6] Leisure-time exercise level was quantified using questionnaires, and PA was calculated on the basis of the type, the frequency, and the duration of listed activities. Participants were classified as exercisers and nonexercisers. None of the 1.6 million SNP satisfied the commonly used threshold of genome-wide significance ($P = 5 \times 10^{-8}$). SNP in three genomic regions indicated *P*-values less than 1×10^{-5}. The strongest evidence of association was located in chromosome 10q23.2 at the $3'$-phosphoadenosine $5'$ phosphosulfate synthase 2 (*PAPSS2*) gene locus: the odds ratio (OR) for an exerciser was 1.32 ($P = 3.81 \times 10^{-6}$) for the common T-allele of SNP rs10887741. *PAPSS2* encodes a protein involved in sulfation of various molecules.[6]

In this study, we briefly overview some practical issues in performing GWAS for PA. We illustrate these practical issues with a GWA data set from the KARE project that was launched in 2007.[7,8] The main objective of KARE was to find genetic factors associated with complex diseases such as type II diabetes and hypertension in the Korean population. The epidemiologic and clinical data for the project were collected from a large-scale general population-based cohort study, called the Korean Genome and Epidemiology study (KoGES), which includes 10,038 participants. The subjects aged from 40 to 69 were recruited from the two communities in the province of South Korea, Ansan and Ansung. There were 5,020 and 5,018 participants from Ansan and Ansung, respectively. These cohorts, established as part of the Korean Genome Epidemiology Study (KoGES) in 2001 provide extensive phenotypic data for over 260 traits. In the KoGES the information on PA can be obtained through questionnaires, as in most genetic association studies for PA.

In order to obtain a reliable association in GWAS, it is important to have a well-defined phenotype. Unfortunately, it is not straightforward to derive PA information from a series of questionnaires. As a first practical issue, we discuss how to define phenotypes of PA appropriately in genetic association studies. The association results would be highly dependent on how to define phenotypes of PA. Sec-ond, we overview some statistical methods for the genetic association studies for PA. Although a number of methods could be used in GWAS, we focus on logistic regression and linear regression, because they are most commonly used. Finally, we discuss some other practical issues such as population stratification, replication, and sample size issues.

GWA data

The data for GWAS are often obtained from cohort study. Both cohorts that we employed for GWAS were designed to allow longitudinal prospective study with repeated follow-up survey. Participants have been examined every two years since the baseline study in 2001. More than 260 traits have been extensively examined through epidemiological surveys, physical examinations, and laboratory tests.

From the total of 10,038 participants, DNA was available for 10,004, all of whom were genotyped with the Affymetrix genome-wide human SNP array 5.0. Genotypes were called using the Bayesian robust linear modeling using the Mahalanobis distance (BRLMM) algorithm and standard quality control procedures were adopted. A total of 38,364 markers were discarded by Hardy–Weinberg equilibrium *P*-value $< 10^{-6}$, 17,926 with genotype call rates below 95% and 92,050 with minor allele frequency (MAF) < 0.01, leaving 352,228 SNPs. After removing the samples with low call rates ($< 96\%$, $n = 401$), sample contamination ($n = 11$), gender inconsistencies ($n = 41$), cryptic relatedness ($n = 608$), and serious concomitant illness ($n = 101$), GWA genotypes from 8,842 individuals were included. Due to missing data of PA, 8,454 individuals were included in our analysis. A total of 8,454 samples consist of 3,898 and 4,556 from Ansung and Ansan, respectively. Some demographic descriptions are given in Table 1. There are some differences between two cohorts. First, there are more female participants in Ansung than Ansan. Second, the mean age of Ansung is higher than that of Ansan. These differences are characterized by the differences between rural and urban areas.

How to define phenotypes of PA for efficient GWAS?

In GWAS, it is important to use a well-defined phenotype because phenotype ambiguity can lead to

Table 1. Descriptive statistics about participants in the Korean GWAS of PA

| | Sex | | Mean age | | |
Area	Male	Female	Male (Mean ± S.D.)	Female (Mean ± S.D.)	Total (Mean ± S.D.)
Ansung (rural)	1,658	2,240	55.92 ± 8.66	55.65 ± 8.81	55.77 ± 8.75
Ansan (urban)	2,337	2,219	48.56 ± 7.44	49.60 ± 8.22	49.07 ± 7.85
	3,995	4,459	51.61 ± 7.44	52.64 ± 9.04	
Total	8,454		52.16 ± 8.92		52.16 ± 8.92

low power. However, it is not easy to quantify PA, because PA information is usually obtained from questionnaires that may not use systematic measurement scheme. Although it is not easy to quantify the amount of PA, it can be possible to digitize PA by using the metabolic equivalent of task (MET) intensity developed by Ainsworth *et al.*[9] MET is defined as the ratio of the work metabolic rate to a standard resting metabolic rate of 1.0 (4.184 kJ)/kg/h. One MET indicates a resting metabolic rate obtained during quiet sitting.[10] MET is the digit-coding intensity unit to measure PA. The METs of PAs range from 0.9 (sleeping) to 18 METs (running at 10.9 mph). Even for the same type of PAs, MET intensities differ depending on the speed or intensity of movement: an adult jogging METs = 8.0 (5 mph) and 10.0 (6 mph).

Haskell *et al.* proposed a simple approach to estimating the total amount of PA calculated by PA intensity × duration.[11] They recommended the minimal amount of total PA in the range of 450–750 MET-min/week to achieve health benefits.

The first GWA study on leisure-time exercise reported the results from two cohort studies: Netherlands Twin Register and Omaha, Nebraska.[6] Leisure-time exercise level was quantified by computing MET-hours on the basis of the type, the frequency, and the duration of reported activities.[6] Subjects who reported at least 4 MET-h/week were classified as exercisers, whereas those with less than 4 weekly MET-h were considered as nonexercisers.

In the Dutch sample, the first question was "Do you participate in exercise regularly?" and in the American sample the question was "Do you take exercise for 60 minutes per week?" The questions could be answered "Yes" or "No"; if the participants responded affirmatively, they were asked to list all voluntary leisure-time exercise activities to indicate the type, frequency, and duration of each activity. A MET value was assigned to each selected activity and the total MET-h per week were calculated. To keep consistent with existing epidemiological studies, individuals were classified as either exercisers or nonexercisers on the basis of a minimal threshold of at least 4 MET-h weekly.[6]

If we compare the first two questions carefully, however, it is clear that "exercise regularly" may not be interpreted equivalently to "take exercise for 60 min per week." Depending on the interpretation of questionnaire, the computed total MET value would vary seriously. Unfortunately, these questions were treated equally in total MET computation, which may have caused low power. Thus, it is important to use a well-defined questionnaire with clear interpretation.

In the KARE study, we focused on finding genetic factors influencing PA in the Korean population. We obtained information on the intensity and duration of daily PA from questionnaires. There were five questions regarding levels of PA: stable (lying except sleeping), sit (typing, playing the instrument, driving, office job, taking a class, etc.), low (walking, doing the laundry, cleaning, entertaining, leisure time ping-pong, etc.), medium (race walking, carpentering, regular exercise, badminton, swimming, tennis, etc.), high (sports competition, climbing, running, logging, farming, forestry, mining, etc.). In each questionnaire, there was information on duration of PA measured in minute per day. Each questionnaire was designed to obtain summarized information for multiple PAs. But it did not have information for the individual PA. Each PA had varying MET intensities. Thus, only the average MET intensity was assigned to each questionnaire. Following Haskell *et al.*'s approach, we calculated the total amount of PA by using PA time and MET, an indicator of activity intensity, as follows:[11]

$$\text{Total amount of daily PA} = \sum [\text{PA intensity}$$
$$(\text{MET}) \times \text{duration (min)} \times \text{day}^{-1}]. \tag{1}$$

Note that our questionnaire does not provide information for individual PA. Thus, this total amount based on the average may dilute MET intensities, which might lead to the low power in our GWA study. Thus, it is important to use a well-defined questionnaire that provides detailed information on each activity.

Statistical methods for GWAS

In this section, we summarize two statistical models that can be used in the GWAS on PA: logistic and linear regression models. Several PA studies classified individuals as exercisers and nonexercisers on the basis of a minimal MET-h threshold (4 MET-h weekly).[2,6,12] In this case, logistic regression can be used. Logistic regression is most widely used to analyze the relationship between a binary response variable and one or more independent variables (e.g., genetic factor, sex, age, etc.). The binary response variable has only two values: 0 and 1 (e.g., nonexerciser and exerciser).

If the binary response variable is used in KARE GWA analysis, the logistic model can be fit with age, gender, area, and body mass index (BMI) as covariates, which is defined as follows:

$$Logit[P(Y = 1|X)] = \beta_0 + \beta_1 Age_j + \beta_2 Gender_j$$
$$+ \beta_3 Area_j + \beta_4 BMI_j + \beta_5 SNP_{ij}, \tag{2}$$

where $P(Y_j = 1)$ represents the probability of being a regular exerciser, where Age_j, $Gender_j$, $Area_j$, BMI_j, and SNP_{ij} represent age, gender, recruitment area (i.e., Ansung and Ansan), BMI, and the number of minor alleles for the ith SNP marker, respectively, $i = 1, 2, \ldots, p$ and p is the number of SNPs under consideration; $j = 1, 2, \ldots, n$ and n is the number of individuals. β_0 denotes intercept, and $\beta_1, \beta_2, \beta_3, \beta_4$ denote the effect sizes of the corresponding covariates. β_5 is the effect size of SNPs. The significance of SNPs can be determined by the Wald test or likelihood ratio test.[13] Its P-value is obtained from the χ^2-distribution with one degree of freedom.

Alternatively, linear regression can be used when the phenotype is quantitative. For KARE GWA anal-

ysis, the linear regression model can be defined in a similar manner as follows:

$$Y_j = \beta_0 + \beta_1 Age_j + \beta_2 Gender_j + \beta_3 Area_j$$
$$+ \beta_4 BMI_j + \beta_5 SNP_{ij} + \varepsilon_j, \tag{3}$$

where Y_j represents the PA trait value and ε_j is the measurement error of the jth individual, $i = 1, 2, \ldots, p, j = 1, 2, \ldots, n$. All other covariates are the same with those in the logistic regression model. The significance of SNPs can be determined by the t-test. Its P-value is obtained from the t-distribution.

For the KARE GWA analysis, regression analysis can be performed for the total sample combining Ansan and Ansung cohort samples and for each cohort sample separately. GWA analyses can be conducted by using PLINK (http://pngu.mgh. harvard.edu/purcell/plink/) and R (www.r-project.org) software. Additional meta-analysis can also be performed by combining the results of Ansung and Ansan cohorts by Fisher's combined P-value method.[14]

As an illustration of regression analysis, we fit logistic and linear regression for "medium (race walking, carpentering, regular exercise, badminton, swimming, tennis, etc.)" of the PA questionnaire in KoGES. The average MET intensity was assigned and total PA was calculated. Figure 1 shows Manhattan plots of logistic and linear regressions. We used different colors to distinguish chromosomes in each model. As can be seen in the two figures, the results were not consistent. The logistic regression model did not provide any SNPs satisfying the GWAS significance level ($1.420 \times 10^{-7} = 0.05/352,228$). On the other hand, in the linear regression model, there was a SNP satisfying the GWAS significance level. This SNP is located in the region of *SLC26A7* gene. The *SLC26A7* gene is a member of a family of sulfate/anion transporter genes. It was reported that deletion of the *Slc26a7* gene results in distal renal tubular acidosis.[15]

Which type of regression model would be better? In general, the quantitative trait may contain more information than the binary trait. However, regression analysis using quantitative traits usually requires the normality assumption that the quantitative trait should follow a normal distribution. If the normality assumption is not satisfied, then the t-test based on the normality assumption would yield false positive or false negative results. On the other hand, the logistic regression model provides

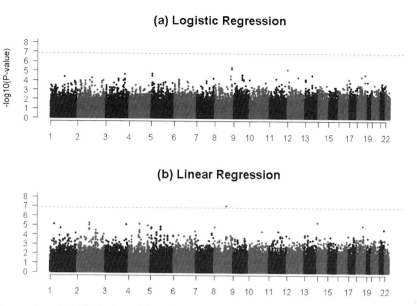

Figure 1. Manhattan plots of PA. The horizontal dotted line presents the GWA significance level 1.420×10^{-7} ($= 0.05/352,228$). The *P*-values from a single SNP association test are indicated in a $-\log10$ scale against each chromosome. Navy and royal blue colors are used to distinguish chromosomes. There was a significant SNP identified by the linear regression model.

a robust result to the normality assumption. If the normality assumption is satisfied, however, then the *t*-test based on the normality assumption would provide higher power. Thus, it would be important to check the normality assumption in order to decide which type of model to use, if a quantitative trait of PA is available. In our data, the normality assumption was well satisfied. Thus, we conclude that the linear regression model provided higher power than the logistic regression model.

Further issues for GWAS of PA

In GWAS, population stratification arises if the underlying population is actually a mix of ancestrally distinct populations with different values of trait prevalence and SNP allele frequency.[16] A widely used approach to evaluate whether confounding due to population stratification exists is to calculate the genomic control λ (λ_{GC}), which is defined as the median x^2 (1 degree of freedom) association statistic across SNPs divided by its theoretical median under the null distribution.[17] A value of $\lambda_{GC} \sim$ (double $\sim$) 1 indicates no stratification, whereas $\lambda_{GC} > 1$ indicates stratification or other confounders, such as family structure, cryptic relatedness, or differential bias. To correct for stratification, some methods that infer genetic ancestry, such as principal compo-

nent analysis (PCA) and structured association, can be used. In our KARE GWA study, λ was estimated as 1.0078 and there is no evidence of population stratification.

It is also important to perform replication studies in GWAS, because it is common that the significant result from a discovery GWA sample is not replicated in the other independent replication GWA sample. In our data, one cohort sample can be used as a discovery data set and the other cohort sample as a replication data set. However, it would not be easy to get consistent results from both cohort areas. If the result is not replicated, it is probably due to false positives in the discovery data set, small sample size in the replication data set, or confounding factors such as population stratification. If the result is not replicated, it would be required to check for all these possibilities.

One other way of confirming the association result is to compare the result with the previously published results from the candidate gene studies or other GWA studies. It would be lucky if the same SNPs were reported in the previous results. We tried to compare our KARE GWA results with those from the candidate gene studies and the first GWA study. However, our data did not have the genotyped SNPs comparable to them. Thus, we could not compare the results. The ugenotyped SNPs in our sample can be imputed using the data from the International Hapmap project (www.hapmap.org).[18] This imputed analysis would be worthy pursuing in the future.

Note that the first GWA analysis on PA did not identify any SNPs in genome-wide significance level either.[6] It is not clear whether it is due to the small sample size or the characteristics of PA. If the effect size of SNP is predictable, the sample size can be easily computed. Some further investigation on the sample size computation is warranted.

Conclusions

In this article, we provide an overview of GWAS for PA. First, it is important to use a well-defined phenotype in GWAS, because phenotype ambiguity can lead to low power. Since PA information is usually obtained from questionnaires, it is not easy to quantify PA from these questionnaires. So far, MET intensity is the most commonly used measure of quantifying PA. We think measuring PA using MET intensity from questionnaire may not provide complete information about PA. It is a rather indirect way of measuring PA. We think a more systematic and direct way for measuring PA needs to be developed. Second, depending on characteristic of response variable, statistical methods can be selected to perform GWAS. In our KARE GWA analysis, linear regression model provided more powerful results with smaller *P*-values than logistic regression model. The lower power of logistic regression might be caused by loss of information in the process of categorizing the quantitative trait into two binary groups. Moreover, regression analysis using quantitative trait requires the normality assumption that the quantitative trait follows a normal distribution. Thus, it would be required to check the normality assumption. Finally, some other practical issues such as population stratification, replication, and sample size issues are also considered to perform efficient GWAS for PA.

To date, there have been extensive GWAS results related to complex diseases such as Type II diabetes and hypertension.[19-23] However, there exist only a few GWAS results for PA. Only the effects of regular PA and sedentary behavior on risk factors for common diseases, health outcomes, and mortality rates have been emphasized.[24-28] Thus, several studies considered PA as an adjusting co-

variate in the genetic association study to identify genetic markers of complex diseases.[11,28-30] Future studies to identify the genetic factors directly influencing health- or fitness-related PA would be desirable. Moreover, since there are severe population diversities in GWAS, a more systematic comparison is required between our Korean results and those from other populations.

Acknowledgments

This work was supported by the National Research Foundation (KRF-2008-313-C00086) and by the Consortium for Large Scale Genome Wide Association Study from the National Institute of Health of Korea (2009-E73007-00). The KARE data analyzed in this study were obtained from the Korean Genome Analysis Project (4845-301) and the epidemiologic data including PA were provided from the KoGES (4851-302) that were funded by a grant from the Ministry for Health and Welfare, Republic of Korea. The authors thank Nam H. Cho (Department of Preventive Medicine, Ajou University, South Korea) and Chol Shin (Department of Internal Medicine, Korea University Ansan Hospital, South Korea) for their great efforts in generating and providing these valuable data.

Conflicts of interest

The authors declare no conflicts of interest.

References

1. Rankinen, T. & C. Bouchard. 2008. Gene-physical activity interactions: overview of human studies. *Obesity* **16**(Suppl 3): S47–S50.
2. Stubbe, J.H. *et al.* 2006. Genetic influences on exercise participation in 37,051 twin pairs from seven countries. *PLoS One.* **1:** e22.
3. Rankinen, T. *et al.* 2010. Advances in exercise, fitness, and performance genomics. *Med. Sci. Sports Exerc.* **42:** 835–846.
4. Hagberg, J.M. *et al.* 2011. Advances in exercise, fitness, and performance genomics in 2010. *Med. Sci. Sports Exerc.* **43:** 743–752.
5. Rankinen, T. *et al.* 2006. The human gene map for performance and health-related fitness phenotypes: the 2005 update. *Med. Sci. Sports Exerc.* **38:** 1863–1888.
6. De Moor, H.M. *et al.* 2009. Genome-wide association study of exercise behavior in Dutch and American adults. *Med. Sci. Sports Exerc.* **41**(10): 1887–1895.
7. Cho, Y.S. *et al.* 2009. A large-scale genome-wide association study of Asian populations uncovers genetic factors influencing eight quantitative traits. *Nat. Genet.* **41**(5): 527–534.

8. Cho, S. *et al.* 2009. Elastic-net regularization approaches for genome-wide association studies of rheumatoid arthritis. *BMC Proc.* **7**(Suppl): S25.

9. Ainsworth, B.E. *et al.* 1993. Compendium of physical activities: energy costs of human movement. *Med. Sci. Sports Exerc.* **25**(1): 71–80.

10. Ainsworth, B.E. *et al.* 2000. Compendium of physical activities: an update of activity codes and MET intensities. *Med. Sci. Sports Exerc.* **32**(9 Suppl): S498–S504.

11. Haskell, W.L. *et al.* 2007. Physical activity and public health: Updated recommendation for adults from the American College of Sports Medicine and the American Heart Association. *Med. Sci. Sports Exerc.* **39**: 1423–1434.

12. Haase, A. *et al.* 2004. Leisure-time physical activity in university students from 23 countries: associations with health beliefs, risk awareness, and national economic development. *Prev. Med.* **39**: 182–190.

13. Bewick, V., L. Cheek & J. Ball. 2005. Statistics review 14: Logistic regression. *Crit. Care.* **9**: 112–118.

14. Hess, A. & H. Iyer. 2007. Fisher's combined p-value for detecting differentially expressed genes using Affymetrix expression arrays. *BMC Genomics* **8**: 96–109.

15. Xu, J. *et al.* 2009. Deletion of the chloride transporter slc26a7 causes distal renal tubular acidosis and impairs gastric acid secretion. *J. Biol. Chem.* **284**: 29470–29479.

16. Lewis, C.M. 2002. Genetic association studies: design, analysis and interpretation. *Brief Bioinform.* **3**: 146–153.

17. Price, A.L. 2010. New approaches to population stratification in genome-wide association studies. *Nat. Rev. Genet.* **11**: 459–463.

18. Servin, B. & M. Stephens. 2007. Imputation-based analysis of association studies: candidate regions and quantitative traits. *PLoS Genet.* **3**: e114.

19. Hong, K.W. *et al.* 2010. Genetic variations in ATP2B1, CSK, ARSG and CSMD1 loci are related to blood pressure and/or hypertension in two Korean cohorts. *J. Hum. Hypertens.* **24**: 367–372.

20. Hong, K.W. *et al.* 2009. Replication of the Wellcome Trust genome-wide association study on essential hypertension in a Korean population. *Hypertens. Res.* **32**: 570–5744.

21. Levy, D. *et al.* 2009. Genome-wide association study of blood pressure and hypertension. *Nat. Genet.* **41**: 677–687.

22. Subirana, I. *et al.* 2009. Genome-wide association study identifies eight loci associated with blood pressure. *Nat. Genet.* **41**(6): 666–676.

23. Diabetes Genetics Initiative of Broad Institute of Harvard and MIT, Lund University, and Novartis Institutes of BioMedical Research, R. Saxena *et al.* 2007. Genome-wide association analysis identifies loci for type 2 diabetes and triglyceride levels. *Science* **316**: 1331–1336.

24. Physical activity and cardiovascular health. 1996. NIH Consensus Development Panel on physical activity and cardiovascular health. *JAMA* **276**: 241–246.

25. Bouchard, C. 2001. Physical activity and health: introduction to the dose-response symposium. *Med. Sci. Sports Exerc.* **33**(6 Suppl): S347–S350.

26. Bouchard, C. & S.N. Blair 1999. Introductory comments for the consensus on physical activity and obesity. *Med. Sci. Sports Exerc.* **31**: S498–S501.

27. Leon, A., Ed. 1997. *Physical Activity and Cardiovascular Health: A National Consensus.* Champaign, IL: Human Kinetics Publishers.

28. US Department of Health & Human Services. 1996. *Physical Activity and Health: A Report of the Surgeon General.* Atlanta, GA: US Department of Health and Human Services, Centers for Disease Control and Prevention, National Center for Chronic Disease Prevention and Health Promotion.

29. Manson, J.E. *et al.* 1999. A prospective study of walking as compared with vigorous exercise in the prevention of coronary heart disease in women. *N. Engl. J. Med.* **341**: 650–658.

30. Manson, J.E. *et al.* 2002. Walking compared with vigorous exercise for the prevention of cardiovascular events in women. *N. Engl. J. Med.* **347**: 716–725.

Ann. N.Y. Acad. Sci. ISSN 0077-8923

The growing challenge of obesity and cancer: an inflammatory issue

Alison E. Harvey,[1] Laura M. Lashinger,[1] and Stephen D. Hursting[1,2]

[1]Department of Nutritional Sciences, University of Texas, Austin, Texas. [2]Department of Molecular Carcinogenesis, University of Texas-MD Anderson Cancer Center, Smithville, Texas

Address for correspondence: Stephen D. Hursting, Ph.D., M.P.H., Department of Nutritional Sciences, Dell Pediatric Research Institute, University of Texas at Austin, 1800 Barbara Jordan Blvd., Austin, TX 78723. shursting@mail.utexas.edu

The prevalence of obesity, an established risk factor for many cancers, has risen steadily for the past several decades in the United States and in many parts of the world. This review synthesizes the evidence on key biological mechanisms underlying the obesity–cancer link, with particular emphasis on the impact of energy balance modulation, such as diet-induced obesity and calorie restriction, on growth factor signaling pathways and inflammatory processes. Particular attention is placed on the proinflammatory environment associated with the obese state, specifically highlighting the involvement of obesity-associated hormones/growth factors in crosstalk between macrophages, adipocytes, and epithelial cells in many cancers. Understanding the contribution of obesity to growth factor signaling and chronic inflammation provides mechanistic targets for disrupting the obesity–cancer link.

Keywords: obesity; cancer; hormones; growth factors; inflammation

Introduction

The prevalence of obesity, defined as having a body mass index (BMI) > 30 kg/m^2, has increased dramatically in the last three decades in the United States[1] and in many parts of the world.[2] As waistlines have expanded, so have the rates of several chronic diseases. Obesity is associated with an increased production of metabolic hormones coupled with a chronic low-grade state of inflammation that is linked to various disease states, such as type II diabetes, cardiovascular disease, and certain types of cancer.[3] In prospective studies such as the Nurses' Health Study,[4] the Health Professionals Follow-up Study,[5] and the Framingham Health Study,[6] individuals who gained weight over a 10- to 15-year period had a significantly increased risk of developing type II diabetes and coronary heart disease. The relationship between obesity and cancer was poorly understood until Calle *et al.*[3] conducted a large prospective study examining the role of obesity or excess adiposity in increasing the risk of dying from most types of cancer. Possible mechanisms underlying the link between obesity and cancer will be discussed below, with an emphasis on hormones, growth factor signaling, and inflammation.

Obesity-related hormones, growth factors, and their signaling pathways

Leptin

Leptin is a peptide hormone produced by adipocytes that is positively correlated with adipose stores and nutritional status.[7] Under normal conditions, leptin functions as an energy sensor and signals the brain to reduce appetite. In the obese state, however, there is an overproduction of leptin by the adipose tissue, and the brain no longer responds to the signal. The release of leptin is stimulated by insulin, glucocorticoids, tumor necrosis factor-alpha (TNF-α), and estrogens.[7] Leptin has direct effects on peripheral tissues, as well as indirect effects on hypothalamic pathways.[7] Leptin also modulates other biological processes including immune function, cytokine production, angiogenesis, and carcinogenesis.[8–10] The leptin receptor has similar homology to class I cytokines that signal through the janus kinase and signal transducer activator of

doi: 10.1111/j.1749-6632.2011.06096.x

transcription (JAK/STAT) pathway that is often dysregulated in cancer.[11,12]

The findings from epidemiological studies have been inconsistent in regard to the association between leptin and cancer.[13–17] *In vitro* studies have shown that leptin has a proliferative effect on human esophageal, breast, and prostate cancers; however, leptin decreased growth of pancreatic cancer cell lines.[18] Additionally, Jaffe *et al.*[19] demonstrated that leptin promoted cell motility and invasiveness in human colon cancer cell lines.

Adiponectin

Adiponectin is a hormone mainly secreted from adipocytes in visceral adipose tissue. Unlike leptin, levels of adiponectin are negatively correlated with adiposity. Adiponectin functions to counter the metabolic profile associated with obesity by modulating glucose metabolism, increasing fatty acid oxidation and insulin sensitivity, and decreasing production of inflammatory cytokines associated with obesity.[20] Following secretion from the adipocyte, adiponectin undergoes posttranslational modifications to generate globular, low and high molecular weight isoforms that bind to one of two adiponectin receptors, adipo1 and adipo2.[21] While both receptors are ubiquitously expressed, adipo1 is found mostly in skeletal muscle and adipo2 is found mostly in the liver.

In addition to its role in metabolism, adiponectin may exert anticancer effects. An inverse relationship between systemic adiponectin concentrations and cancer risk has been observed in colon, prostate, gastric, endometrial, and renal cancers in multiple case-controlled studies.[22–25] The potential mechanisms through which adiponectin exerts it anticancer effects include increasing insulin sensitivity, decreasing insulin/insulin-like growth factor (IGF)-1 and mTOR signaling via activation of 5′AMP-activated protein kinase (AMPK), and reducing proinflammatory cytokine expression via the inhibition of nuclear factor kappa-light-chain-enhancer of activated B cells (NF-κB).[26]

Insulin

Insulin is a peptide hormone produced by the beta cells of the pancreas and released in response to elevated blood glucose. BMI correlates with serum insulin levels, and obesity is linked to the development of insulin resistance, hyperglycemia, hyperinsulinemia, and type II diabetes.[27–29] In the obese state, blood glucose levels increase and trigger the pancreas to increase insulin production, resulting in hyperinsulinemia and insulin resistance. The development of insulin resistance is associated with aberrant glucose metabolism, chronic inflammation, and production of other metabolic hormones, such as adiponectin and IGF-1.[30–32] Additionally, hyperinsulinemia and type II diabetes increase the risk for colorectal, kidney, breast, endometrial, and pancreatic cancers, independent of obesity.[33–38] Insulin promotes cancer development through binding of the insulin receptor and initiating signal transduction in extracellular signal–regulated kinase (ERK) and phosphtidylinositol-3 kinase (PI3K) pathways.[39] In contrast to the glucose metabolism effects that occur at physiologic levels of insulin, the mitogenic effect of insulin occurs mainly at supraphysiological levels, and proliferative effects of insulin are believed to take place indirectly through increasing levels of bioavailable IGF-1.[39]

IGF-1

IGF-1 is a hormone and growth factor produced primarily by the liver following stimulation by signals received from the central nervous system. It plays an important role in regulating growth and development of many tissues, particularly in prenatal growth.[40] Similar to insulin, levels of IGF-1 correspond to energy status and are often elevated in obese individuals.[41,42] IGF-1 in circulation is typically bound to IGF-binding proteins (IGF-BPs), which function to regulate free IGF-1 levels, controlling the availability of IGF-1 to bind to its receptor.[41] Insulin can influence IGF-1 synthesis and reduce IGFBPs, thereby increasing the amount of bioavailable IGF-1 that interacts with the IGF-1 receptor (IGF-1R). Binding of IGF-1 to its receptor activates downstream signaling pathways such as ERK and PI3K, modulating transcription factors that control gene expression related to cancer development.

The role of IGF-1 as a risk factor for cancer has been established in many cancer types.[11,43–46] Experimentally, transactivation of the IGF-1 receptor and leptin receptor was demonstrated in human breast cancer cells.[47] The synergistic effects of IGF-1 and leptin receptor activation on breast cancer cell proliferation suggest that obesity is likely promoting cancer development through multiple metabolic hormones and pathways.[47] Additionally, tumor volume and multiplicity were decreased in IGF-1–deficient mouse models of colon[48] and pancreatic cancer (Lashinger *et al.*, personal communication) compared to wild-type mice.

Lessons from calorie restriction research

Calorie restriction (CR), a dietary regimen involving a reduction in total energy (typically 20–40%), is an effective way to increase life span of mammals and inhibit carcinogenesis.[49] Among many activities, CR has been shown to modulate the hormones discussed above, as well as to increase antioxidant defense mechanisms, increase DNA repair processes, and decrease expression and production of inflammatory cytokines.[50] Energy balance modulation, ranging from CR to diet-induced obesity regimens, impacts circulating levels of IGF-1, insulin, adiponectin, and leptin, all of which function as a network of messengers to regulate metabolism and inflammation and are intimately involved with several aspects of tumor development, as discussed above. Given how difficult it is for many people to adopt a low-calorie diet for an extended period, the identification of drugs or natural products that could either complement or even reproduce the anticancer effects of CR without drastic changes in diet and lifestyle is a goal for many investigators and pharmaceutical companies. Thus far, promising data have emerged for mTOR inhibitors, such as rapamycin and metformin, or sirtuin modulators, such as resveratrol, as CR mimetics.[49]

Obesity and chronic inflammation

Adipocytes, macrophages, and inflammatory cytokines

Obesity is associated with a chronic low-grade state of inflammation that is attributed to increased fatty acids, inflammatory cytokine production, and an influx of immune cells, such as macrophages, that also produce inflammatory mediators. Adipocytes can transdifferentiate into macrophages *in vivo*, highlighting the role of adipose tissue as an immune organ in addition to an energy storage depot.[51] Adipocytes can enlarge past the point of effective oxygen diffusion, which results in hypoxia, inflammation, and increased macrophage infiltration. Enlarged adipocytes produce more inflammatory cytokines and exhibit greater insulin resistance than smaller adipocytes. Furthermore, adipocytes have a limited amount of storage capacity, and when

exceeded and in the context of excess lipids, there are increases in circulating free fatty acids that deposit in other tissues and result in diabetes, hypertension, and fatty liver disease.[52] Adipose tissue can be classified as subcutaneous and visceral adipose tissue, the latter being more predictive of obesity-related comorbities and mortality.[53] Visceral adipose tissue also exhibits increased insulin resistance, lipolysis, and inflammatory cytokine expression relative to subcutaneous adipose tissue. Visceral adipose tissue is in close proximity to the portal vein; this proximity allows drainage of excess free fatty acids and inflammatory mediators directly to the liver, which in turn creates additional inflammation and affecting metabolism.[52]

In addition to adipokine hormones such as leptin and adiponectin, adipose tissue produces inflammatory cytokines such as TNF-α, interleukin (IL)-6, IL-1β, and monocyte chemoattractant protein (MCP)-1. In acute inflammatory conditions, these mediators are present for short periods of time, typically in response to bacterial or viral stimuli. It is through a negative feedback loop initiated by the production of antiinflammatory cytokines that proinflammatory cytokine levels return back to normal. Obesity is associated with a chronic state of inflammation because a major source of inflammatory mediators is the expanding adipose tissue. Furthermore, as a result of the inflammatory environment present in adipose tissue, macrophages are recruited to the site and in turn produce additional proinflammatory mediators. Adipose-derived macrophages are more prevalent in obese individuals and correlate with BMI. Subbaramaiah *et al.* showed that fatty acids released from adipocytes are able to stimulate release of TNF-α, IL-1β, and the inflammatory inducible enzyme, cyclooxygenase (COX)-2, from a human monocyte–derived cell line, further demonstrating the underlying complexity of diverse cell types and their crosstalk present in adipose tissue.[54]

In addition to its role in inflammation, TNF-α contributes to insulin resistance through downregulation of insulin receptors and glucose transporters. Recently, IL-6 has been shown to contribute to systemic insulin resistance.[55] In addition, plasma IL-6 levels are higher in the portal vein than in peripheral artery blood in obese individuals, suggesting that inflammatory cytokines are elevated in visceral fat compared to subcutaneous fat.[56] Fenton *et al.*[57] demonstrated that IL-6 induced proliferation of preneoplastic colon epithelial cells, leptin increased cell proliferation via an IL-6–dependent mechanism, and leptin increased IL-6 secretion from preneoplastic colon cells in a time- and dose-dependent manner. These findings suggest a link between adipose-derived hormones and inflammatory cytokines in cancer development.

Inflammatory signaling regulated by NF-κB

NF-κB is a transcription factor that is activated in response to bacterial and viral stimuli, growth factors, and inflammatory molecules, such as TNF-α, IL-6, and IL-1β. In addition, NF-κB is responsible for inducing gene expression associated with cell proliferation, apoptosis, inflammation, metastasis, and angiogenesis. The NF-κB complex is made up of five subunits (Rel A/p65, c-Rel, Rel-B, p105/p50, and p100/p52) that have the ability to form multiple homo- and/or heterodimers depending on the stimulus. NF-κB typically remains sequestered in the cytoplasm, but upon activation by upstream activators IκB kinase α and β (IKK-α and IKK-β), the inhibitor of kappa B-α (IκB-α) is degraded, allowing NF-κB to translocate to the nucleus and initiate gene transcription.[58] Activation of NF-κB is associated with insulin resistance and is upregulated in many types of cancers.[39]

Metabolic hormones, such as leptin, insulin, and IGF-1, have also been shown to modulate NF-κB signaling when their systemic levels are altered in response to energy balance modulation. Once bound to their cognate receptor, IGF-1, insulin, and leptin activate Akt, which is an established upstream kinase of the IKK complex. Subsequently, the activated IKK complex targets IκB-α for degradation and allows the p50/p65 subunits to translocate to the nucleus and initiate gene transcription. Leptin-stimulated activation of NF-κB has been demonstrated *in vitro* in human preneoplastic and neoplastic colonic epithelial cells.[57,59] Insulin has been shown to activate NF-κB signaling *in vitro* and *in vivo* in HEK293 kidney cells and in aged kidneys harvested from overweight rats; furthermore, this activation was attenuated in rats administered a 40% CR diet.[60] Mitsiades and colleagues[61] showed that IGF-1 increased NF-κB DNA binding activity comparable to that of TNF-α, and induced expression of FLIP, XIAP, cIAP-2, Al/Bfl-1, and survivin, all downstream genes mediated by NF-κB.[61]

Inflammation and cancer

The link between chronic inflammation and cancer development was first noticed over 100 years ago by Rudolph Virchow when he observed an abundance of leukocytes in neoplastic tissue.[62] Since then, the role of chronic inflammation as a precursor to cancer development has been observed in multiple cancer types, some of which include gastritis and gastric cancer, inflammatory bowel disease (IBD) and colon cancer, and pancreatitis and pancreatic cancer.[63,64] In various mouse models of human cancers, inflammation has also been shown to influence tumor promotion and progression.[65–67]

Like adipose tissue, tumor microenvironments are composed of multiple cell types including epithelial cells, fibroblasts, mast cells, and cells of the innate and adaptive immune system that favor a proinflammatory, protumorigenic environment.[68–70] Furthermore, tumor cells as well as stromal cells increase expression of COX-2 in neoplastic tissues. COX-2 is considered an indicator of poor prognosis in multiple cancer types,[71] and population-based studies have shown that long-term use of nonsteroidal anti-inflammatories (NSAIDS) and COX-2 inhibitors decreases colon cancer risk by 50%, gastric and esophageal cancer risk by 40%, and breast cancer risk by 20%.[72] TNF-α is produced by tumor cells and stromal cells and is believed to enhance tumor development through NF-κB–induced gene transcription.[73] TNF-α has been linked to the development of skin, liver, and colon cancer, and treatment with a TNA-α antagonist during the promotion stage inhibited the progression of hepatocellular carcinoma.[73] IL-6 promotes cell growth, inhibits apoptosis, and is associated with the development of Kaposi sarcoma, multiple myeloma, and Hodgkin's lymphoma. In addition, high circulating levels of IL-6 are correlated with IBD and risk for colon carcinogenesis.[74]

Contributing to the proinflammatory tumor environment is the presence of tumor-associated macrophages (TAMs). The recruitment of TAMs to the tumor microenvironment is largely dependent on the MCP-1. Levels of MCP-1 in tumor tissue are highly correlated with the accumulation of TAMs in ovarian, breast, and pancreatic cancer.[75] TAMs are capable of polarizing into what is known as an M1, a classically activated cytotoxic macrophage, or an M2, an immunosuppressive macrophage. The cytokines produced by each type of macrophage are what distinguish an M1 from an M2, and tumor tissue typically contains a larger quantity of M2 type macrophages.[75] In addition to producing cytokines and chemokines, TAMs also produce growth factors that enhance proliferation, angiogenesis, and contribute to deposition and dissolution of connctive tissue.[76] There is also some evidence to suggest that NF-κB plays a role in mediating TAM transcriptional programs and by extension, protumorigenic effects of TAMs.[76–78]

Targeting inflammation for cancer prevention

Current approaches to inhibit inflammation center on targeting various intermediates of the NF-κB pathway and sensitizing tumors to chemotherapeutic agents. NSAIDS such as aspirin have been studied extensively for their ability to modulate NF-κB activity. Prolonged treatment of colon cancer cells with aspirin has been shown to inhibit translocation of NF-κB to the nucleus resulting in apoptosis.[79] Experimentally, the use of COX-2 inhibitors has proven to be effective at preventing pancreatic lesions in a transgenic mouse model of pancreatitis and pancreatic dysplasia,[80] as well as inhibiting growth and promoting apoptosis in pancreatic cancer cells.[81] However, results from human studies suggest combining COX-2 inhibitors with the standard chemotherapeutic drugs Gemcitabine or Cisplatin does not increase the therapeutic response relative to the chemotehrapeutic drugs used alone.[82] Sulindac (another NSAID) has been shown to decrease colon cancer cell proliferation, and sulindac combined with parthenolide has been demonstrated to inhibit NF-κB and pancreatic cancer cell growth.[83,84]

The proteasome inhibitor, PS-341, more commonly known as Bortezomib, is currently approved for clinical use in the treatment of mantle cell lymphoma and multiple myeloma through increased stabilization of the IκBα subunit and decreased NF-κB activity. It has been shown to facilitate growth arrest and apoptosis in lung cancer cells and has been shown to increase effectiveness of chemotherapy drugs in patients with multiple myeloma.[85] In addition to pharmacological inhibitors, dietary components have also been studied for their ability to inhibit inflammation. Curcumin is a spice often used in Asia that has potent antioxidant, antiinflammatory, and anticancer effects.[86] Multiple studies have shown *in vitro* and *in*

vivo that curcumin inhibits NF-κB signaling in various cell types. In genetically obese mice, curcumin was shown to prevent macrophage accumulation in adipose tissue in addition to inhibiting NF-κB activation in the liver.[87] Experimentally, curcumin has been shown to decrease cancer proliferation in breast.[88] and pancreatic cancer cells, as well as to decrease DNA binding of NF-κB, reduce COX-2 protein levels, and inhibit PGE_2 production in multiple pancreatic cancer cell lines.[89] In mouse models, curcumin has been shown to inhibit cancers of the skin,[90] breast,[91] liver,[92] and colon.[60] Curcumin inhibits TNF-α–induced phosphorylation and degradation of the IκBα subunit and also prevents hydrogen peroxide–mediated activation of NF-κB activation.[93] Curcumin can also suppress steady-state signaling through the mTOR pathway in multiple tissues, which, as discussed above, likely contributes to the anticancer effects of cucumin. The main obstacles that prevent broader use of curcumin as a therapeutic or preventive agent are its low water solubility and limited bioavailability.[94]

Conclusion

Multiple signals associated with the obese state contribute to inflammatory and growth factor signaling, and components of these interacting pathways represent promising targets for breaking the obesity–cancer link.

Conflicts of interest

The authors declare no conflicts of interest.

References

1. Hedley, A.A., C.L. Ogden, C.L. Johnson, *et al.* 2004. Prevalence of overweight and obesity among US children, adolescents, and adults, 1999–2002. *JAMA* **291**: 2847–2850.
2. Hossain, P., B. Kawar, & M. El Nahas. 2007. Obesity and diabetes in the developing world – a growing challenge. *N. Engl. J. Med.* **356**: 213–215.
3. Calle, E.E., C. Rodriguez, K. Walker-Thurmond & M.J. Thun. 2003. Overweight, obesity, and mortality from cancer in a prospectively studied cohort of U.S. adults. *N. Engl. J. Med.* **348**: 1625–1638.
4. Haffner, S.M. 2006. Relationship of metabolic risk factors and development of cardiovascular disease and diabetes. *Obesity* **14**(Suppl 3): 121S–127S.
5. Colditz, G.A., W.C. Willett, A. Rotnitzky & J.E. Manson. 1995. Weight gain as a risk factor for clinical diabetes mellitus in women. *Ann. Int. Med.* **122**: 481–486.
6. Wilson, P.W., W.B. Kannel, H. Silbershatz & R.B. D'Agostino. 1999. Clustering of metabolic factors and coronary heart disease. *Arch. Int. Med.* **159**: 1104–1109.

7. Kershaw, E.E. & J.S. Flier. 2004. Adipose tissue as an endocrine organ. *J. Clin. Endocrinol. Metab.* **89:** 2548–2556.

8. Margetic, S., C. Gazzola, G.G. Pegg & R.A. Hill. 2002. Leptin: a review of its peripheral actions and interactions. *Int. J. Obes. Relat. Metab. Disord.* **26:** 1407–1433.

9. Lord, G.M., G. Matarese, J.K. Howard, *et al.* 1998. Leptin modulates the T-cell immune response and reverses starvation-induced immunosuppression. *Nature* **394:** 897–901.

10. Somasundar, P., D. Riggs, B. Jackson, *et al.* 2003. Leptin stimulates esophageal adenocarcinoma growth by nonapoptotic mechanisms. *Am. J. Surg.* **186:** 575–578.

11. Yu, H., D. Pardoll & R. Jove. 2009. STATs in cancer inflammation and immunity: a leading role for STAT3. *Nature Rev.* **9:** 798–809.

12. Houseknecht, K.L., C.A. Baile, R.L. Matteri & M.E. Spurlock. 1998. The biology of leptin: a review. *J. Anim. Sci.* **76:** .

13. Chang, S., S.D. Hursting, J.H. Contois, *et al.* 2001. Leptin and prostate cancer. *Prostate* **46:** 62–67.

14. Stattin, P., S. Soderberg, G. Hallmans, *et al.* 2001. Leptin is associated with increased prostate cancer risk: a nested case-referent study. *J. Clin. Endocrinol. Metab.* **86:** 1341–1345.

15. Vona-Davis, L. & D.P. Rose. 2007. Adipokines as endocrine, paracrine, and autocrine factors in breast cancer risk and progression. *Endocr.-Relat. Cancer* **14:** 189–206.

16. Stattin, P., R. Palmqvist, S. Soderberg, *et al.* 2003. Plasma leptin and colorectal cancer risk: a prospective study in Northern Sweden. *Oncol. Rep.* **10:** 2015–2021.

17. Stattin, P., A. Lukanova, C. Biessy, *et al.* 2004. Obesity and colon cancer: does leptin provide a link? *Int. J. Cancer* **109:** 149–152.

18. Somasundar, P., A.K. Yu, L. Vona-Davis & D.W. McFadden. 2003. Differential effects of leptin on cancer in vitro. *J. Surg. Res.* **113:** 50–55.

19. Jaffe, T. & B. Schwartz. 2008. Leptin promotes motility and invasiveness in human colon cancer cells by activating multiple signal-transduction pathways. *Int. J. Cancer* **123:** 2543–2556.

20. Havel, P.J. 2002. Control of energy homeostasis and insulin action by adipocyte hormones: leptin, acylation stimulating protein, and adiponectin. *Curr. Opin. Lipidol.* **13:** 51–59.

21. Byeon, J.-S., J.-Y. Jeong, M.J. Kim, *et al.* 2010. Adiponectin and adiponectin receptor in relation to colorectal cancer progression. *Int. J. Cancer* **127:** 2758–2767.

22. Rzepka-Gorska, I., R. Bedner, A. Cymbaluk-Ploska & A. Chudecka-Glaz. 2008. Serum adiponectin in relation to endometrial cancer and endometrial hyperplasia with atypia in obese women. *Eur. J. Gynaecol. Oncol.* **29:** 594–597.

23. Tian, Y.F., C.H. Chu, M.H. Wu, *et al.* 2007. Anthropometric measures, plasma adiponectin, and breast cancer risk. *Endocr.-Relat. Cancer* **14:** 669–677.

24. Wei, E.K., E. Giovannucci, C.S. Fuchs, W.C. Willett & C.S. Mantzoros. 2005. Low plasma adiponectin levels and risk of colorectal cancer in men: a prospective study. *J. Natl. Cancer Inst.* **97:** 1688–1694.

25. Sher, D.J., W.K. Oh, S. Jacobus, *et al.* 2008. Relationship between serum adiponectin and prostate cancer grade. *Prostate* **68:** 1592–1598.

26. Barb, D. *et al.* Adiponectin in relation to malignancies: a review of existing basic research and clinical evidence. *Am. J. Clin. Nutr.* **86:** 858S–866S.

27. Godsland, I.F. 2010. Insulin resistance and hyperinsulinaemia in the development and progression of cancer. *Clin. Sci.* **118:** 315–332.

28. Kahn, B.B. & J.S. Flier. 2000. Obesity and insulin resistance. *J. Clin. Invest.* **106:** 473–481.

29. Pisani, P. 2008. Hyper-insulinaemia and cancer, meta-analyses of epidemiological studies. *Arch. Physiol. Biochem.* **114:** 63–70.

30. Jazet, I.M., H. Pijl & A.E. Meinders. 2003. Adipose tissue as an endocrine organ: impact on insulin resistance. *Neth. J. Med.* **61:** 194–212.

31. Kahn, S.E., R.L. Hull & K.M. Utzschneider. 2006. Mechanisms linking obesity to insulin resistance and type 2 diabetes. *Nature* **444:** 840–846.

32. Shoelson, S.E., J. Lee & A.B. Goldfine. 2006. Inflammation and insulin resistance. *J. Clin. Invest.* **116:** 1793–1801.

33. Larsson, S.C., L. Bergkvist & A. Wolk. 2006. Consumption of sugar and sugar-sweetened foods and the risk of pancreatic cancer in a prospective study. *Am. J. Clin. Nutr.* **84:** 1171–1176.

34. Huxley, R., A. Ansary-Moghaddam, A. Berrington de Gonzalez, *et al.* 2005. Type-II diabetes and pancreatic cancer: a meta-analysis of 36 studies. *Br. J. Cancer* **92:** 2076–2083.

35. Lindblad, P., W.H. Chow, J. Chan, *et al.* 1999. The role of diabetes mellitus in the aetiology of renal cell cancer. *Diabetologia* **42:** 107–112.

36. Friberg, E., C.S. Mantzoros, & A. Wolk. 2007. Diabetes and risk of endometrial cancer: a population-based prospective cohort study. *Cancer Epidemiol. Biomarkers Prev.* **16:** 276–280.

37. Kaaks, R. 1996. Nutrition, hormones, and breast cancer: is insulin the missing link? *Cancer Causes Control* **7:** 605–625.

38. Stoll, B.A. 1999. Premalignant breast lesions: role for biological markers in predicting progression to cancer. *Eur. J. Cancer* **35:** 693–697.

39. Renehan, A.G., D.L. Roberts & C. Dive. 2008. Obesity and cancer: pathophysiological and biological mechanisms. *Arch. Physiol. Biochem.* **114:** 71–83.

40. LeRoith, D. & C.T. Roberts. 2003. The insulin-like growth factor system and cancer. *Cancer Lett.* **195:** 127–137.

41. Calle, E.E. & M.J. Thun. 2004. Obesity and cancer. *Oncogene* **23:** 6365–6378.

42. Frystyk, J. 2004. Free insulin-like growth factors – measurements and relationships to growth hormone secretion and glucose homeostasis. *Growth Horm. IGF Res.* **14:** 337–375.

43. Wolk, A., C.S. Mantzoros, S.O. Andersson, *et al.* 1998. Insulin-like growth factor 1 and prostate cancer risk: a population-based, case-control study. *J. Natl. Cancer Inst.* **90:** 911–915.

44. Cutting, C.W., C. Hunt, J.A. Nisbet, *et al.* 1999. Serum insulin-like growth factor-1 is not a useful marker of prostate cancer. *BJU Int.* **83:** 996–999.

45. Hankinson, S.E., W.C. Willett, G.A. Colditz, *et al.* 1998. Circulating concentrations of insulin-like growth factor-I and risk of breast cancer. *Lancet* **351:** 1393–1396.

46. Ma, J., M.N. Pollak, E. Giovannucci, *et al.* 1999. Prospective study of colorectal cancer risk in men and plasma levels of insulin-like growth factor (IGF)-I and IGF-binding protein-3. *J. Natl. Cancer Inst.* **91:** 620–625.

47. Saxena, N.K., L. Taliaferro-Smith, B.B. Knight, *et al.* 2008. Bidirectional crosstalk between leptin and insulin-like growth factor-I signaling promotes invasion and migration of breast cancer cells via transactivation of epidermal growth factor receptor. *Cancer Res.* **68:** 9712–9722.

48. Olivo-Marston, S.E., S.D. Hursting, J. Lavigne, *et al.* 2009. Genetic reduction of circulating insulin-like growth factor-1 inhibits azoxymethane-induced colon tumorigenesis in mice. *Mol. Carcinog.* **48:** 1071–1076.

49. Hursting, S.D., S.M. Smith, L.M. Lashinger. 2010. Calories and carcinogenesis: lessons learned from 30 years of calorie restriction research. *Carcinogenesis* **31:** 83–89.

50. Bhattacharya, A., B. Chandrasekar, M.M. Rahman, *et al.* 2006. Inhibition of inflammatory response in transgenic fat-1 mice on a calorie-restricted diet. *Biochem. Biophys. Res. Commun.* **349:** 925–930.

51. Charriere, G., B. Cousin, E. Arnaud, *et al.* 2003. Preadipocyte conversion to macrophage. Evidence of plasticity. *J. Biol. Chem.* **278:** 9850–9855.

52. O'Rourke, R.W. 2009. Inflammation in obesity-related diseases. *Surgery* **145:** 255–259.

53. Carey, D.G., G.J. Cowin, G.J. Galloway, *et al.* 2002. Effect of rosiglitazone on insulin sensitivity and body composition in type 2 diabetic patients [corrected]. *Obes. Res.* **10:** 1008–1015.

54. Subbaramaiah, K., L.R. Howe, P. Bhardwaj, *et al.* 2011. Obesity is associated with inflammation and elevated aromatase expression in the mouse mammary gland. *Cancer Prev. Res.* **4:** 329–346.

55. Kim, T., S. Choi, E. Ha, *et al.* 2011. IL-6 induction of TLR-4 gene expression via STAT3 has an effect on insulin resistance in human skeletal muscle. *Acta Diabetologica* 1–12.

56. Fontana, L., J.C. Eagon, M.E. Trujillo, *et al.* 2007. Visceral fat adipokine secretion is associated with systemic inflammation in obese humans. *Diabetes* **56:** 1010–1013.

57. Fenton, J.I., S.D. Hursting, S.N. Perkins & N.G. Hord. 2006. Interleukin-6 production induced by leptin treatment promotes cell proliferation in an Apc (Min/+) colon epithelial cell line. *Carcinogenesis* **27:** 1507–1515.

58. Dolcet, X., D. Llobet, J. Pallares & X. Matias-Guiu. 2005. NF-kB in development and progression of human cancer. *Virchows Arch.* **446:** 475–482.

59. Rouet-Benzineb, P., T. Aparicio, S. Guilmeau, *et al.* 2004. Leptin counteracts sodium butyrate-induced apoptosis in human colon cancer HT-29 cells via NF-kappaB signaling. *J. Biol. Chem.* **279:** 16495–16502.

60. Kim, D.H., J.Y. Kim, B.P. Yu & H.Y. Chung. 2008. The activation of NF-kappaB through Akt-induced FOXO1 phosphorylation during aging and its modulation by calorie restriction. *Biogerontology* **9:** 33–47.

61. Mitsiades, C.S., N. Mitsiades, V. Poulaki, *et al.* 2002. Activation of NF-kappaB and upregulation of intracellular anti-apoptotic proteins via the IGF-1/Akt signaling in human multiple myeloma cells: therapeutic implications. *Oncogene* **21:** 5673–5683.

62. Balkwill, F. & A. Mantovani. 2001. *Lancet.* **357:** 539–545.

63. Foltz, C.J., J.G. Fox, R. Cahill, *et al.* 1998. *Helicobacter.* **3:** 69–78.

64. Coussens, L.M. & Z. Werb. 2002. Inflammation and cancer. *Nature* **420:** 860–867.

65. Balkwill, F., K.A. Charles & A. Mantovani. 2005. Smoldering and polarized inflammation in the initiation and promotion of malignant disease. *Cancer Cell.* **7:** 211–217.

66. Karin, M. 2005. Inflammation and cancer: the long reach of Ras. *Nature Med.* **11:** 20–21.

67. Karin, M. 2006. Nuclear factor-kappaB in cancer development and progression. *Nature* **441:** 431–436.

68. Ishigami, S., S. Natsugoe, K. Tokuda, *et al.* 2000. Prognostic value of intratumoral natural killer cells in gastric carcinoma. *Cancer* **88:** 577–583.

69. Ribatti, D., M.G. Ennas, A. Vacca, *et al.* 2003. Tumor vascularity and tryptase-positive mast cells correlate with a poor prognosis in melanoma. *Eur. J. Clin. Invest.* **33:** 420–425.

70. Leek, R.D., R.J. Landers, A.L. Harris & C.E. Lewis. 1999. Necrosis correlates with high vascular density and focal macrophage infiltration in invasive carcinoma of the breast. *Br. J. Cancer* **79:** 991–995.

71. Koki, A., N.K. Khan, B.M. Woerner, *et al.* 2002. Cyclooxygenase-2 in human pathological disease. *Adv. Exp. Med. Biol.* **507:** 177–184.

72. Tlsty, T.D. & L.M. Coussens. 2006. Tumor stroma and regulation of cancer development. *Ann. Rev. Pathol.* **1:** 119–150.

73. Lin, W.W. & M. Karin. 2007. A cytokine-mediated link between innate immunity, inflammation, and cancer. *J. Clin. Invest.* **117:** 1175–1183.

74. Hosokawa, T., K. Kusugami, K. Ina, *et al.* 1999. Interleukin-6 and soluble interleukin-6 receptor in the colonic mucosa of inflammatory bowel disease. *J. Gastroenterol. Hepatol.* **14:** 987–996.

75. Allavena, P., A. Sica, C. Garlanda & A. Mantovani. 2008. The yin-yang of tumor-associated macrophages in neoplastic progression and immune surveillance. *Immunol. Rev.* **222:** 155–161.

76. Mantovani, A., S. Sozzani, M. Locati, *et al.* 2002. Macrophage polarization: tumor-associated macrophages as a paradigm for polarized M2 mononuclear phagocytes. *Trends Immunol.* **23:** 549–555.

77. Greten, F.R., L. Eckmann, T.F. Greten, *et al.* 2004. IKKbeta links inflammation and tumorigenesis in a mouse model of colitis-associated cancer. *Cell* **118:** 285–296.

78. Pikarsky, E., R.M. Porat, I. Stein, *et al.* 2004. NF-kappaB functions as a tumour promoter in inflammation-associated cancer. *Nature* **431:** 461–466.

79. Stark, L.A., F.V. Din, R.M. Zwacka & M.G. Dunlop. 2001. Aspirin-induced activation of the NF-kappaB signaling pathway: a novel mechanism for aspirin-mediated apoptosis in colon cancer cells. *FASEB J.* **15:** 1273–1275.

80. Colby, J.K., R.D. Klein, M.J. McArthur, *et al.* 2008. *Neoplasia, N.Y.* **10:** 782–796.

81. El-Rayes, B.F., S. Ali, F.H. Sarkar & P.A. Philip. 2004. Cyclooxygenase-2-dependent and -independent effects of celecoxib in pancreatic cancer cell lines. *Mol. Cancer Ther.* **3:** 1421–1426.

82. Cascinu, S., R. Berardi, R. Labianca, *et al.* 2008. Cetuximab plus gemcitabine and cisplatin compared with gemcitabine and cisplatin alone in patients with advanced pancreatic cancer: a randomised, multicentre, phase II trial. *Lancet Oncol.* **9:** 39–44.

83. Yamamoto, Y., M.J. Yin, K.M. Lin & R.B. Gaynor. 1999. Sulindac inhibits activation of the NF-kappaB pathway. *J. Biol. Chem.* **274:** 27307–27314.

84. Yip-Schneider, M.T., H. Nakshatri, C.J. Sweeney, *et al.* 2005. Parthenolide and sulindac cooperate to mediate growth suppression and inhibit the nuclear factor-kappa B pathway in pancreatic carcinoma cells. *Mol. Cancer Ther.* **4:** 587–594.

85. Ma, M.H., H.H. Yang, K. Parker, *et al.* 2003. The proteasome inhibitor PS-341 markedly enhances sensitivity of multiple myeloma tumor cells to chemotherapeutic agents. *Clin. Cancer Res.* **9:** 1136–1144.

86. Shishodia, S., H.M. Amin, R. Lai & B.B. Aggarwal. 2005. Curcumin (diferuloylmethane) inhibits constitutive NF-kappaB activation, induces G1/S arrest, suppresses proliferation, and induces apoptosis in mantle cell lymphoma. *Biochem. Pharmacol.* **70:** 700–713.

87. Weisberg, S.P., R. Leibel & D.V. Tortoriello. 2008. Dietary curcumin significantly improves obesity-associated inflammation and diabetes in mouse models of diabesity. *Endocrinology* **149:** 3549–3558.

88. Chen, H., Z.S. Zhang, Y.L. Zhang & D.Y. Zhou. 1999. Curcumin inhibits cell proliferation by interfering with the cell cycle and inducing apoptosis in colon carcinoma cells. *Anticancer Res.* **19:** 3675–3680.

89. Li, L., B.B. Aggarwal, S. Shishodia, *et al.* 2004. Nuclear factor-kappaB and IkappaB kinase are constitutively active in human pancreatic cells, and their down-regulation by curcumin (diferulolylmethane) is associated with the suppression of proliferation and the induction of apoptosis. *Cancer* **101:** 2351–2362.

90. Limtrakul, P., S. Lipigorngoson, O. Namwong, *et al.* 1997. Inhibitory effect of dietary curcumin on skin carcinogenesis in mice. *Cancer Lett.* **116:** 197–203.

91. Huang, M.T., H.L. Newmark & K. Frenkel. 1997. Inhibitory effects of curcumin on tumorigenesis in mice. Journal of cellular biochemistry. *J. Cell. Biochem.* **27:** 26–34.

92. Chuang, S.E., A.L. Cheng, J.K. Lin & M.L. Kuo. 2000. Inhibition by curcumin of diethylnitrosamine-induced hepatic hyperplasia, inflammation, cellular gene products and cell-cycle-related proteins in rats. *Food Chem. Toxicol.* **38:** 991–995.

93. Singh, S. & B.B. Aggarwal. 1995. Activation of transcription factor NF-kappa B is suppressed by curcumin (diferuloylmethane) [corrected]. *J. Biol. Chem.* **270:** 24995–25000.

94. Pandelidou, M., K. Dimas, A. Georgopoulos, *et al.* 2011. Preparation and characterization of lyophilised EGG PC liposomes incorporating curcumin and evaluation of its activity against colorectal cancer cell lines. *J. Nanosci. Nanotechnol.* **11:** 1259–1266.

Ann. N.Y. Acad. Sci. ISSN 0077-8923

ANNALS OF THE NEW YORK ACADEMY OF SCIENCES

Issue: *Nutrition and Physical Activity in Aging, Obesity, and Cancer*

Metabolic approaches to overcoming chemoresistance in ovarian cancer

Dong Hoon Suh,[1] Mi-Kyung Kim,[1] Jae Hong No,[4] Hyun Hoon Chung,[1] and Yong Sang Song[1,2,3]

[1]Department of Obstetrics and Gynecology, Seoul National University College of Medicine, Seoul, Republic of Korea. [2]Cancer Research Institute, Seoul National University College of Medicine, Seoul, Republic of Korea. [3]Major in Biomodulation, World Class University, Seoul National University, Seoul, Republic of Korea. [4]Department of Obstetrics and Gynecology, Seoul National University Bundang Hospital, Seongnam, Republic of Korea

Address for correspondence: Yong Sang Song, Department of Obstetrics and Gynecology, Seoul National University College of Medicine, Seoul 110-744, Republic of Korea. yssong@snu.ac.kr

The poor prognosis in the treatment of ovarian cancer is mainly attributed to chemoresistance. The development of new strategies is urgently necessary to overcome chemoresistance because of the low efficacy of the current standard chemotherapy in ovarian cancer. Metabolic alterations have been suggested to have a crucial role in cancer development. The key metabolic changes in cancer include aerobic glycolysis and macromolecular synthesis, causing antiapoptosis in cancer cells. Therefore, the manipulation of the metabolic derangement could be an effective strategy to overcome chemoresistance in ovarian cancer. In this review, we will discuss metabolic interventions as promising anticancer strategies in ovarian cancer, focusing on the glycolytic, mitochondrial apoptotic, and necrotic pathways. In addition, the role of p53 in relation to metabolic alterations in cancer will be mentioned.

Keywords: ovarian cancer; chemoresistance; metabolic interventions; aerobic glycolysis; antiapoptosis

Introduction

Ovarian carcinoma is the most lethal gynecological malignancy in the United States. The 5-year survival rate for patients with ovarian cancer is just 45%.[1] Patients usually respond to initial therapy and cytoreductive surgery followed by adjuvant chemotherapy with platinum and paclitaxel.[2] However, approximately 70% of patients with the advanced stage experience recurrence, which is incurable mainly due to the development of chemoresistance.[3,4] In order to overcome chemoresistance in ovarian cancer, establishment of new treatment strategies is essential because the current chemotherapy does not seem to be effective for inducing cancer cell death in chemoresistant cells.[1,5,6]

A cell has multiple death mechanisms. Apoptosis is an efficient programmed cell death process regulated by an intrinsic or extrinsic pathway.[7] It is now well documented that most chemotherapeutic agents work through the induction of apoptosis.[8]

Thus, the disruption of apoptotic pathways can reduce the sensitivity of tumor cells to treatment.[7,9] Necrosis is another cell death mechanism where cells die by a loss of physical integrity.[10] It occurs in apoptosis-defective tumor cells under the condition of energy deprivation. Metabolic stress is a potent trigger for both apoptosis and necrosis, suggesting that metabolism is an alternative therapeutic target. Furthermore, cancer cell metabolism is considered a more attractive target due to an inherent weakness from the unrelenting energy demand for the rapid proliferation of cancer cells.

In 1926, Otto Warburg proposed that "aerobic glycolysis," high glycolysis even in the presence of oxygen, was at the heart of cancer development.[11] Metabolic changes in cancer are now reemerging issues along with a growing realization that metabolic transformation can have a crucial role in tumorigenesis. Many researchers have shown that glycolysis plays a far more important role in ATP generation in cancer than it does in normal tissue.[12] The fact

doi: 10.1111/j.1749-6632.2011.06095.x

that tumors prefer glycolysis to convert glucose to ATP formed the basis of tumor imaging by fluorine-18 fluorodeoxyglucose ($[^{18}F]FDG$) positron emission tomography (PET),[13] of which the clinical usefulness was well demonstrated in ovarian cancer.[14] In this review, we focus on metabolic intervention to overcome chemoresistance in ovarian cancer.

Metabolic dysfunction in cancer

Aerobic glycolysis

Aerobic glycolysis is a key hallmark of many cancers.[15] Although the causal relationship between the Warburg effect and cancer progression is still not clear, the metabolic derangement is triggered by oncogene activation, inactivation of the tumor suppressor gene, and hypoxia in the tumor microenvironment.[7] As a tumor expands, it outgrows its local blood supply, leading to hypoxia and stabilization of hypoxia-inducible transcription factor 1 (HIF-1). HIF-1 upregulates glycolysis, although it prevents the mitochondria from functioning properly in ATP production. Oxidative phosphorylation in mitochondria is much more efficient than glycolysis in producing ATP; however, the latter is much faster than the former.

More importantly, an excessive rate of glycolysis ultimately results in the generation of lactic acid via lactate dehydrogenase (LDH). The resultant acidity compromises an immune response while preparing surrounding tissues to favor tumor invasion and even metastasis.[16,17] In addition, the glycolytic shift in tumor cells not only compensates for mitochondrial dysfunction but also provides the acquired resistance to apoptotic cell death.[18]

Macromolecular synthesis through the mTOR pathway

The mammalian target of rapamycin (mTOR) is in the middle of signaling pathways that are involved in the energy metabolism and cell growth/division through the synthesis of macromolecules, such as protein and lipid. As a key regulator of cell growth, mTOR promotes cell growth and proliferation, suppresses the induction of autophagy, and ultimately results in tumor development.[11,19]

There are two influential regulators of mTOR. One is the mTOR activator, Akt, which promotes anabolic, energy-consuming pathways like fatty acid synthesis. The other is the mTOR repressor, AMPK, which drives catabolic, energy-producing responses like fatty acid oxidation.

Activation of Akt enhances glycolytic activity and is commonly observed in cancer cells, including ovarian cancer.[20–22] This constitutive activation of Akt, which leads to the cell growth and inhibits autophagy, may be the inherent weakness of tumor cells because it renders them difficult to adapt to nutrient and growth factor limitation.[7]

Metabolic pathways associated with chemoresistance

There are two major apoptotic pathways, the extrinsic (death receptor–mediated apoptosis) and intrinsic pathways (mitochondria-mediated apoptosis). The latter involves permeabilization of the outer mitochondrial membrane (OMM), a key event during the early phase of the apoptosis.[23] Then it is followed by the release of cytochrome c from the intermembrane space of mitochondria.[18] The defects of the intrinsic pathway not only contribute to carcinogenesis in normal cells but also serve as mechanisms of chemoresistance in tumor cells.[5]

OMM permeabilization consists of three pore systems. One is the voltage-dependent anion channel (VDAC) in the OMM. To date, it is not clear whether the closed or the open conformations of VDAC are involved in promoting apoptosis.[24,25] Another is mitochondrial permeability transition pore (MPTP), a nonspecific pore in the inner mitochondrial membrane. Mitochondria in tumor cells are relatively less susceptible to Ca^{2+}-induced mitochondrial permeability transition (MPT) than those in normal cells. The other pore mechanism is mitochondrial apoptosis-induced channel (MAC), a specific pore in the OMM.[26]

OMM permeabilization resulting from these three pore systems requires the oligomeric form of Bax. During apoptosis, tBid (the truncated form of the BH3-only protein Bid)-mediated oligomerization of Bax causes OMM permeabilization, whereas Bcl-2, an antiapoptotic protein, interacts with Bax to prevent its oligomerization to inhibit apoptosis. Therefore, it is not surprising that all three pore mechanisms are directly or indirectly regulated by Bcl-2 family proteins.[24,27,28] The antiapoptotic protein, Bcl-X_L, prevents apoptosis by interacting with VDAC directly and closing it, whereas Bax and Bad interact with VDAC to accelerate its opening (Fig. 1A).[15] Bcl-2 overexpression in the tumor cells

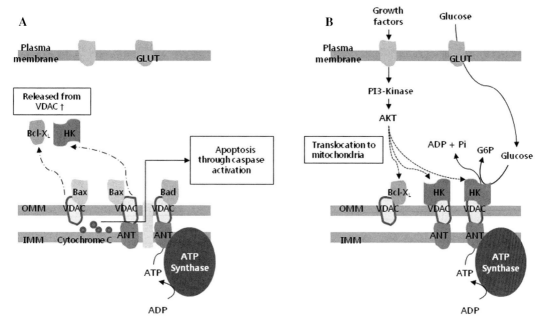

Figure 1. HK II binding to VDAC is critical for preventing the induction of apoptosis. (A) In normal cells, apoptosis is induced when HK II is released from VDAC. Proapoptotic Bcl-2 family proteins (Bax and Bad) interact with VDAC and are likely to activate the mitochondrial permeability transition pore (MPTP) complex in the OMM, through which cytochrome c is released. (B) In tumor cells, the activated PI3-kinase/Akt pathway facilitates the translocation of Bcl-X_L and HK II to VDAC on OMM, preventing apoptosis. Bcl-X_L interacts with VDAC directly to close it, while HK II inhibits apoptosis by occupying the binding sites for Bax and Bad on VDAC. HK, hexokinase; VDAC, voltage-dependent anion channel; ANT, adenine nucleotide transporter; GLUT, glucose transporter; OMM, outer mitochondrial membrane; IMM, inner mitochondrial membrane. Modified and adapted by permission from Mathupala *et al.*[15]

is shown to be related to the sensitivity of MPTP and MACs.[18]

Interestingly, HK, which catalyzes the essentially irreversible first step of the glycolytic pathway where glucose is phosphorylated to glucose-6-phosphate, is often upregulated in tumors. The predominant isoform in malignant tumors, HK II, plays a major role in preventing tumor apoptosis. HK II preoccupies the VDAC binding sites for proapoptotic proteins, such as Bax and Bad, preventing their oligomerization, which is necessary for activation of the MPTP. HK II also prevents formation of a MPTP by altering the conformation of the VDAC-adenine nucleotide transporter (ANT) protein complex to reduce OMM permeabilization (Fig. 1B).[15,29]

In addition, there is a growing body of evidence that Akt could enhance OMM stability and protect cells from apoptosis.[30] Akt phosphorylates the proapoptotic protein Bad to inhibit the function of Bad and inhibits p53-mediated expression or oligomerization of Bax, thus preventing OMM permeabi-

lization.[31–33] Akt was also shown to facilitate the translocation of Bcl-X_L and HK II to mitochondria, allowing them to interact with VDAC.[18] The binding sites for proapoptotic proteins on the OMM are occupied by HK II through the HK II-VDAC interaction, and thereby apoptosis is impeded (Fig. 1B).[34]

Metabolic pathways and chemoresistance in ovarian cancer

Despite the endless list of metabolic targets being investigated in various cancers, the studies in ovarian cancer were only a few.[35] A glucose analog, 2-deoxyglucose (DG), competes with native glucose for entry into the glycolytic pathway not to be further metabolized. The resultant deprivation of ATP was shown to induce apoptosis with various levels from just slowdown of the proliferation to massive apoptosis.[36] The combination of cisplatin and 2-DG, or cisplatin and rapamycin significantly increased the proportion of apoptotic cells compared with cisplatin, 2-DG, or rapamycin alone.[37] This

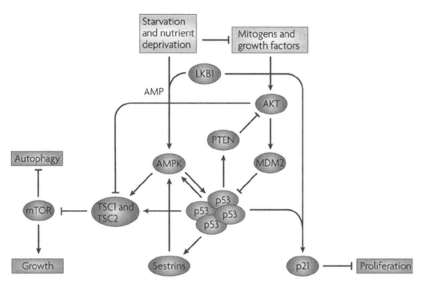

Figure 2. The activation of p53 in response to a lack of nutrients signals through the activation of AMPK and the inhibition of AKT. p53 further induces AMPK (both directly and indirectly through the sestrins) and activates the expression of tuberous sclerosis 2 (TSC2), resulting in the inhibition of mTOR. This leads to a decrease in cell growth, which coordinates with the inhibition of proliferation that is also mediated through the activation of p53, together with LKB1. This pathway also contributes to p53-mediated activation of autophagy. Under hypoxic conditions, reduced MDM2, a ubiquitin ligase that mediates the degradation of p53, activates p53 through alleviating the autoregulatory negative feedback on p53. AMPK, AMP-activated protein kinase; LKB1, liver kinase B1; mTOR, mammalian target of rapamycin. Adapted by permission from Vousden and Ryan.[11]

study also demonstrated that the combination of cisplatin and 2-DG not only activated the intrinsic apoptotic pathway with caspase-9 being activated, but also induced nonapoptotic necrotic cell death.

On the other hand, p53, a well-known tumor suppressor protein, plays a central role in the metabolic pathways (Fig. 2). The TP53 mutation is reported in 60–80% of both sporadic and familial cases of ovarian carcinoma, more frequently in advanced stage than in early stage, and is associated with poor survival.[8,38,39] The poor prognosis associated with TP53 alteration has been thought to be due to not only more aggressive phenotype, but also resistance to chemotherapy-induced apoptosis.[40–48] Interestingly, increased glucose metabolism caused by the upregulated HK II was reported to suppress p53 activity, suggesting that the high levels of glycolysis in cancers may help evade the tumor-suppressive effects of p53.[49]

Metabolic intervention in anticancer therapy

Targeting aerobic glycolysis
Glycolysis is a series of enzyme reactions that convert a molecule of glucose into lactate with

the generation of two molecules of ATP.[35] Apart from 2-DG mentioned above, many glycolytic inhibitors, including lonidamine (a derivative of indazole-3-carboxylic acid) and methyl jasmonate on HK, 3-(3-pyridinyl)-1-(4-pyridinyl)-2-propen-1-one (3-PO) on phosphofructokinase (PFK), iodoacetate on glyceraldehydes-3-phosphate dehydrogenase (GAPDH), and TLN-232 on pyruvate kinase (PK), have been under preclinical or clinical development.[50–52]

PFK is the enzyme of the rate-limiting step in glycolysis. HK II also set the pace of glycolysis. Therefore, these two steps are likely to be considered effective metabolic targets for driving tumor cells to the state of metabolic crisis (Fig. 3).

Lonidamine inhibits HK II in relatively hypoxic conditions, although the mechanism of action is still obscure.[53] In a phase I clinical trial, lonidamine was shown to be active and tolerable in the treatment of advanced ovarian cancer when used in combination with cisplatin/paclitaxel.[54] Lonidamine has been clinically approved for use in Europe in some cancer therapeutic protocols.[50]

Another HK inhibitor, methyl jasmonate, binds to mitochondrial HK II and detaches it from VDAC.

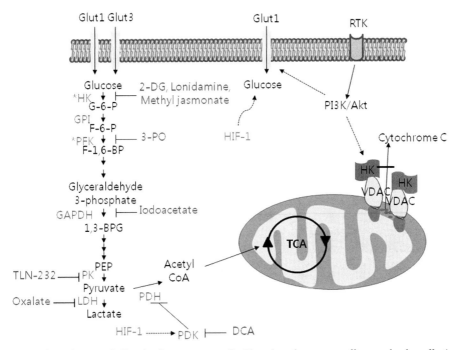

Figure 3. Increased gycolysis is a hallmark of most cancer cells. There have been many efforts to develop effective glycolytic inhibitors at each step. In particular, PFK, the rate-limiting enzyme in glycolysis, and HK II, the enzyme regulating the pace of glycolysis, are the most interesting targets. Besides the aerobic glycolysis, the apoptotic machinery of the mitochondria also serves as the target for anticanacer therapy. Oncogenic alterations (PI3K/Akt) and HIF-1 stabilization result in increased expression of glucose transporters and glycolytic enzymes. PI3K/Akt also facilitates the translocation and binding of HK II to VDAC, which prevent cytochrome c and further apoptosis.* = key enzymes in the glycolytic pathway. HK, hexokinase; GPI, glucose-6-phosphate isomerase; PFK, phosphofructokinase; GAPDH, glyceraldehyde-3-phosphate dehydrogenase; PK, pyruvate kinase; LDH, lactate dehydrogenase; PDH, pyruvate dehydrogenase; PDK, pyruvate dehydrogenase kinase; HIF-1, hypoxia-inducible transcription factor; 2-DG, 2-deoxyglucose; 3-PO, 3-(3-pyridinyl)-1-(4-pyridinyl)-2-propen-1-one; DCA, dichloroacetate; RTK, receptor tyrosine kinase; VDAC, voltage-dependent anion channel; TCA, tricarboxylic acid cycle; G-6-P, glucose-6-phosphate; F-6-P, fructose-6-phosphate; F-1,6-BP, fructose-1,6-bisphophate; 1,3-BPG, 1,3-bisphosphoglycerate; PEP, phosphoenol pyruvate. Modified and with permission from Ref. 62.

The dissociation of HK II from mitochondria triggers a concomitant release of cytochrome c.[35] Although very little is known about methyl jasmonate in ovarian cancer, it is expected to be a promising molecule because it facilitates the mitochondrial apoptotic pathway as well as a significant degree of ATP depletion.

3-PO inhibits 6-phophofructo-2-kinase/fructose-2, 6-bisphophatase 3 (PFKFB3), which is the key enzyme regulating the activity of PFK1, suppressing glycolytic flux and tumor growth in several human cancer cell lines.[55] This small molecule is still being tested *in vitro* and in animal models. It is thought to have a considerable antineoplastic effect in ovarian cancer because PFK regulates the highly exergonic and irreversible step of glycolysis regardless of the cancer type.

Pyruvate dehydrogenase (PDH) converts pyruvate to acetyl-CoA, which enters the Krebs cycle and goes through the oxidative phosphorylation in mitochondria. LDH catalyzes the conversion of pyruvate to lactate. Pyruvate dehydrogenase kinase (PDK) phosphorylates and inactivates PDH, thus resulting in the suppression of the Krebs cycle and mitochondrial respiration.[18] Recent studies have shown that induction of PDK3 by HIF-1 promotes chemoresistance to conventional anticancer drugs like cisplatin and paclitaxel.[56] Dichloroacetate (DCA), a pyruvate analog, was shown to shift metabolism from glycolysis to oxidative phosphorylation by inhibition of PDK. However, this approach would work only in cancer cells with functionally impaired mitochondria because otherwise diverted energy sources could compensate for the inhibited glycolysis through the competent mitochondria. Therefore, the combination of DCA with an inhibitor of mitochondrial ATP synthase, apoptolidin, might be a highly effective strategy in ovarian cancer, regardless of the functional status of mitochondria.[50]

Control of the mitochondrial apoptotic pathway

Because the induction of MPT is the sentinel, irreversible event in the intrinsic apoptotic pathway, agents modulating MPT seem to be of great use for apoptotic cell death. Furanonapthoquinone (FNQ) targets VDAC1 to induce apoptosis via ROS production at the OMM, causing collapse of the membrane potential and cytochrome c release.[57] Bongkrekic acid and atractyloside modulate MPT and induce mitochondrial swelling through binding to the ANT, the inner membrane component of the MPTP system.[58]

Detachment of HK II from the mitochondria potentiates cisplatin-induced mitochondrial injury and cytotoxicity through facilitating Bak oligomerization.[59] Clotrimazole is capable of displacing HK II from its mitochondrial biding site in both isolated mitochondria and intact cells.[60] Clotrimazole combined with cisplatin results in a synergistic effect of cisplatin-induced cytotoxicity.

In addition, several strategies designed for targeting the Bcl-2 family proteins have been developed to block the abnormally increased antiapoptotic proteins in cancers, such as anti-Bcl-2 antibody, anti-Bcl-2 ribozyme, and Bak BH3 peptide. Small molecule inhibitors that bind the BH3 binding site of Bcl-2 have been developed to block the interaction of Bcl-2 with proapoptotic proteins and thus promote apoptosis, for example, ABT-263.[61]

Targeting the necrotic pathway

Various kinds of cancer cells constitutively activate the PI3K/Akt pathway, outgrowing the nutrient supply. It makes the microenvironment hostile because tumor cells demand an unrelenting supply of energy. On the other hand, the main ATP source in tumor cells is shifted from oxidative phosphorylation to glycolysis. Furthermore, autophagy, an alternative energy source, is inhibited by the activation of mTOR in tumor cells. Thus, the tumor cells often go through "metabolic crisis" to end up with necrotic cell death.[62–65] A necrotic pathway as a default cell death mechanism can be considered a po-

tential therapeutic approach, in particular, to many chemoresistant cancers.[7] Cell necrosis can be induced through "metabolic crisis" by way of angiogenesis inhibition, accelerated ATP consumption, and autophagy inhibition together with metabolic deprivation and glycolysis inhibition.

Conclusions

Cell fate is directly related to cell metabolism. Increased glycolysis with mitochondrial dysfunction characterizes metabolic alterations in many types of cancer, causing inhibition of apoptosis and a resultant unrelenting demand of energy. Thus, metabolic starvation may affect the cancer cells significantly. Considering the high incidence of chemoresistance and the rapid spread of disease in ovarian cancer, metabolic approaches are rational strategies to improve the poor prognosis of ovarian cancer. Induction of a metabolic starvation through glycolysis inhibition and other metabolic stresses and targeting mitochondrial apoptotic machinery appear to be promising strategies. In particular, the combination of anticancer chemotherapeutics and metabolic modulators can cause a synergistic effect to overcome chemoresistance.

Considerable efforts still should be put into basic and clinical research to elucidate the biomolecular mechanisms of metabolic changes and chemoresistance in ovarian cancer. It will lead us to the development of the new molecules targeting metabolic derangement so that we can achieve significant improvement in the management of ovarian cancer.

Acknowledgments

This work was supported by the Priority Research Centers Program through the National Research Foundation of Korea (NRF) funded by the Ministry of Education, Science and Technology (2009-0093820). This research was also supported by the WCU (World Class University) program through the Korea Science and Engineering Foundation funded by the Ministry of Education, Science and Technology (R31-2008-000-10056-0).

Conflicts of Interest

The authors declare no conflicts of interest.

References

1. McLean, K., N.A. VanDeVen, D.R. Sorenson, *et al.* 2009. The HIV protease inhibitor saquinavir induces endoplasmic

reticulum stress, autophagy, and apoptosis in ovarian cancer cells. *Gynecol. Oncol.* **112:** 623–630.

2. Omura, G., J.A. Blessing, C.E. Ehrlich, *et al.* 1986. A randomized trial of cyclophosphamide and doxorubicin with or without cisplatin in advanced ovarian carcinoma. A gynecologic oncology group study. *Cancer* **57:** 1725–1730.

3. Matsuo, K., M.L. Eno, D.D. Im, *et al.* 2010. Clinical relevance of extent of extreme drug resistance in epithelial ovarian carcinoma. *Gynecol. Oncol.* 116: 61–65.

4. Salani, R., R.J. Kurman, R. Giuntoli, 2nd, *et al.* 2008. Assessment of TP53 mutation using purified tissue samples of ovarian serous carcinomas reveals a higher mutation rate than previously reported and does not correlate with drug resistance. *Int. J. Gynecol. Cancer* 18: 487–491.

5. Kaufmann, S.H. & D.L. Vaux. 2003. Alterations in the apoptotic machinery and their potential role in anticancer drug resistance. *Oncogene* **22:** 7414–7430.

6. Fraser, M., B. Leung, A. Jahani-Asl, *et al.* 2003. Chemoresistance in human ovarian cancer: the role of apoptotic regulators. *Reprod. Biol. Endocrinol.* **1:** 66.

7. Jin S., R.S. DiPaola, R. Mathew, *et al.* 2007. Metabolic catastrophe as a means to cancer cell death. *J. Cell. Sci.* **120:** 379–383.

8. Bast, R.C., Jr., B. Hennessy & G.B Mills. 2009. The biology of ovarian cancer: new opportunities for translation. *Nat. Rev. Cancer* **9:** 415–428.

9. Pennington, K., H. Pulaski, M. Pennington, *et al.* 2010. Too much of a good thing: suicide prevention promotes chemoresistance in ovarian carcinoma. *Curr. Cancer Drug Targets* **10:** 575–583.

10. Thompson, C.B., D.E. Bauer, J.J. Lum, *et al.* 2005. How do cancer cells acquire the fuel needed to support cell growth? *Cold Spring Harb. Symp. Quant. Biol.* **70:** 357–362.

11. Vousden, K.H. & K.M. Ryan. 2009. p53 and metabolism. *Nat. Rev. Cancer* **9:** 691–700.

12. Gottlieb, E., K.H. Vousden. 2010. p53 regulation of metabolic pathways. *Cold Spring Harb. Perspect. Biol.* **2:** a001040.

13. Zhang, Z., H. Li, Q. Liu, *et al.* 2004. Metabolic imaging of tumors using intrinsic and extrinsic fluorescent markers. *Biosens. Bioelectron.* **20:** 643–650.

14. Chung, H.H., W.J. Kang, J.W. Kim, *et al.* 2007. Role of [18F]FDG PET/CT in the assessment of suspected recurrent ovarian cancer: correlation with clinical or histological findings. *Eur. J. Nucl. Med. Mol. Imaging* **34:** 480–486.

15. Mathupala, S.P., Y.H. Ko & P.L. Pedersen. 2006. Hexokinase II: cancer's double-edged sword acting as both facilitator and gatekeeper of malignancy when bound to mitochondria. *Oncogene* **25:** 4777–4786.

16. Gatenby, R.A., E.T. Gawlinski. 2003. The glycolytic phenotype in carcinogenesis and tumor invasion: insights through mathematical models. *Cancer Res.* **63:** 3847–3854.

17. Gillies R.J., I. Robey, R.A. Gatenby. 2008. Causes and consequences of increased glucose metabolism of cancers. *J. Nucl. Med.* **49**(Suppl 2): 24S–42S.

18. Gogvadze, V., S. Orrenius, B. Zhivotovsky. 2008. Mitochondria in cancer cells: what is so special about them? *Trends Cell. Biol.* **18:** 165–173.

19. Fogarty, S. & D.G. Hardie. 2010. Development of protein kinase activators: AMPK as a target in metabolic disorders and cancer. *Biochim. Biophys. Acta* **1804:** 581–591.

20. Plas, D.R. & C.B. Thompson. 2005. Akt-dependent transformation: there is more to growth than just surviving. *Oncogene* **24:** 7435–7442.

21. Elstrom, R.L., D.E. Bauer, M. Buzzai, *et al.* 2004. Akt stimulates aerobic glycolysis in cancer cells. *Cancer Res.* **64:** 3892–3889.

22. Bellacosa, A., D. de Feo, A.K. Godwin, *et al.* 1995. Molecular alterations of the AKT2 oncogene in ovarian and breast carcinomas. *Int. J. Cancer* **64:** 280–285.

23. Gogvadze, V., S. Orrenius, B. Zhivotovsky. 2006. Multiple pathways of cytochrome c release from mitochondria in apoptosis. *Biochim. Biophys. Acta* **1757:** 639–647.

24. Shimizu, S., Y. Shinohara, Y. Tsujimoto. 2000. Bax and Bcl-xL independently regulate apoptotic changes of yeast mitochondria that require VDAC but not adenine nucleotide translocator. *Oncogene* **19:** 4309–4318.

25. Vander Heiden M.G., X.X. Li, E. Gottlieb, *et al.* 2001. Bcl-xL promotes the open configuration of the voltage-dependent anion channel and metabolite passage through the outer mitochondrial membrane. *J. Biol. Chem.* **276:** 19414–19419.

26. Kinnally, K.W. & B. Antonsson. 2007. A tale of two mitochondrial channels, MAC and PTP, in apoptosis. *Apoptosis* **12:** 857–868.

27. Evtodienko, Y.V., V.V. Teplova, T.S. Azarashvily, *et al.* 1999. The Ca2+ threshold for the mitochondrial permeability transition and the content of proteins related to Bcl-2 in rat liver and Zajdela hepatoma mitochondria. *Mol. Cell. Biochem.* **194:** 251–256.

28. Pavlov, E.V., M. Priault, D. Pietkiewicz, *et al.* 2001. A novel, high conductance channel of mitochondria linked to apoptosis in mammalian cells and Bax expression in yeast. *J. Cell. Biol.* **155:** 725–731.

29. Majewski, N., V. Nogueira, R.B. Robey, *et al.* 2004. Akt inhibits apoptosis downstream of BID cleavage via a glucose-dependent mechanism involving mitochondrial hexokinases. *Mol. Cell. Biol.* **24:** 730–740.

30. Franke T.F., D.R. Kaplan, L.C. Cantley. 1997. PI3K: downstream AKTion blocks apoptosis. *Cell* **88:** 435–437.

31. del Peso, L, M. Gonzalez-Garcia, C. Page, *et al.* 1997. Interleukin-3-induced phosphorylation of BAD through the protein kinase Akt. *Science* **278:** 687–689.

32. Yamaguchi, A., M. Tamatani, H. Matsuzaki, *et al.* 2001. Akt activation protects hippocampal neurons from apoptosis by inhibiting transcriptional activity of p53. *J. Biol. Chem.* **276:** 5256–5264.

33. Mookherjee, P., R. Quintanilla, M.S. Roh, *et al.* 2007. Mitochondrial-targeted active Akt protects SH-SY5Y neuroblastoma cells from staurosporine-induced apoptotic cell death. *J. Cell. Biochem.* **102:** 196–210.

34. Pastorino, J.G., N. Shulga & J.B. Hoek. 2002. Mitochondrial binding of hexokinase II inhibits Bax-induced cytochrome c release and apoptosis. *J. Biol. Chem.* **277:** 7610–7618.

35. Pathania, D., M. Millard & N. Neamati. 2009. Opportunities in discovery and delivery of anticancer drugs targeting mitochondria and cancer cell metabolism. *Adv. Drug Deliv. Rev.* **61:** 1250–1275.

36. Zhang, X.D., E. Deslandes, M. Villedieu, *et al.* 2006. Effect of 2-deoxy-D-glucose on various malignant cell lines in vitro. *Anticancer Res.* **26:** 3561–3566.

37. Loar, P., H. Wahl, M. Kshirsagar, *et al.* 2010. Inhibition of glycolysis enhances cisplatin-induced apoptosis in ovarian cancer cells. *Am. J. Obstet. Gynecol.* **202:** 371 e1–8.

38. Havrilesky, L., M. Darcy, H. Hamdan, *et al.* 2003. Prognostic significance of p53 mutation and p53 overexpression in advanced epithelial ovarian cancer: a Gynecologic Oncology Group study. *J. Clin. Oncol.* **21:** 3814–3825.

39. Lavarino, C., S. Pilotti, M. Oggionni, *et al.* 2000. p53 gene status and response to platinum/paclitaxel-based chemotherapy in advanced ovarian carcinoma. *J. Clin. Oncol.* **18:** 3936–45.

40. van der Zee, A.G., H. Hollema, A.J. Suurmeijer, *et al.* 1995. Value of P-glycoprotein, glutathione S-transferase pi, c-erbB-2, and p53 as prognostic factors in ovarian carcinomas. *J. Clin. Oncol.* **13:** 70–78.

41. Berns, E.M., J.G. Klijn, W.L. van Putten, *et al.* 1998. p53 protein accumulation predicts poor response to tamoxifen therapy of patients with recurrent breast cancer. *J. Clin. Oncol.* **16:** 121–127.

42. Geisler, J.P., H.E. Geisler, M.C. Wiemann, *et al.* 1997. Quantification of p53 in epithelial ovarian cancer. *Gynecol. Oncol.* **66:** 435–438.

43. Marks, J.R., A.M. Davidoff, B.J. Kerns, *et al.* 1991. Overexpression and mutation of p53 in epithelial ovarian cancer. *Cancer Res.* **51:** 2979–2984.

44. Brown, R., C. Clugston, P. Burns, *et al.* 1993. Increased accumulation of p53 protein in cisplatin-resistant ovarian cell lines. *Int. J. Cancer* **55:** 678–684.

45. Righetti, S.C., G. Della Torre, S. Pilotti, *et al.* 1996. A comparative study of p53 gene mutations, protein accumulation, and response to cisplatin-based chemotherapy in advanced ovarian carcinoma. *Cancer Res.* **56:** 689–693.

46. Perego, P., M. Giarola, S.C. Righetti, *et al.* 1996. Association between cisplatin resistance and mutation of p53 gene and reduced bax expression in ovarian carcinoma cell systems. *Cancer Res.* **56:** 556–562.

47. Buttitta, F., A. Marchetti, A. Gadducci, *et al.* 1997. p53 alterations are predictive of chemoresistance and aggressiveness in ovarian carcinomas: a molecular and immunohistochemical study. *Br. J. Cancer* **75:** 230–235.

48. Reles, A., W.H. Wen, A. Schmider, *et al.* 2001. Correlation of p53 mutations with resistance to platinum-based chemotherapy and shortened survival in ovarian cancer. *Clin. Cancer Res.* **7:** 2984–2997.

49. Zhao, Y., J.L. Coloff, E.C. Ferguson, *et al.* 2008. Glucose metabolism attenuates p53 and Puma-dependent cell death upon growth factor deprivation. *J. Biol. Chem.* **283:** 36344–36353.

50. Brawer, M.K. 2005. Lonidamine: basic science and rationale for treatment of prostatic proliferative disorders. *Rev. Urol.* **7**(Suppl 7): S21–S26.

51. Giaccone, G., E.F. Smit, M. de Jonge, *et al.* 2004. Glufosfamide administered by 1-hour infusion as a second-line treatment for advanced non-small cell lung cancer; a phase II trial of the EORTC-New Drug Development Group. *Eur. J. Cancer* **40:** 667–672.

52. Scatena, R., P Bottoni, A. Pontoglio, *et al.* 2008. Glycolytic enzyme inhibitors in cancer treatment. *Expert Opin. Investig. Drugs* **17:** 1533–1545.

53. Floridi, A., M.G. Paggi, M.L. Marcante, *et al.* 1981. Lonidamine, a selective inhibitor of aerobic glycolysis of murine tumor cells. *J. Natl. Cancer Inst.* **66:** 497–499.

54. De Lena, M., V. Lorusso, A. Latorre, *et al.* 2001. Paclitaxel, cisplatin and lonidamine in advanced ovarian cancer. A phase II study. *Eur. J. Cancer* **37:** 364–368.

55. Clem, B., S. Telang, A. Clem, *et al.* 2008. Small-molecule inhibition of 6-phosphofructo-2-kinase activity suppresses glycolytic flux and tumor growth. *Mol. Cancer Ther.* **7:** 110–120.

56. Lu, C.W., S.C. Lin, K.F. Chen, *et al.* 2008. Induction of pyruvate dehydrogenase kinase-3 by hypoxia-inducible factor-1 promotes metabolic switch and drug resistance. *J. Biol. Chem.* **283:** 28106–28114.

57. Simamura, E., K. Hirai, H. Shimada, *et al.* 2006. Furanon-aphthoquinones cause apoptosis of cancer cells by inducing the production of reactive oxygen species by the mitochondrial voltage- dependent anion channel. *Cancer Biol. Ther.* **5:** 1523–1529.

58. Zamzami, N. & G. Kroemer. 2001. The mitochondrion in apoptosis: how Pandora's box opens. *Nat. Rev. Mol. Cell. Biol.* **2:** 67–71.

59. Shulga, N., R. Wilson-Smith, J.G. Pastorino. 2009. Hexokinase II detachment from the mitochondria potentiates cisplatin induced cytotoxicity through a caspase-2 dependent mechanism. *Cell Cycle* **8:** 3355–3364.

60. Majewski, N., V. Nogueira, P. Bhaskar, *et al.* 2004. Hexokinase-mitochondria interaction mediated by Akt is required to inhibit apoptosis in the presence or absence of Bax and Bak. *Mol. Cell* **16:** 819–830.

61. Lessene, G., P.E. Czabotar, P.M. Colman. 2008. BCL-2 family antagonists for cancer therapy. *Nat. Rev. Drug Discov.* **7:** 989–1000.

62. Degenhardt, K., R. Mathew, B. Beaudoin, *et al.* 2006. Autophagy promotes tumor cell survival and restricts necrosis, inflammation, and tumorigenesis. *Cancer Cell.* **10:** 51–64.

63. Jin, S. & E. White. 2007. Role of autophagy in cancer: management of metabolic stress. *Autophagy* **3:** 28–31.

64. Zong, W.X. & C.B. Thompson. 2006. Necrotic death as a cell fate. *Genes Dev.* **20:** 1–15.

65. Zong, W.X., D. Ditsworth, D.E. Bauer, *et al.* 2004. Alkylating DNA damage stimulates a regulated form of necrotic cell death. *Genes Dev.* **18:** 1272–1282.

Ann. N.Y. Acad. Sci. ISSN 0077-8923

ANNALS OF THE NEW YORK ACADEMY OF SCIENCES
Issue: *Nutrition and Physical Activity in Aging, Obesity, and Cancer*

Obesity-induced metabolic stresses in breast and colon cancer

Mi-Kyung Sung,[1,2] Jee-Young Yeon,[1] Shin-Young Park,[1] Jung Han Yoon Park,[2,3] and Myung-Sook Choi[2,4]

[1]Department of Food and Nutrition, Sookmyung Women's University, Seoul, Korea. [2]Center for Food and Nutritional Genomics, Kyungpook National University, Daegu, Korea. [3]Department of Food Science and Nutrition, Hallym University, Chuncheon, Korea. [4]Department of Food Science and Nutrition, Kyungpook National University, Daegu, Korea

Address for correspondence: Mi-Kyung Sung, Department of Food and Nutrition, Sookmyung Women's University, 52 Hyochangwon-gil, Yongsan-gu, Seoul 140-742, Korea. mksung@sm.ac.kr

Epidemiological studies have suggested that excess body weight gain may be a major risk factor for colon and breast cancer. A positive energy balance creates metabolic stresses, including the excess production of reactive oxygen species (ROS), hyperinsulinemia, the elevated adipokine secretion, and increased gut permeability. Obesity is a risk factor for breast cancer in postmenopausal women, and overweight women are more likely to have poor outcomes. The higher circulating concentration of insulin-like growth factor 1 (IGF-1) in overweight and obese women is thought to be an important mediator to promote cell proliferation and survival via the activation of phosphatidylinositol 3-kinase (PI3K)/Akt and mitogen-activated protein kinase (MAPK)/p38 signaling pathways. In an animal model of colon carcinogenesis, overweight mice fed a high-fat diet exhibited a greater number of colon tumors than lean animals. The increased abdominal fat was associated with higher concentrations of leptin, insulin, and IGF-1, which possibly mediate tumor growth. These data suggest that the metabolic burden created by excess adiposity accelerates uncontrolled cell growth and survival, thereby increasing the risk of developing breast and colon cancer.

Keywords: obesity; breast cancer; colon cancer

Introduction

It has recently been reported that there are an estimated 12.7 million new cancer cases worldwide and that 7.6 million cancer deaths occurred in 2008.[1] Lung cancer is the most common cancer and is followed by breast and colorectal cancer. There are indications that global cancer incidence will continue to increase, and cancer prevention strategies including nutritional habits and physical activity will be very important. However, despite a great effort to reduce cancer deaths by implementing dietary modifications, limited progress has been made possibly due to the very complicated nature of the diet and difficulties in behavioral modifications.

Experimental studies have suggested that plant food components exert beneficial effects to suppress cancer development through a variety of different mechanisms. However, from human intervention trials, rather subtle data concerning plant food components and cancer have been obtained.[2–4] Recent epidemiological studies have strongly suggested that excess body weight gain may be a major risk factor in many cancers, especially cancers of the colon and breast. A summary report of the World Cancer Research Fund and the American Institute of Cancer Research indicated that the maintenance of a healthy weight (body mass index [BMI] between 21 and 23) throughout the life span is one of the most important ways to protect against cancer.[5]

Unfortunately, the percentage of adults who are overweight or obese has greatly increased worldwide. The National Center for Health Statistics of the United States indicated that the age-adjusted prevalence of obesity was 33.8% in 2007–2008, and the corresponding prevalence estimates for overweight and obesity combined were 68.0%.[6] The National Health and Nutrition Examination Surveys of

doi: 10.1111/j.1749-6632.2011.06094.x
Ann. N.Y. Acad. Sci. 1229 (2011) 61–68 © 2011 New York Academy of Sciences.

Korea have reported that the percentage of adults with a BMI $\geq$ 25 was 31.7% in 2008. The steady increases in obesity and an overweight population are attributed to increases in energy consumption and decreases in physical activity, creating an energy imbalance contributing to the steady increases in cancer incidence. In this review, the current understanding of obesity, metabolic stresses, and cancer development, in particular, breast and colorectal cancer, is summarized.

Metabolic stress and energy imbalance

Energy supply is a vital component of life. Dietary macronutrients including carbohydrates, fat, and protein provide energy as chemical energy and heat. Metabolic stresses are derived from an excess metabolic burden, mostly energy overload. Categories of metabolic stresses related to excess energy intake and obesity include excess production of reactive oxygen species (ROS), hyperinsulinemia, elevated adipokine secretion, and increased gut permeability (Fig. 1).

The tricarboxylic acid (TCA) cycle oxidizes the metabolites of macronutrients to form the reduced nicotinamide adenine dinucleotide (NADH $+ H^+$) and the reduced flavin adenine dinucleotide (FADH$_2$). High-energy electrons from NADH and FADH$_2$ enter the electron transport chain and produce ATP. This process is called oxidative phosphorylation, and macronutrients supplied in excess of the body's energy needs are converted to fat and stored in the adipose tissue. During this oxidation process, two electrons are transferred and combined with $1/2$ O_2 to form H_2O. In the meantime, incomplete oxidation also occurs, producing superoxide ($O_2{}^-$), which is a source of ROS. The most common ROS include superoxide anion, hydroxyl radicals, and hydrogen peroxide. ROS are extremely reactive to cellular components and cause DNA, protein, and lipid modifications. In normal circumstances, endogenous antioxidant enzymes, including superoxide dismutase, glutathione peroxidase, catalase, as well as exogenous antioxidants, such as vitamin C, vitamin E, and polyphenols, effectively scavenge ROS. However, the elevated level of ROS and/or defective defense mechanisms increase oxidative stress and cellular damage, which are closely related to aging and the development of chronic diseases, including cancer. Recent studies have suggested that ROS regulate cell survival and cell death

via the activation of major signaling pathways.[7,8] ROS have been shown to activate nuclear factor-kappa B (NF-κB), which is a central coordinator of immunity, inflammation, cell differentiation, and survival.[9]

Energy metabolism is subject to tight hormonal regulation. Insulin and glucagon are the most representative hormones exerting opposite metabolic effects. The postprandial increase in insulin accelerates the tissue uptake of glucose and drives the metabolism toward the synthesis of glycogen and fat. Nutrient overload, followed by an increase in adipose tissue mass, creates hyperinsulinemia, which stimulates receptor-mediated signaling of insulin, including the activation of MAPK cascades and related modulation of gene expression. The activation of inflammatory NF-κB pathway is shown to be a key mediating signal to produce inflammatory cytokines followed by insulin resistance.[10] Additionally, obesity is related to excess production of free fatty acids and inflammatory cytokines, which, in turn, induce insulin resistance.

Metabolic stresses induced by excess energy intake are also caused by increases in body fat mass. It has been shown that dynamic crosstalk exists between the adipocytes and immune cells, which suggests that fat tissue is an important mediator of inflammatory responses in many chronic disease conditions. Adipose tissue comprises adipocytes, preadipocytes, macrophages, lymphocytes, and endothelial cells, which enable the tissue to be metabolically and immunologically active. Adipocytes produce adipocytokines (leptin, adiponectin, resistin), cytokines (tumor necrosis factor [TNF]-α, interleukine [IL]-6, IL-1) and chemokines (CC-chemokine ligand 2 [CCL2]).[11] CCL2 contributes to macrophage infiltration into adipose tissue.[12] Adipose tissue also expresses toll-like receptor (TLR) subsets, which are linked to the activation of NF-κB followed by the production of proinflammatory cytokines and chemokines.[13]

More recently, the interrelationship among gut flora, gut permeability, and obesity has received attention. Alteration in the intestinal barrier has been proposed to be associated with intestinal and liver disorders, autoimmune diseases, and diabetes. Evidence suggests that a leaky gut might be a causative factor predisposing one to inflammatory disease development,[14] although no clear explanation has been provided. The increased gut permeability

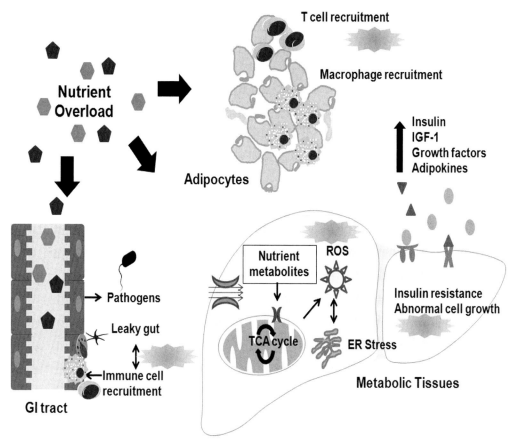

Figure 1. Energy overload and metabolic stresses. Metabolic stresses are derived from nutrient overload, which supplies excess energy. Metabolic tissues including the liver oxidize macronutrients through the TCA cycle, and incomplete oxidation produces ROS, which increase oxidative stresses. The excess energy is converted to fat and stored in adipocytes. The accumulation of fat increases circulating concentrations of insulin, IGF-1, and adipokines, which lead to insulin resistance and abnormal cell growth. Increases in fat mass actively attract immune cells, thereby creating inflammatory conditions. Nutrient overload also increases intestinal cell membrane permeability, possibly through changes in gut flora composition followed by immune cell recruitment. Abbreviations: TCA (tricarboxylic acid), ROS (reactive oxygen species), ER (endoplasmic reticulum), IGF-1(insulin-like growth factor-1), GI tract (gastrointestinal tract).

allows the passage of luminal antigens, which induce autoimmune reactions in a target tissue, such as insulin-producing β cells.[15] Additionally, the increased intestinal permeability exerts local inflammatory type responses contributing to systemic inflammation followed by metabolic alterations such as insulin resistance. Other studies have also indicated that diet-induced obesity or dietary fat feeding increases metabolic inflammation by increasing intestinal permeability through changes in gut flora populations.[16,17]

Metabolic stress in breast cancer

The incidence of breast cancer in women is increasing in most countries, particularly in countries where the incidence used to be relatively low.[18,19] Breast cancer development is closely related to hormonal and genetic factors. Lactation is suggested as a strong protective factor against breast cancer. Lactation is associated with lower exposure to endogenous sex hormones and increased elimination of breast epithelial cells by apoptosis at the end of lactating period.

A great deal of effort has been made for many years to explain the relationship between diet and breast cancer. Dietary fat is a source of endogenous estrogen and has been suggested as a possible risk factor. However, prospective cohort studies have shown inconsistent effects, suggesting that dietary fat per se may not increase the risk.[20] In contrast to the inconclusive relationship between dietary components and breast cancer, convincing data have shown that body fatness increases the risk of breast cancer in postmenopausal women.[5] A pooled analysis of seven prospective cohort studies comprised 337,819 women, and 4,385 incident invasive breast cancer cases indicated that the pooled relative risk of breast cancer was 1.26 (95% CI: 1.09–1.46) when a BMI > 28 kg/m^2 was used as the highest category in the categorical analyses in postmenopausal women.[21] However, the inverse association was found in premenopausal women. Being overweight or obese is also associated with poorer prognosis and increased recurrence. Among 34 studies looking at the relationship between survival/recurrence and obesity/weight gain in early-stage breast cancer patients, 26 studies found significantly positive associations.[22]

Estrogen production in premenopausal women occurs mainly in the ovaries, while the ovarian production of estrogen is replaced by adipose tissue in postmenopausal women.[23] Epidemiological data have suggested that serum estrogen concentration is a risk factor for breast cancer in postmenopausal women.[24] Therefore, the cancer-promoting role of body fat has been attributed to the higher local production of estrogen, thereby providing an explanation for the connection between postmenopausal breast cancer risk and body fatness. However, an inverse association between body fatness and breast cancer risk in premenopausal women may not be fully justified by the previous explanations. Experimental studies have suggested that estrogen deprivation decreases insulin sensitivity and increases atopic fat accumulation in high fat–fed mice, suggesting a protective role of estrogen in metabolic alteration.[25–27] Therefore, the increased breast cancer risk in obese postmenopausal women may be partly explained by hyperinsulinemia resulting from estrogen depletion and excess accumulation of fat tissue (Fig. 2).

IGF-1, an insulin-related protein, is known to function as a growth factor for mammary epithelium.[28] Epidemiological studies have shown that women with elevated blood concentrations of IGF-1 exhibit an increased risk of breast cancer.[29,30] The elevated circulating level of insulin indirectly affects tumorigenesis by regulating IGF-1 synthesis, a mechanism that has been implicated in the regulation of cell cycles and apoptosis.[31] The IGF-1 receptor (IGF-1R) and insulin receptor (IR) have been reported to be overexpressed in breast cancer cells and tissue specimens.[32] Insulin receptor substrate (IRS)-1, a major substrate for IR and IGF-1R, activates survival signaling via the PI3K/Akt and MAPK/p38 pathways promoting cancer cell proliferation and survival.[33,34]

Rodent studies have also indicated an association between serum IGF-1 concentration and mammary cancer risk. LID mice carrying a hepatic IGF-1 gene deletion showed a dramatic reduction in serum circulating IGF-1 levels and the delayed onset of chemically and genetically induced mammary tumors.[35] Rats fed a calorie-restricted diet exhibited decreased serum insulin and IGF-1 concentrations, which may be related to the suppression of mammary tumor growth in these animals.[36] Therefore, increases in circulating IGF-1, which results from excess dietary energy intake, may be one of the major key links between excess energy supply and breast cancer risk.

The higher circulating concentrations of pro-inflammatory cytokines are suggested to have a close relationship with breast cancer risk.[37] We have also found that proinflammatory IL-1β and IL-6 concentrations are significantly higher in breast cancer patients compared to those of the age-matched control subjects.[38] Insulin resistance has been associated with the increased production of TNF-α and IL-6.[39–41] These cytokines are shown to promote tumor cell growth by regulating the expression of antiapoptotic and angiogenic proteins.[42,43] In highly metastatic breast cancer cells (MDA-MB231), AP-1 and NF-κB are shown to have a prominent role in IL-6 gene transcription.[44] These cytokines are also inducers of aromatase and possibly increase the circulating estrogen concentration.[45]

Metabolic stress in colon cancer

Excess body fat and abdominal fatness have been reported as convincing risk factors of colorectal cancer (CRC).[5] The risk of CRC is reported to increase by 7% as BMI increases by 2.[46] The results of one meta-analysis also revealed a 5% increased risk of CRC per inch of waist circumference, an indication of abdominal fatness.[5] Abdominal fatness is associated with the circulating concentrations of hormones, growth factors, and inflammatory cytokines, which accelerates uncontrolled cell growth, possibly leading to the development of cancer.

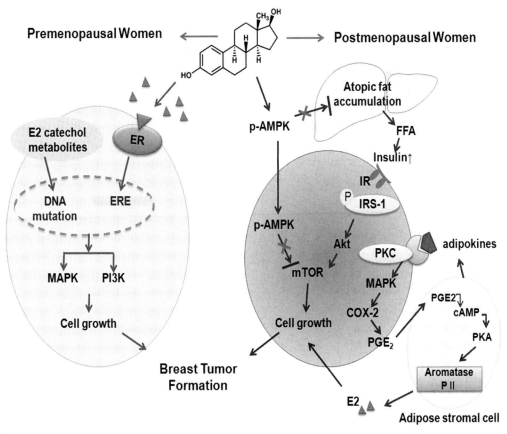

Figure 2. Two faces of estrogen. Estrogen promotes breast tumor growth by receptor-mediated cellular signaling pathways such as MAPK and PI3K signals. Estrogen metabolites induce DNA mutation, thereby initiating carcinogenesis. In postmenopausal women, estrogen deprivation blocks AMPK activation inducing atopic fat accumulation followed by IR-mediated activation of Akt and mTOR, possibly accelerating abnormal cell growth. On the other hand, the postmenopausal body fat accumulation induces the activation of adipocyte stromal cell aromatase through PKC-mediated signaling and produces estradiol, promoting breast tumor formation. Abbreviations: E_2 (estradiol), ER (estrogen receptor), ERE (estrogen-responsive element), MAPK (mitogen-activated protein kinase), PI3K (phophoinositide 3-kinase), p-AMPK (phosphorylated AMP-activated protein kinase), mTOR (mammalian target of rapamycin), FFA (free fatty acid), IR (insulin receptor), IRS-1 (insulin receptor substrate-1), PKC (protein kinase C), COX-2 (cyclooxygenase-2), PGE_2 (prostaglandin E_2), cAMP (cyclic adenine monophosphate), PKA (protein kinase A).

Hyperinsulinemia in relation to colon cancer development has been reported. Epidemiological studies suggested hyperinsulinemia assessed by measuring plasma C-peptide is related to an increased risk of colon cancer.[47] Type 2 diabetes patients are shown to have three times higher risk of developing colon cancer.[48] *In vitro* studies have demonstrated that insulin promotes colon cancer cell proliferation.[49,50] Hyperinsulinemia decreases the concentration of the IGF-1 binding protein (IGFBP-1), which increases circulating free IGF-1.[51] IGF-1, as a key mitogen to accelerate cell cycle progression, increases the risk of cellular transformation due to rapid cell turnover.[52] The binding of insulin to its receptor phosphorylates insulin receptor substrates, IRS-1 or IRS1/4, thereby stimulating the downstream signaling.[53] The activation of IRS-1 and IRS1/4 is shown to stimulate the RAS/RAF/MEK/extracellular signal-regulated kinase (ERK) signaling pathway and the PI3K/Akt signaling pathway, respectively, regulating cell proliferation, survival, growth, and motility processes that are critical for colon tumorigenesis.[51,54,55] Leptin, an adipocyte-derived peptide hormone, belongs to the cytokine family and controls appetite to modulate energy balance. It is produced proportional to body fat, and obese subjects showed chronically elevated levels of circulating leptin.[56] The synthesis of leptin in adipose tissue is influenced by insulin,[57] and this may also contribute to the high leptin concentration in obesity. Despite a lack of direct evidence that an increased leptin concentration is a risk factor for colon cancer, studies have proposed that higher leptin concentrations may be a possible link between obesity and the development of colorectal cancer.[58,59] *In vitro* studies have provided evidence that leptin modulates the proliferation of LS174T and HM7 colon adenocarcinoma cells.[60]

As the colon is not generally considered as a major target tissue for the insulin action, few experimental studies have been conducted to determine whether obesity-induced hyperinsulinemia contributes to colon tumor development. We have recently conducted a study to investigate molecular mechanisms of diet-induced obesity in colon carcinogenesis in a mouse model of colitis-associated colon cancer.[61] In this study, animals were fed either a high-fat diet (HFD; 45% of total calories from fat) or a normal diet (ND; 15% of calories from fat) for 12 weeks. The colon tumor was induced by a single intraperitoneal injection of azoxymenthane (10 mg/kg body weight) followed by two one-week cycles of disodium sulfate supply. Results from this study clearly demonstrated that the HFD feeding increased the number of colonic tumors, two times higher than that in animals fed the ND. The HFD-induced epididymal fat deposition was associated with increases in circulating insulin, IGF-1, and leptin, as well as the mRNA levels of epididymal fat pad leptin and colonic leptin receptor (Ob-R). Additionally, the animals fed the HFD showed higher levels of the Ob-R, IR, phosphorylated Akt, phosphorylated ERK, Bcl-xL, and cyclin D1 proteins in the colon. From these results, it can be speculated that obesity facilitates colon tumor formation, possibly through increases in blood insulin, IGF-1, and leptin, which induce activation of their corresponding receptors in the colon and subsequently induce PI3K/Akt and ERK1/2 pathways.

Obesity is associated with chronic low-grade systemic inflammation. As in the case of obesity-related breast cancer risk, adipocyte-derived factors have been suggested to mediate inflammatory responses in colon cancer. Adipocyte-derived leptin increases TNF-α production,[62] and insulin was shown to increase IL-6 expression of adipocytes.[63] Because TNF-α and IL-6 are proinflammatory cytokines promoting cell proliferation and survival,

these data clearly suggest that obesity increases the risk of colon cancer by inducing chronic inflammation and activating downstream cellular signaling.

Conclusion

It is only in recent years that body fatness has been suggested as a most convincing risk factor for developing cancer of the breast and colon. At the same time, adipocytes, which had been considered an inert storage organ, are receiving attention as a center of metabolic intergration. So far we only have pieces of information that have not been pulled together to create a complete picture. Nevertheless, it is clear from the existing evidence that adipocytes induce metabolic stress in coordination with immune cells, which may explain accelerated cell growth and survival in cancerous tissues. Further studies to elucidate the signaling network between adipokines and mediators of immune responses are required in order to establish intervention targets.

Acknowledgments

This study was supported by a National Research Foundation of Korea (NRF) Grant funded by the Korea government (MEST) (2008-0060833), and by the Basic Science Research Program through the National Research Foundation of Korea (NRF) funded by the Ministry of Education, Science and Technology (2010-0001886).

Conflicts of interest

The authors declare no conflict of interest.

References

1. Ferlay, J., H.R. Shin, F. Bray, *et al.* 2010. Estimates of worldwide burden of cancer in 2008: GLOBOCAN 2008. *Int. J. Cancer* **127:** 2893–2917.

2. Albanes, D., O.P. Heinonen, P.R. Taylor, *et al.* 1996. Alpha-Tocopherol and beta-carotene supplements and lung cancer incidence in the alpha-tocopherol, beta-carotene cancer prevention study: effects of base-line characteristics and study compliance. *J. Natl. Cancer Inst.* **88:** 1569–1570.

3. Lippman, S.M., E.A. Klein, P.J. Goodman, *et al.* 2009. Effect of selenium and vitamin E on risk of prostate cancer and other cancers: the Selenium and Vitamin E Cancer Prevention Trial (SELECT). *JAMA* **310:** 39–51.

4. Pierce, J.P., L. Natarajan, B.J. Caan, *et al.* 2007. Influence of a diet very high in vegetables, fruit, and fiber and low in fat on prognosis following treatment for breast cancer: the Women's Healthy Eating and Living (WHEL) randomized trial. *JAMA* **298:** 289–298.

5. World Cancer Research Fund/ American Institute for Cancer Research. 2007. *Food, Nutrition, Physical Activity and the Prevention of Cancer: A Global Perspective.* AICR. Washington, DC.

6. Flegal, K.M., M.D. Carroll, C.L. Ogden & L.R. Curtin. 2010. Prevalence and trends in obesity among US adults, 1999–2008. *JAMA* **303:** 235–241.

7. Curtin, J.F., M. Donovan & T.G. Cotter. 2002. Regulation and measurement of oxidative stress in apoptosis. *J. Immunol. Methods* **265:** 49–72.

8. Martindale, J.L., & N.J. Holbrook. 2002. Cellular response to oxidative stress: signaling for suicide and survival. *J. Cell. Physiol.* **192:** 1–15.

9. Bubici, C., S. Papa, K. Dean & G. Franzoso. 2006. Mutual cross-talk between reactive oxygen species and nuclear factor-kappa B: molecular basis and biological significance. *Oncogene* **25:** 6731–6748.

10. Tanti, J.F. & J. Jager. 2009. Cellular mechanisms of insulin resistance: role of stress-regulated serine kinase and insulin receptor substrates (IRS) serine phosphorylation. *Curr. Opin. Pharmacol.* **9:** 753–762.

11. Tilg, H. & A.R. Moschen. 2006. Adipocytokines: mediators linking adipose tissue, inflammation and immunity. *Nat. Rev. Immunol.* **6:** 772–783.

12. Kanda, H., S. Tateya, Y. Tamori, *et al.* 2006. MCP-1 contributes to macrophage infiltration into adipose tissue, insulin resistance, and hepatic steatosis in obesity. *J. Clin. Invest.* **116:** 1494–1505.

13. Schäffler, A. & J. Schölmerich. 2010. Innate immunity and adipose tissue biology. *Trends Immunol.* **31:** 228–235.

14. Arrieta, M.C., L. Bistritz & J.B. Meddings. 2006. Alterations in intestinal permeability. *Gut* **55:** 1512–1520.

15. de Kort, S., D. Keszthelyi & A.A. Masclee. 2011. Leaky gut and diabetes mellitus: what is the link? *Obes. Rev* **15:** 449–458. doi:10.111/j.1467-798X.2010.00845.x

16. Cani, P.D., R. Bibiloni, C. Knauf, *et al.* 2008. Changes in gut microbiota control metabolic endotoxemia-induced inflammation in high-fat diet-induced obesity and diabetes in mice. *Diabetes* **57:** 1470–1481.

17. Suzuki, T. & H. Hara. 2010. Dietary fat and bile juice, but not obesity, are responsible for the increase in small intestinal permeability induced through the suppression of tight junction protein expression in LETO and OLETF rats. *Nutr. Metab.* **7:** 19.

18. Parkin, D.M., F. Bray, J. Ferlay & P. Pisani. 2005. Global cancer statistics, 2002. *CA Cancer J. Clin.* **55:** 74–108.

19. The Ministry of Health, Welfare and Family Affairs of Korea/National Cancer Control. 2009. *Cancer Facts & Figures 2009.*

20. Smith-Warner, S.A., D. Spiegelman, H.O. Adami, *et al.* 2001. Types of dietary fat and breast cancer: a pooled analysis of cohort studies. *Int. J. Cancer* **92:** 767–774.

21. van den Brandt, P.A., D. Spiegelman, S.S. Yaun, *et al.* 2000. Pooled analysis of prospective cohort studies on height, weight, and breast cancer risk. *Am. J. Epidemiol.* **152:** 514–527.

22. Chlebowski, R.T., E. Aiello & A. McTiernan. 2002. Weight loss in breast cancer patient management. *J. Clin. Oncol.* **20:** 1128–1143.

23. Lorincz, A.M., S. Sukumar. 2006. Molecular links between obesity and breast cancer. *Endocr. Relat. Cancer* **13:** 279–292.

24. Cleary, M.P. & M.E. Grossmann. 2009. Minireview: obesity and breast cancer: the estrogen connection. *Endocrinology* **150:** 2537–2542.

25. Paquette, A., M. Shinoda, R.R. Lhoret, D. Prud'homme, & J.M. Lavoie. 2007. Time course of liver lipid infiltration in ovariectomized rats: impact of a high-fat diet. *Maturitas* **58:** 182–190.

26. Bryzgalova, G., L. Lundholm, N. Portwood, *et al.* 2008. Mechanisms of antidiabetogenic and body weight-lowering effects of estrogen in high-fat diet-fed mice. *Am. J. Physiol. Endocrinol. Metab.* **295:** E904–E912.

27. Riant, E., A. Waget, H. Cogo, *et al.* 2009. Estrogens protect against high-fat diet-induced insulin resistance and glucose intolerance in mice. *Endocrinology* **150:** 2109–2117.

28. Lautenbach, A., A. Budde, C.D. Wrann, *et al.* 2009. Obesity and the associated mediators leptin, estrogen and IGF-I enhance the cell proliferation and early tumorigenesis of breast cancer cells. *Nutr. Cancer* **61:** 484–491.

29. Schernhammer, E.S., J.M. Holly, M.N. Pollak & S.E. Hankinson. 2005. Circulating levels of insulin-like growth factors, their binding proteins, and breast cancer risk. *Cancer Epidemiol. Biomarkers Prev.* **14:** 699–704.

30. Toniolo, P., P.F. Bruning, A. Akhmedkhanov, *et al.* 2000. Serum insulin-like growth factor-I and breast cancer. *Int. J. Cancer* **88:** 828–832.

31. Pollak, M. 2008. Insulin and insulin-like growth factor signalling in neoplasia. *Nat. Rev. Cancer* **8:** 915–928.

32. Lann, D. & D. LeRoith. 2008. The role of endocrine insulin-like growth factor-I and insulin in breast cancer. *J. Mammary Gland Biol. Neoplasia.* **13:** 371–379.

33. Surmacz, E. 2000. Function of the IGF-I receptor in breast cancer. *J. Mammary Gland Biol. Neoplasia.* **5:** 95–105.

34. Bartucci, M., C. Morelli, L. Mauro, *et al.* 2001. Differential insulin-like growth factor I receptor signaling and function in estrogen receptor (ER)-positive MCF-7 and ER-negative MDA-MB-231 breast cancer cells. *Cancer Res.* **61:** 6747–6754.

35. Wu, Y., K. Cui, K. Miyoshi, *et al.* 2003. Reduced circulating insulin-like growth factor I levels delay the onset of chemically and genetically induced mammary tumors. *Cancer Res.* **63:** 4384–4388.

36. Ruggeri, B. A., D.M. Klurfeld, D. Kritchevsky & R.W. Furlanetto. 1989. Caloric restriction and 7,12-dimethylbenz(a) anthracene-induced mammary tumor growth in rats: alterations in circulating insulin, insulin-like growth factors I and II, and epidermal growth factor. *Cancer Res.* **49:** 4130–4134.

37. Rose, D.P., D. Komninou & G.D. Stephenson. 2004. Obesity, adipocytokine, and insulin resistance in breast cancer. *Obes. Rev.* **5:** 153–165.

38. Yeon, J.-Y., Y.-J. Suh, S.-W. Kim, *et al.* 2011. Evaluation of dietary factors in relation to the biomarkers of oxidative stress and inflammation in breast cancer risk. *Nutrition.* doi:10.1016/j.nut.2010.10.012.

39. Kern, P.A., S. Ranganathan, C. Li, *et al.* 2001. Adipose tissue tumor necrosis factor and interleukin-6 expression in human obesity and insulin resistance. *Am. J. Physiol. Endocrinol. Metab.* **280:** E745–E751.

40. Hotamisligil, G.S., P. Arner, J.F. Car, *et al.* 1995. Increased adipose tissue expression of tumor necrosis-α in human obesity and insulin resistance. *J. Clin. Invest.* **95:** 2409–2415.

41. Miyazaki, Y., R. Pipek, L.J. Mandarino & R.A. DeFronzo. 2003. Tunor necrosis factor-α and insulin resistance in obese type 2 diabetic patients. *Int. J. Obes. Relat. Metab. Disord.* **27:** 88–94.

42. Nicolini, A., A. Carpi & G. Rossi. 2006. Cytokines in breast cancer. *Cytokine Growth Factor Rev.* **17:** 325–337.

43. Pantschenko, A.G., I. Pushkar, K.H. Anderson, *et al.* 2003. The interleukin-1 family of cytokines and receptors in human breast cancer: implications for tumor progression. *Int. J. Oncol.* **23:** 269–284.

44. Ndlovu, M.N., C. Van Lint, K. Van Wesemael, *et al.* 2009. Hyperactivated NF-{kappa}B and AP-1 transcription factors promote highly accessible chromatin and constitutive transcription across the interleukin-6 gene promoter in metastatic breast cancer cells. *Mol. Cell. Biol.* **29:** 5488–5504.

45. Purohit, A., S.P. Newman & M.J. Reed. 2002. The role of cytokines in regulating estrogen synthesis: implications for the etiology of breast cancer. *Breast Cancer Res.* **4:** 65–69.

46. Calle, E.E. & R. Kaaks. 2004. Overweight, obesity and cancer: epidemiological evidence and proposed mechanisms. *Nat. Rev. Cancer* **4:** 579–591.

47. Giovannucci, E. & D. Michaud. 2007. The role of obesity and related metabolic disturbances in cancers of the colon, prostate and pancreas. *Gastroenterology* **132:** 2208–2225.

48. Khaw, K.T., N. Wareham, S. Bingham, *et al.* 2004. Preliminary communication: glycated hemoglobin, diabetes, and incident colorectal cancer in men and women: a prospective analysis from the European prospective investigation into cancer-Norfolk study. *Cancer Epidemiol. Biomarkers Prev.* **13:** 915–919.

49. Shi, B., L. Sepp-Lorenzino, M. Prisco, *et al.* 2007. Micro RNA 145 targets the insulin receptor substrate-1 and inhibits the growth of colon cancer cells. *J. Biol. Chem.* **282:** 32582–32590.

50. Watkins, L.F., L.R. Lewis & A.E. Levine. 1990. Characterization of the synergistic effect o finsulin and transferrin and the regulation of their receptors on a human colon carcinoma cell line. *Int. J. Cancer* **45:** 372–375.

51. Huang, X.-F. & Chen, J.-Z. 2009. Obesity, the PI3K/Akt signal pathway and colon cancer. *Obes. Rev.* **10:** 610–616.

52. Pais, R., H. Silaghi, A.C. Silaghi, *et al.* 2009. Metabolic syndrome and risk of subsequent colorectal cancer. *World J. Gastroenterol.* **15:** 5141–5148.

53. Becker, S., L. Dossus & R. Kaaks. 2009. Obesity related hyperinsulinaemia and hyperglycaemia and cancer development. *Arch. Physiol. Biochem.* **115:** 86–96.

54. Tu, Y., A. Gardner & A. Lichtenstein. 2000. The phosphatidylinositol 3-kinase/AKT kinase pathway in multiple myeloma plasma cells: roles in cytokine-dependent survival and proliferative responses. *Cancer Res.* **60:** 6763–6770.

55. Wang, L., X.X. Cao, Q. Chen, *et al.* 2009. DIXDC1 targets p21 and cyclin D1 via PI3K pathway activation to promote colon cancer cell proliferation. *Cancer Sci.* **100:** 1801–1808.

56. Chu, N.F., D. Spiegelman, J. Yu, *et al.* 2001. Plasma leptin concentrations and four-year weight gain among US men. *Int. J. Obes. Relat. Metab. Disord.* **25:** 346–353.

57. Fantuzzi, G. 2005. Adipose tissue, adipokines, and inflammation. *J. Allergy Clin. Immunol.* **115:** 911–919.

58. Stattin, P., A. Lukanova, C. Biessy, *et al.* 2004. Obesity and colon cancer: does leptin provide a link? *Int. J. Cancer* **109:** 149–152.

59. Chia, V.M., P.A. Newcomb, J.W. Lampe, *et al.* 2007. Leptin concentrations, leptin receptor polymorphisms, and colorectal adenoma risk. *Cancer Epidemiol. Biomarkers Prev.* **16:** 2697–2703.

60. Jaffe, T. & B. Schwartz. 2008. Leptin promotes motility and invasiveness in human colon cancer cells by activating multiple signal-transduction pathways. *Int. J. Cancer* **123:** 2543–2556.

61. Park, S.-Y., J.-S. Kim, Y.-R. Seo & M.-K. Sung. 2011. Effects of diet-induced obesity on colitis-associated colon tumor formation in A/J mice. *Int. J. Obes.* doi:10.1038/ijo.2011.83

62. Molina, A., J. vendrell, C. Gutierrez, *et al.* 2003. Insulin resistance, leptin and TNF-alpha system in morbidly obese women after gastric bypass. *Obes. Surg.* **13:** 615–621.

63. LaPensee, C.R., E.R. Hugo & N. Ben-Jonathan. 2008. Insulin stimulates interleukin-6 expression and release in LS14 human adipocytes through multiple signaling pathways. *Endocrinology* **149:** 5415–5422.

Ann. N.Y. Acad. Sci. ISSN 0077-8923

ANNALS OF THE NEW YORK ACADEMY OF SCIENCES

Issue: *Nutrition and Physical Activity in Aging, Obesity, and Cancer*

Avian biomodels for use as pharmaceutical bioreactors and for studying human diseases

Gwonhwa Song and Jae Yong Han

WCU Biomodulation Major, Department of Agricultural Biotechnology, Seoul National University, Seoul, Korea

Address for correspondence: Jae Yong Han, Department of Agricultural Biotechnology, Seoul National University, 599 Gwanak-ro, Gwanak-gu, Seoul 151-921, Korea. jaehan@snu.ac.kr

Animal-based biotechnologies involve the use of domestic animals for the production of pharmaceuticals and various proteins in milk and eggs, as disease models, as tools for stem cell research and animal cloning, and as sources of organs for xenotransplantation into humans. Avian species offer several advantages over mammalian models, and they have been used historically to advance the fields of embryology, immunology, oncology, virology, and vaccine development. In addition, avian species can be used for studying the etiology of human ovarian cancer and other human diseases such as disorders based on the abnormal metabolism of lipids and as unique mechanisms for the biosynthesis and transport of cholesterol. This review integrates recent progress and insight into the molecular and physiologic mechanisms associated with transgenic birds and gives an overview of the use of avian models as pharmaceutical bioreactors and as tools for studying human diseases.

Keywords: avian; germ cells; transgenesis; bioreactor; biomodel

Introduction

Substantial efforts have been made to overcome disease and to enhance the quality of human life through advances in medicine and biotechnologies. Since the completion of the human genome project, there has been intense interest in mining the human genome database for genomic signatures of disease for diagnosis and drug development. Many researchers use animal models to understand human disease, and the results of these studies have helped to reduce morbidity and mortality. An animal model can be defined as a living organism that is closely related phylogenetically to humans and that can be used to study shared biological systems in relation to health and disease. Thus, the genetic similarities among animals in a taxonomic system are validated on the bases of comparative DNA and RNA analyses. A range of approaches are needed to develop and refine animal models for transgenic applications. Currently, transgenic animals are valuable models for assessing therapeutics for humans. Animal disease models that allow long-term assessment of alternative therapies are also necessary. This

is especially true for animal models that are developed or customized to study specific diseases, so as to elucidate the biological pathways implicated in those diseases. Although rodent models have proven useful in the past in revealing disease etiology and developing treatments, avian models are emerging as important alternatives. This review presents an integrated view of recent progress and new insights into the molecular and physiologic mechanisms that are relevant to the use of avian models as bioreactors for the production of therapeutics and for studies of human diseases.

History of avian models

Avian embryos have been used for many basic and translational studies because they develop *in ovo* independently of most environmental factors. Aristotle used chick embryos to monitor organ development through various stages and concluded that life is generated spontaneously. William Harvey monitored the formation of arteries, veins, capillaries, and vessels in developing chick embryos. In the early 1800s, Malphigi paved the way for studies of animal

doi: 10.1111/j.1749-6632.2011.06087.x

development by monitoring neural tube and somite formation in chick embryos.[1] In 1911, Rous first demonstrated that tumors could be induced by a virus (thereafter called *Rous sarcoma virus*; RSV), and Temin discovered the retrovirus and, subsequently, the function of reverse transcriptase in 1970. These advances led to the establishment of major concepts in modern virology.[2] In addition, the avian immune system has been used for studying the differentiation and function of B and T lymphocytes. Chick embryos are commonly used to study body axis formation, neurogenesis, limb generation, ocular development, and muscle differentiation.[1] Chick embryos are also potential research models for studies of oncogenesis, viral disease, vaccine development, and human diseases, as well as for the development and testing of therapeutic agents. The full potential of avian species as research models will be realized through studies in the agricultural, biomedical, and industrial fields.

Advantages of avian models

Avian embryos have many advantages as a research model, because they develop independent of maternal influences, thereby facilitating multiple experimental procedures *in ovo*. Manipulations of postgastrulation stage embryos (e.g., isolation, transplantation, and gene transfer into various cells) allow experimental procedures and various types of analyses of living cells. Avian embryos also permit monitoring of organogenesis, because the distinct characteristics of development can be observed as the embryonic organs form and develop.

The estimated total number of genes in the chicken is similar to that in humans, although the chick genome is only half the size of the human genome. The chicken genome was the first nonvertebrate amniote genome to be sequenced.[3] Therefore, recent results regarding the evolutionary correlations between humans and chickens provide information on the general aspects of the evolution of animal genomes.

Avian models are appropriate for research in the basic scientific disciplines. Moreover, these models can be further utilized for biotechnological and agricultural applications. Birds have well-developed, economically important traits, such as egg laying, weight gain, and lipid metabolism. Furthermore, the genetic pathways in chickens that regulate these traits may be used in human research to, for example, identify the etiologies of cardiovascular disease, obesity, and chronic wasting syndromes.[4] In the chicken, reproductive traits are controlled by photoperiodicity, and a laying hen can produce more than 300 eggs annually. Moreover, the chicken is regarded as an optimal bioreactor system owing to its many biologically active nutrients and the fact that the egg proteins are structurally simple.[5,6] Because hens ovulate almost daily and are highly susceptible to developing ovarian cancer once the egg-laying period is finished, they are more valuable for studying human ovarian cancer than are rodent or human models, in which ovulation is less frequent or must be stimulated.[7] Moreover, many hens can be maintained and managed in a limited amount of space, and one can expect to find various lesions from hens with ovarian cancer or other diseases.

Technological advances in the production of transgenic birds

The transfer of a gene construct into the pronucleus of a zygote is the most commonly used method for producing transgenic mammals. After the production of the first transgenic mice, pronuclear injection became the method of choice for producing transgenic animals.[8] Spurred on by the accomplishments in mammals, similar efforts to produce transgenic birds in the mid-1990s revealed that pronuclear injection was not feasible in avian zygotes.[9,10] Pronuclear injection in avian species is technologically demanding because the rapid development of the embryo hinders the selection of suitable embryos for gene insertion. In addition, it is not easy to collect zygotes from the hen oviduct using surgical procedures, and the presence of a nontranslucent yolk surrounding the embryos interferes with the precise positioning of the pipette tip to deliver the gene constructs into the zygote. The most efficient method for producing transgenic avian species is to introduce retroviral gene constructs into the embryos immediately after oviposition, i.e., the laying of the egg.

The embryos of freshly laid eggs have two embryonic layers that contain 40,000–60,000 undifferentiated cells. After genes are introduced into these structures, they are transduced into the somatic and germ cells and a genetically mosaic chick is produced. This bird is bred at sexual maturity to produce a mosaic bird that is crossed with its wild-type counterpart to obtain G1 transgenic offspring. It has been demonstrated that retroviral constructs transferred into embryos at this stage create transgenic germ cells.[11] More recently, the production of transgenic chickens that carry the β-lactamase gene in their genomes was accomplished using avian leukosis virus (AVL)-based retroviral vectors.[12] Remarkably, the gene construct was successfully transmitted to the next generation without altering expression of the target gene. That study was the first to indicate the feasibility of producing biopharmaceuticals in a hen bioreactor system. Thereafter, various retroviral vector systems were developed. However, it is now clear that the expression of target genes transferred by retroviral vectors can be altered in various tissues and at various developmental stages.[13,14] To overcome these limitations, multiple classes of lentiviral vectors are used to produce transgenic birds (Fig. 1).[15–18] An alternative method is to transfer the retroviral concentrates into the circulation of chick embryos incubated for 53h ∼ 55h to prevent gene silencing via a mechanism that involves transgene variegation but that is currently not well defined.[19]

Despite the many technological advances and several failures, the search continues for new methods to produce transgenic birds. Some major obstacles need to be overcome. First, the retroviral construct integrates randomly into the host chromosome, which can lead to transgene expression at various developmental stages and in various tissues. This is caused by neighboring chromosomal elements that act as negative regulators of transgene expression. Such epigenetically regulated phenomena are called "position effects" and may be overcome by including additional regulatory elements in the delivered transgene construct. Second, the rate of germline transmission of proviral constructs can be quite low, thereby complicating the process of establishing transgenic lines in birds. Third, proviral constructs can become oncogenic due to the presence of innate retroviral elements.

Primordial germ cells (PGCs) are the precursors of functional sperm and oocytes. PGCs have unique translocation and migration abilities during embryonic development and they ultimately colonize the urogenital ridge of the embryo. The PGCs in birds originate from the epiblasts and translocate into the hypoblast during incubation. After approximately 16 h, the PGCs congregate in the anterior extra-embryonic area called the "germi-

nal crescent." Thereafter, with the development of the embryonic cardiovascular system, the PGCs migrate, enter into the circulation, and eventually colonize the urogenital ridges. Exploiting this unique developmental sequence, the transfer of PGCs from donor to recipient embryos results in the production of germline chimeras, and ultimately, transgenic chicks are derived from the retrovirally transduced PGCs.[20,21] However, the usefulness of PGCs as a vehicle for gene transfer is limited by the low number of PGCs that can be extracted from the germinal crescent and that are suitable for gene transfer. Attempts have been made to overcome these limitations by using cultured PGCs. Embryonic germ cells are pluripotent stem cells that are derived from PGCs through an extended culturing period.[22] Park and Han were the first to succeed in producing embryonic germ cells by culturing PGCs harvested from embryonic gonads.[23] They demonstrated that these cells differentiate into three germ layers, the origins of which are developmentally distinct. These pluripotent cells can be used to create chimeric recipient embryos, and they differentiate into gametes.[24] It is noteworthy that PGCs that were cultured, transfected, and transferred to a recipient embryo successfully generated a transgenic chick and a transgenic quail (Fig. 1).[18,25]

Because avian PGCs are transported via the blood vessels during embryonic growth, they colonize the urogenital ridges and give rise to germline chimeras in birds, as a means of conserving the species in ecosystems. Currently, there are hundreds of species of birds at risk of extinction. The generation of germline chimeric poultry by transferring PGCs from endangered bird species is an ideal method for restoring depleted populations of bird species. This idea has been validated by the reported production of viable pheasants using chickens, which demonstrates that this technique can be used to produce wild birds via germ cell transplantation.[26]

Tissue sources other than embryonic blood or gonads can also be used for generating germline chimeric birds. Spermatogonial stem cells (SSCs) are progenitors of sperm that reside on the peripheral boundaries of Sertoli cells. SSCs give rise to differentiated spermatogonial cells, plus an identical SSC as a mechanism for self-renewal. In chickens, PGCs are collected from early embryos (embryos from 2.5 to 5.5 days), whereas SSCs are harvested from the differentiated testes of male chicks that

A

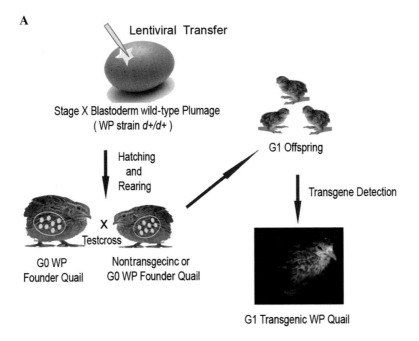

Lentiviral Transfer

Stage X Blastoderm wild-type Plumage
(WP strain d+/d+)

Hatching
and
Rearing

G1 Offspring

Transgene Detection

G0 WP
Founder Quail

X
Testcross

Nontransgecinc or
G0 WP Founder Quail

G1 Transgenic WP Quail

B

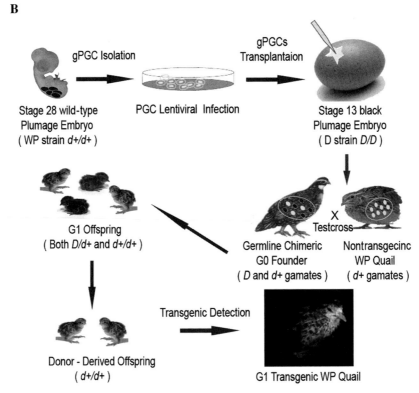

gPGC Isolation

gPGCs
Transplantaion

Stage 28 wild-type
Plumage Embryo
(WP strain d+/d+)

PGC Lentiviral Infection

Stage 13 black
Plumage Embryo
(D strain D/D)

G1 Offspring
(Both D/d+ and d+/d+)

Germline Chimeric
G0 Founder
(D and d+ gamates)

X
Testcross

Nontransgecinc
WP Quail
(d+ gamates)

Donor - Derived Offspring
(d+/d+)

Transgenic Detection

G1 Transgenic WP Quail

Figure 1. Schematic of the production of transgenic birds. (A) Production of transgenic birds by lentiviral transduction of stage X embryos. (B) Production of transgenic birds using lentivirus-transduced primordial germ cells (adapted from Shin *et al.* [18]).

are several weeks old. SSCs can be used to produce donor-derived offspring, because high numbers of cells can be harvested and there is no requirement to wait until the male recipient chicks become sexually mature. One of our research interests includes developing a novel method for reproduction in birds.[27] Given the potential of SSCs to give rise to germline stem cells (GSCs), the production of transgenic offspring from SSCs would replace the conventional embryo-mediated transgenesis systems developed during the last few decades.[28] Such efforts will be helpful for studying the mechanisms that control pluripotency and dedifferentiation in germ cells.

Future prospects for avian models

Technologies for producing transgenic birds have evolved significantly over the last few decades, although the potential applications have not been thoroughly explored. A self-contained avian embryo undergoing development offers numerous advantages as an animal biomodel.[29] The chick is free from maternal effects, which allows accurate assessments of the responses to various treatments, including environmental chemicals and physical stress. This unique *in vitro*-like—but in fact *in vivo*—system allows the monitoring of developmental events over time via eggshell windows, and the use of well-established surrogate systems for incubating embryos so that they have high rates of survival and normal developmental patterns. This classical embryologic model has been used to study developmental processes such as aging as well as hematopoiesis and the development of muscles and neurons.[30–32] The chicken is also a good model for studying human diseases such as lymphoma and for regenerative medicine.[33,34] Chickens are especially valuable models of ovarian cancer due to their unique physiologic traits.[35–39] The murine model is not suitable for studying this disease because, in the mouse, ovarian cancer originates mainly from granulosa cells or germ cells and not from the epithelium of the ovary.[35] Although epithelial ovarian cancer can be artificially induced by carcinogens, the overexpression of the SV40 large T antigen, or through the use of xenografts, these modes do not support efforts to identify the etiology of human epithelial ovarian cancer.[40] The physiologic characteristics of epithelial ovarian cancer in chickens are similar to those of the cancer in humans. Convincing evidence exists that human epithelial ovarian cancer

results from the accumulation of DNA damage in the ovarian epithelium due to incessant ovulation.[41] In humans, the incidence of epithelial ovarian cancer tends to increase dramatically after menopause or when the regular cycles of ovulation cease due to the hormones of pregnancy or the use of oral contraceptives.[41] The chicken is an excellent model for studying epithelial ovarian cancer because hens ovulate almost daily and produce about 300 eggs annually. Other studies have reported that continuous DNA damage occurs in the ovarian epithelial cells while the laying hen produces eggs, which is consistent with the major risk factors for human epithelial ovarian cancer.[42] In conjunction with the established transgenic techniques, avian biomodeling systems will advance the development of human disease models and will promote research approaches to improve human health and well-being.

Eggs contain lipids, proteins, carbohydrates, minerals, and other nutrients, and can be used in cooking and in further processing. Although eggs have clear nutritional value, persons who are suffering from atherosclerosis or who have a family history of hyperlipidemia may need to limit their intake of eggs, which contain high levels of cholesterol. To reduce the cholesterol content of eggs, hens are managed so as to modify their lipid sources, e.g., through fiber-rich feed or by adjusting the intake of micronutrients. However, such efforts are not sustainable because they are not cost-effective for poultry operations engaged in the large-scale production of eggs. In hens, cholesterol is synthesized in the liver and transported to peripheral tissues, including the ovary, in the form of very low-density lipoproteins.[43] Several key regulators of cholesterol synthesis have been identified, and it seems likely that the lipid content of eggs can be reduced.

Major pharmaceutical companies have concentrated on developing novel drugs because the potential for success is greater than for other applications. The overall market value of recombinant proteins was US$18.8 billion in 1997, and it is expected to be more than US$57 billion by 2010. However, major technological advances have been made using *Escherichia coli*, insect cells, fungi, yeast, and mammalian cells to produce therapeutic molecules that are subsequently used in translational or clinical studies of human disease. Conventional cell culturing systems entail high maintenance costs, and the products are often not suitable for therapeutic purposes due to the lack of appropriate structural modifications. Opportunities for the mass production of biopharmaceuticals in egg-white proteins are significant. When this becomes feasible, the pharmaceutical industry will undergo a revolutionary change.

Conclusions

In this review, we have focused on the roles of transgenic avian species in the past, as well as on the current procedures in manufacturing and biotechnology to produce products of importance to the agricultural, academic, and industrial sectors. Avian models are currently being used to study human diseases and to assess the efficacies of candidate therapeutics. Considering that the major concepts underlying studies of aging, stress responses, cell differentiation and dedifferentiation, and metabolic syndrome have been established in lower vertebrates, the use of avian models is expected to expand and intensify as efforts are made to elucidate the physiologic states of health and disease. Furthermore, avian models can be developed for industrial purposes to produce human proteins, therapeutics, and foodstuffs. Future studies are expected to result in the development of advanced transgenic technologies that exploit and enhance the advantages of avian models for basic and translational research.

Acknowledgments

This research was funded by the World Class University (WCU) program (R31-10056) through the National Research Foundation of Korea (NRF), funded by the Ministry of Education, Science, and Technology, and by a grant from the Next-Generation BioGreen 21 Program, Rural Development Administration, Republic of Korea.

Conflicts of interest

The authors declare no conflicts of interest.

References

1. Stern, C.D. 2005. The chick: a great model system becomes even greater. *Dev. Cell.* **8:** 9–17.
2. Temin, H.M. & S. Mizutani. 1970. RNA-dependent DNA polymerase in virions of Rous sarcoma virus. *Nature* **226:** 1211–1213.
3. Hillier, L.W. *et al.* International Chicken Genome Sequencing Consortium. 2004. Sequence and comparative analysis of the chicken genome provide unique perspectives on vertebrate evolution. *Nature* **432:** 695–716.
4. Sato, K., A. Ohuchi, S.H. Sook, *et al.* 2003. Changes in mRNA expression of 3-hydroxy-3-methylglutaryl coenzyme A reductase and cholesterol 7 alpha-hydroxylase in chickens. *Biochim. Biophys. Acta.* **1630:** 96–102.
5. Han, J.Y. 2009. Germ cells and transgenesis in chickens. *Comp. Immunol. Microbiol. Infect. Dis.* **32:** 61–80.
6. Song, G., T.S. Park, T.M. Kim & J.Y. Han. 2010. Avian biotechnology: insights from germ cell-mediated transgenic system. *J. Poult. Sci.* **47:** 197–207.
7. Fredrickson, T.N. 1987. Ovarian tumors of the hen. *Environ. Health Perspect.* **73:** 35–51.
8. Brinster, R.L., H.Y. Chen, R. Warren, *et al.* 1982. Regulation of metallothionein-thymidine kinase fusion plasmids injected into mouse eggs. *Nature* **296:** 39–42.
9. Love, J., C. Gribbin, C. Mather & H. Sang. 1994. Transgenic birds by DNA microinjection. *Biotechnology* **12:** 60–63.
10. Naito, M., E. Sasaki, M. Ohtaki & M. Sakurai. 1994. Introduction of exogenous DNA into somatic and germ cells of chickens by microinjection into the germinal disc of fertilized ova. *Mol. Reprod. Dev.* **37:** 167–171.
11. Salter, D.W., E.J. Smith, S.H. Hughes, *et al.* 1986. Gene insertion into the chicken germ line by retroviruses. *Poult. Sci.* **65:** 1445–1458.
12. Harvey, A.J., G. Speksnijder, L.R. Baugh, J.A. Morris & R. Ivarie. 2002. Expression of exogenous protein in the egg white of transgenic chicken. *Nat. Biotechnol.* **19:** 396–399.
13. Mizuarai, S., K. Ono, K. Yamaguchi, *et al.* 2001. Production of transgenic quails with high frequency of germ-line transmission using VSV-G pseudotyped retroviral vector. *Biochem. Biophys. Res. Commun.* **286:** 456–463.
14. Mozdziak, P.E., S. Borwornpinyo, D.W. McCoy & J.N. Petitte. 2003. Development of transgenic chickens expressing bacterial beta-galactosidase. *Dev. Dyn.* **226:** 439–445.
15. McGrew, M.J., A. Sherman, F.M. Ellard, *et al.* 2004. Efficient production of germline transgenic chickens using lentiviral vectors. *EMBO Rep.* **5:** 728–733.
16. Chapman, S.C., A. Lawson, W.C. Macarthur, *et al.* 2005. Ubiquitous GFP expression in transgenic chickens using a lentiviral vector. *Development* **132:** 935–940.
17. Lillico, S.G., A. Sherman, M.J. McGrew, *et al.* 2007. Oviduct-specific expression of two therapeutic proteins in transgenic hens. *Proc. Natl. Acad. Sci. USA* **104:** 1771–1776.
18. Shin, S.S., T.M. Kim, S.Y. Kim, *et al.* 2008. Generation of transgenic quail through germ cell-mediated germline transmission. *FASEB J.* **22:** 2435–2444.
19. Kamihira, M., K. Ono, K. Esaka, K. Nishijima, *et al.* 2005. High-level expression of single-chain Fv-Fc fusion protein in serum and egg white of genetically manipulated chickens by using a retroviral vector. *J. Virol.* **79:** 10864–10874.
20. Wentworth, B.C., H. Tsai, J.H. Hallett, *et al.* 1989. Manipulation of avian primordial germ cells and gonadal differentiation. *Poult. Sci.* **68:** 999–1010.
21. Vick, L., Y. Li & K. Simkiss. 1993. Transgenic birds from transformed primordial germ cells. *Proc. Biol. Sci.* **251:** 179–182.
22. Matsui, Y., K. Zsebo & B.L. Hogan. 1992. Derivation of pluripotential embryonic stem cells from murine primordial germ cells in culture. *Cell* **70:** 841–847.

23. Park, T.S. & J.Y. Han. 2000. Derivation and characterization of pluripotent embryonic germ cells in chicken. *Mol. Reprod. Dev.* **56:** 475–482.

24. Park, T.S., Y.H. Hong, S.C. Kwon, *et al.* 2003. Birth of germline chimeras by transfer of chicken embryonic germ (EG) cells into recipient embryos. *Mol. Reprod. Dev.* **65:** 389–395.

25. Park, S.H., J.N. Kim, T.S. Park, *et al.* 2010. CpG methylation modulates tissue-specific expression of a transgene in chickens. *Theriogenology* **74:** 805–816.

26. Kang, S.J., J.W. Choi, S.Y. Kim, *et al.* 2008. Reproduction of wild birds via interspecies germ cell transplantation. *Biol. Reprod.* **79:** 931–937.

27. Lee, Y.M., J.G. Jung, J.N. Kim, *et al.* 2006. A testis-mediated germline chimera production based on transfer of chicken testicular cells directly into heterologous testes. *Biol. Reprod.* **75:** 380–386.

28. Jung, J.G., Y.M. Lee, T.S. Park, *et al.* 2007. Identification, culture, and characterization of germline stem cell-like cells in chicken testes. *Biol. Reprod.* **76:** 173–182.

29. Rashidi, H. & V. Sottile. 2009. The chick embryo: hatching a model for contemporary biomedical research. *Bioessays* **31:** 459–465.

30. Holmesa, D.J. & M.A. Ottinger. 2003. Birds as long-lived animal model for the study of aging. *Exp. Gerontol.* **38:** 1365–1375.

31. Dieterlen-Lievre, F. & N.M. Le Douarin. 2004. From the hemangioblast to self-tolerance: a series of innovations gained from studies on the avian embryo. *Mech. Dev.* **121:** 1117–1128.

32. Stern, C.D. 2006. Neural induction: 10 years on since the 'default model'. *Curr. Opin. Cell Biol.* **18:** 692–697.

33. Burgess, S.C., J.R. Young, B.J. Baaten, *et al.* 2004. Marek's disease is a natural model for lymphomas overexpressing Hodgkin's disease antigen (CD30). *Proc. Natl. Acad. Sci. USA* **101:** 13879–13884.

34. Coleman, C.M. 2008. Chicken embryo as a model for regenerative medicine. *Birth Defects Res. C.* **84:** 245–256.

35. Vanderhyden, B.C., T.J. Shaw & J.F. Ethier. 2003. Animal models of ovarian cancer. *Reprod. Biol. Endocrin.* **1:** 67–77.

36. Johnson, P.A. & J.R. Giles. 2006. Use of genetic strains of chickens in studies of ovarian cancer. *Poult. Sci.* **85:** 246–250.

37. Ahn, S.E., J.W. Choi, H.W. Seo, *et al.* 2010. Increased expression of cysteine cathepsins in ovarian tissue from chickens with ovarian cancer. *Reprod. Biol. Endocrin.* **8:** 100–107.

38. Seo, H.W., D. Rengaraj, J.W. Choi, *et al.* 2010. Claudin 10 is a glandular epithelial marker in the chicken model as human epithelial ovarian cancer. *Int. J. Gynecol. Cancer.* **20:** 1465–1473.

39. Seo, H.W., D. Rengaraj, J.W. Choi, *et al.* 2011. The expression profile of apoptosis-related genes in the chicken as a human epithelial ovarian cancer model. *Oncol. Rep.* **25:** 49–56.

40. Garson, K., T.J. Shaw, K.V. Clark, *et al.* 2005. Models of ovarian cancer-are we there yet? *Mol. Cell. Endocrinol.* **239:** 15–26.

41. Johnson, K.A. 2009. The standard of perfection: thoughts about the laying hen model of ovarian cancer. *Cancer Prev. Res.* (Phila) **2:** 97–99.

42. Murdoch, W.J., E.A. Van Kirk & B.M. Alexander. 2005. DNA damages in ovarian surface epithelial cells of ovulatory hens. *Exp. Biol. Med.* **230:** 429–433.

43. Schneider, W.J. 2009. Receptor-mediated mechanisms in ovarian follicle and oocyte development. *Gen. Comp. Endocrinol.* **163:** 18–23.

Ann. N.Y. Acad. Sci. ISSN 0077-8923

ANNALS OF THE NEW YORK ACADEMY OF SCIENCES
Issue: *Nutrition and Physical Activity in Aging, Obesity, and Cancer*

Telomere dynamics: the influence of folate and DNA methylation

Carly J. Moores,[1,2] Michael Fenech,[1] and Nathan J. O'Callaghan[1]

[1]CSIRO Food and Nutritional Sciences Division, Adelaide, South Australia. [2]School of Medicine, Flinders University of South Australia, Bedford Park, South Australia

Address for correspondence: Michael Fenech, CSIRO Food and Nutritional Sciences, PO Box 10041, Adelaide 5000, South Australia. michael.fenech@csiro.au

Since the suggestion of their existence, a wealth of literature on telomere biology has emerged aimed at solving the DNA end-underreplication problem identified by Olovnikov in 1971. Telomere shortening/dysfunction is now recognized as increasing degenerative disease risk. Recent studies have suggested that both dietary patterns and individual micronutrients—including folate—can influence telomere length and function. Folate is an important dietary vitamin required for DNA synthesis, repair, and one-carbon metabolism within the cell. However, the potential mechanisms by which folate deficiency directly or indirectly affects telomere biology has not yet been reviewed comprehensively. The present review summarizes recent published knowledge and identifies the residual knowledge gaps. Specifically, this review addresses whether it is plausible that folate deficiency may (1) cause accelerated telomere shortening, (2) intrinsically affect telomere function, and/or (3) cause increased telomere-end fusions and subsequent breakage–fusion–bridge cycles in the cell.

Keywords: folate; telomeres; epigenetics; DNA methylation; diet

Folate

Folate, a water-soluble B group vitamin (vitamin B9), is required for the vital metabolic processes of DNA methylation and nucleotide biosynthesis, including conversion of dUMP to dTTP.[1,2] Such essential cellular pathways are affected by total dietary intake of folate and its metabolic cofactors, and certain genetic variants.[3] Folate can occur in various metabolic forms (Fig. 1); and some of these, such as 5-methyltetrahydrofolate (5-MeTHF) and 5,10-methylenetetrahydrofolate (5,10-MeTHF), can donate methyl groups to other molecules. In a folate-deficient state, a cell is limited in 5,10-MeTHF required for conversion of dUMP to dTTP by methylation, and hence the ratio of dUMP:dTTP increases, leading to inadvertent incorporation of uracil in the DNA of dividing cells.[4] 5-MeTHF is required to synthesize methionine from homocysteine, and this reaction requires vitamin B12 as a cofactor and zinc at the catalytic site to activate homocysteine.[5,6] Methionine is then converted to

S-adenosyl methionine, the universal methyl donor employed for methylation of histones and cytosine in mammalian DNA[7] (Fig. 1). When folate is deficient, maintenance of methylation of histones and cytosine may be inadequate.[8]

Homocysteine accumulates in response to folate- and B12-deficient conditions, as there is insufficent 5-MeTHF to provide methyl groups to reform methionine. A high plasma level of homocysteine has been shown to increase risk of adverse cardiovascular events[9] and is associated with increased chromosome damage.[10] Periconceptional exposure to elevated folate has long been recognized to prevent neural tube defects in the developing fetus,[11,12] and use of a folate supplement before and during early pregancy is now considered "best practice" in the Western world.[13] Additionally, suboptimal folate status has been associated with an increased risk of many cancer types such as colorectal cancer, adenoma, esophageal, and gastric cancer[14] as well as cardiovascular disease.[15]

doi: 10.1111/j.1749-6632.2011.06101.x

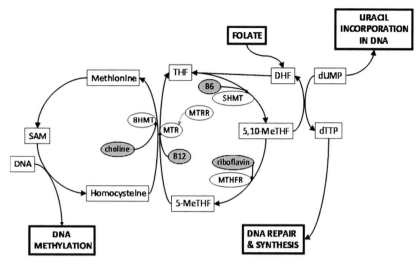

Figure 1. Folate metabolism: folate, along with choline, methionine, cobalamin, pyridoxine, and riboflavin, is involved in several essential metabolic processes within the cell, in particular DNA synthesis, repair, and methylation. Folate is also essential as a methyl donor in the maintenance of dUMP:dTTP ratios within the cell. When the ratio of dUMP:dTTP is increased, there is an increased incorporation of uracil into the DNA. Image modified from Ref. 78. 5-MeTHF, 5-methyltetrahydrofolate; 5,10-MeTHF, 5,10-methylenetetrahydrofolate; B6, pyridoxine; B12, cobalamin; BHMT, betaine homocysteine methyltransferase; DHF, dihydrofolate; DNA, deoxyribonucleic acid; dUMP, deoxyuridine monophosphate; dTTP, deoxythymidine triphosphate; MTHFR, methylenetetrahydrofolate reductase; MTR, methionine synthase; MTRR, methionine synthase reductase; SAM, S-adenosyl methionine; SHMT, serine hydroxymethyltransferase; THF, tetrahydrofolate.

Telomeres and cellular aging

Telomeres are repeats of the hexamer sequence $(TTAGGG)_n$, which, with the associated shelterin protein complex, cap the end of all mammalian chromosomes. As the ends of the double-helical DNA of linear chromosomes are unable to be entirely replicated during each cycle of nuclear division, telomeric DNA is sacrificed to ensure that the coding genetic sequence is not lost from the extremities of the chromosome, known as the end-replication problem or marginotomy.[16–18] As a consequence of the end-replication problem, telomeric sequence repeats abridge by approximately 30–200 bp during each cycle of cell division in most somatic cells.[19] Telomere attrition occurs naturally during the aging process;[20,21] however, it is accelerated in certain premature aging syndromes such as ataxia telangiectasia (Fig. 2). The length of the telomeric sequence declines with age until the telomere becomes critically short, typically signaling cellular senescence and resulting in programmed cell death.[22–25] Telomere length is regarded as an indicator of the biological age of a cell or its ability to undergo additional mitotic divisions.[26] Since telomere length changes are also known to be induced by

various environmental, physiological, and psychological stressors,[27] such variations in telomere length may suggest that aside from the effect of the end-replication problem, other factors may contribute to telomere shortening.

Telomeres and disease

Short telomeres have been widely investigated for use as a potential biomarker in determining increased risk of many diseases, particularly those with age-associated manifestations. Studies have determined that truncated telomeric repeats are associated with increased risk of cancer,[28] Alzheimer's disease,[29] Parkinson's disease,[30] rheumatoid arthritis,[31] cardiovascular disease,[32] and progression of liver cirrhosis.[33] Telomere length dynamics, however, appear to be complex, with long telomere length not consistently a sign of healthy cellular status. Recently Svenson *et al.* reported that an increased telomere length in peripheral blood cells was associated with negative prognosis in breast cancer patients.[34] Furthermore, it has been observed that offspring born to older parents have a longer telomere length[35–38] and, in isolation, that increased parental age at birth can increase the risk of adult-onset non-Hodgkin's

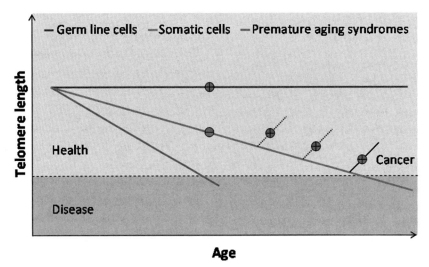

Figure 2. Telomere attrition with aging: the erosion of telomeric sequence accumulates with age in normal somatic cells; however, telomere attrition is greatly accelerated in premature aging syndromes such as ataxia telangiectasia. The length of telomeres in germ cells is stable due to the activity of telomerase (+). Somatic cells express basal levels of telomerase (−) unless they become transformed, cancerous (+). Image modified from Ref. 154.

lymphoma,[39] and breast[40–42] and prostate[43] cancers in the progeny. These observations suggest that the telomere length alone may not be an adequate predictor of degenerative disease risk and that, perhaps, the quality and functionality of telomeres should also be an important consideration.

Telomere structure and telomeric dysfunction

The terminal end of the telomere consists of both a double stranded and single stranded DNA region, which loops back on itself to form a cap at the end of the chromosome.[44] This lariat structure contains a larger, double-stranded telomere-duplex loop (t-loop) into which the long 3′ G-rich single-strand overhang, the displacement loop (D-loop), is inserted.[44,45] The D-loop-t-loop lariat and associated proteins, including the shelterin complex, serve to eliminate "free ends" of DNA that may be processed as double- or single-stranded DNA breaks. The structure prevents the triggering of an apoptotic response within the cell that is otherwise induced at broken chromosome loci.[46] Whether the deficiency of folate or other dietary methyl donors might affect telomeric structure and cause chromosomal dysfunction within the cell has been suggested previously but remains indefinite.[47] It is a possibility that folate deficiency and resulting uracil incorpo-

ration, DNA hypomethylation, or both, could affect the assembly of the D-loop-t-loop structure at the telomere end and/or the binding of telomere-associated proteins.

The shelterin complex and chromosomal stability

Telomeres and their shelterin complex additionally serve to prevent chromosome end-to-end fusions or other chromosomal rearrangements.[48] The mammalian shelterin complex consists of six protein subunits (TRF1, TRF2, POT1, Rap1, TIN2, and TPP1) that are in part responsible for telomere length maintenance and shaping the telomere cap.[49–51] Telomere binding proteins may reduce the likelihood of nucleolytic degradation and increase chromosomal stability as well as influence the access of the telomerase enzyme to the telomeric sequence.[52] Furthermore, the core protein components of the shelterin complex are involved in an assortment of intracellular signaling pathways.[53] Probing the interaction networks of the shelterin compartments and their activities has permitted the construction of an intricate shelterin interactome.[50,53] The composition and localization of the shelterin complex serves to prevent the recognition of telomeric DNA termini as double-stranded breaks and, as such, vetoing DNA damage response pathways.[49] However,

DNA damage response proteins have been observed at telomeres and appear to be essential for telomere replication, protection, and function.[54,55]

Telomere dysfunction within a cell has been measured as telomere end-to-end associations, telomere aggregates, telomere doublets, nucleoplasmic bridges (NPB), telomere clusters, or telomeric chromatid concatenates, and these have been associated with disease states or predisease conditions. Recent evidence is emerging to show that such telomeric dysfunction is increased under conditions of tumourigenesis and oxidative stress.[56,57] Telomere aggregates can be visualized using 2-D fluorescence microscopy and may represent telomere-end fusions that later could potentially become involved in breakage–fusion–bridge (BFB) cycles.[58] Folate deficiency has been shown to induce NPB formation;[59,60] however, it is not clear whether these events are caused by telomere end fusion, misrepair of DNA breaks in telomeres or anywhere else along the chromosome.[61] Telomere doublets or telomeric DNA-containing double-minute chromosomes (TDMs) are characterized by multiple telomere signals at a lone chromatid end.[62] These TDMs are postulated to be formed through recombination events between telomeric sequence and interstitial telomere-like sequences,[63] such as those located in subtelomeric regions.[64]

Cellular senescence, crisis, and immortality

The *in vitro* culture of normal somatic cells provides evidence of a limited replicative potential, whereby cells enter a state of senescence, mortality stage 1 (M1), or the Hayflick limit.[65] The Hayflick limit of cellular division is the number of population doublings determined by continued and accumulative telomere erosion.[66,67] Continued cellular proliferation following bypass or inactivation of the M1 mechanism induces the mortality stage 2 (M2) or crisis mechanism. *In vitro* escape from this M2 stage results in the emergence of an immortal cell line[68] by telomerase expression[69] and/or via the alternative lengthening of telomeres (ALT) mechanism.[70] A study by Counter *et al.* showed that unlike M1 cells, M2 cells had a reduced mean telomere length (1.5 kb content) and an increased number of dicentric chromosomes due to telomere end-fusions, resulting in greater genomic instability.[69]

For some time it has been recognized that the telomere length is polymorphic or heterogeneous across chromosomes, with senescence, likely the result of a critical telomere loss to just one or a few chromosomes.[71] The chromosome 17p telomere is noted as the critical telomere in humans because of its comparatively short-telomeric sequence.[72] High frequency loss of heterozygosity of 17p—the arm that houses p53 and potentially other tumor suppressor genes such as *HIC1*[73–76]—is one of the most common genetic modifications in cancer.[77] As folate is required for DNA repair, nucleotide biosynthesis, and conversion of dUMP to dTTP, it is undoubtedly important for accurate nuclear division and cellular proliferation. It is not known whether folate deficiency or excess affects 17p-specific telomere loss. Even so, given the tendency for folate deficiency to cause chromosomal breaks, it is plausible that insufficient folate could cause global telomere attrition, including at 17p by DNA strand break induction, while surplus folate could accelerate cellular proliferation,[78] with both scenarios resulting in "unexclusive" telomere loss.

Telomerase and the ALT mechanism

Unlike somatic cells that express very low or basal levels of telomerase transcripts, stem and germ cells have greatly upregulated telomerase expression in order to maintain telomere length. Somatic cells become immortal by activating expression of the human telomerase reverse transcriptase (hTERT) enzyme or by an ALT recombination-based mechanism of telomere elongation. hTERT adds *de novo* $(TTAGGG)_n$ hexamer repeats to the $3'$ G-rich end of the telomere[79] and appears to operate, such that short telomeric sequences are preferentially elongated.[80] Both telomerase and ALT recombination-based[81–83] mechanisms of telomere elongation are dysregulated during tumorigenesis. A large majority of tumors express telomerase, while approximately 10–15% of tumors are ALT positive.[81] Epidemiologic evidence suggests that deficiency of folate is potentially procarcinogenic,[84] perhaps as increased cellular dUMP:dTTP ratios in low-folate conditions cause a halt or collapse of DNA replication forks, as well as intermediates of base excision repair, and subsequently DNA strand breaks.[85] The processing of these DNA double-stranded breaks by homologous recombination can induce a variety of changes in the genetic material.[85]

While folate deficiency is purported to cause increased recombination in the cell for this reason, whether folate could influence ALT-associated recombination is unknown. It is also plausible that low dTTP in folate-deficient cells could influence the action and/or efficiency of the *de novo* addition of $(TTAGGG)_n$ to the chromosome ends by hTERT. In addition, the recent observation that methionine restriction causes a reversible induction of ALT-associated promyelocytic leukemia bodies (APBs) in the nucleus suggests that it may be possible that deficiency in folate, which is required for methionine synthesis, may indirectly influence ALT mechanisms of telomere lengthening in ALT-positive cells.[86]

The Breakage–Fusion–Bridge cycle

Along with telomere loss, BFB cycles are a central mechanism in carcinogenesis.[87] BFB cycles may ensue when a dicentric chromosome is formed either through an incorrect repair of DNA double-stranded breaks, or when fusion occurs between telomeric regions. During the anaphase, spindle fibers may guide this dicentric chromosome to opposite poles of the cell, which results in asymmetrical and unordered breakage of the chromosome; thus daughter cells might contain deletions or duplications of the chromosomal complement. Chromatids that lack telomere sequence after dicentric chromosome breakage that is likely fuse again following DNA replication during the S-phase, forming a dicentric chromosome and further perpetuating the BFB cycle.[88–90] These BFB cycles contribute to deletions, gene amplification, and nonreciprocal translocations.[57] Deficiency in dietary methyl donor folate induces NPB formation[60] and is consistent with observations that loss of DNA methylation results in increased telomeric recombination.[91] Though substantial progress has been made in understanding the molecular mechanisms behind NPB formation,[61] the influence of folate deficiency still requires definition. It is unresolved whether NPBs in folate-deficient cells are induced by misrepair of DNA-stranded breaks or by dysfunctional telomeres that could cause telomere sequence amplification and telomere-end fusions.

Epigenetics, DNA methylation, and folate

While telomerase and ALT mechanisms actively govern telomere length, epigenetic modification at or near the telomere also influences the length of the repeat.[92–96] The epigenetic state of a DNA sequence is both heritable and reversible, involving higher order control of gene transcription while the underlying DNA sequence remains unchanged.[97] Epigenetic mechanisms of gene expression control include histone modifications, DNA methylation, and small noncoding RNA sequences. The former two mechanisms contribute to the remodeling of chromatin into an active or inactive state, while the latter modulates gene expression by binding target RNA transcripts (mRNA) and negatively regulating efficiency of protein translation and stability of these translation products.[98]

Perhaps the most important function of dietary folate in genome integrity maintenance is its role as a methyl donor for epigenetic control of gene expression by DNA methylation. Vertebrate DNA methylation is the addition of a methyl group (CH_3) to cytosine residues resulting in the modified base 5-methylcytosine (m^5C). A family of DNA methyltransferase (DNMT) enzymes is responsible for catalyzing methylation of cytosine bases in mammals. DNMT3A and DNMT3B enzymes catalyze primarily *de novo* methylation,[99] while DNMT1 is the principal enzyme involved in maintenance methylation of hemimethylated DNA following semiconservative DNA replication.[100] It is purported that approximately 4% of cytosine bases are methylated in vertebrates,[101] with these modified residues largely occurring at CpG dinucleotides located within promoter regions.[102] As gene promoter regions are typically rich in these CpG dinucleotides, they are known as CpG islands. CpG islands are also in large abundance in human gene exons. Gene-specific DNA methylation can cause gene silencing and expression via hyper- or hypomethylation, respectively. Both global (genome-wide) and local (gene-specific) DNA methylation patterns are modified by micronutrients such as folate, and these methylation patterns are often altered in cancer cells.[103]

Subtelomere DNA methylation and telomere length

Unlike the repeat unit of the telomere, which is highly conserved, the subtelomeric region (refer to Fig. 3 for schematic diagram) of the chromosome is variable,[104,105] with human subtelomere assemblies differing across all chromosome ends.[64,106,107] These subtelomeric assemblies contain segmental tandem repeats sourced from other sequences

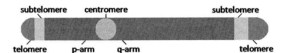

Figure 3. Schematic image of a chromosome: the mammalian chromosome includes the following distinct regions, from left to right: the telomere region (blue) contains tandem repeats of the hexamer $(TTAGGG)_n$ in humans; the subtelomere (light blue); chromosomal coding DNA (gray); the centromere (light gray). N.B.: schematic not to scale.

within the genome,[108] $(TTAGGG)_n$-like sequences, single-copy regions, and subtelomeric repeat sequences.[64,107,109] While mammalian telomeric hexamer repeats are devoid of DNA methylation substrates (CpG), the subtelomere contains a high proportion of CpG dinucleotides, which are methylated in human somatic cells.[104,110,111] Analogous subtelomeric regions in mice have high-CpG methylation that has been shown to taper when DNMT is abrogated.[91] Since global hypomethylation is a hallmark of cancer cells, it was hypothesized that reduced methylation may mediate telomere elongation.[7] Inadequate folate in the diet *in vivo*, as well as in *in vitro* models, has been consistently shown to be result in reduced DNA methylation.[112]

Maintenance (DNMT1) and *de novo* (DNMT3A and DNMT3B) DNA methyltransferases negatively regulate telomere length[91] through methylation of cytosine on a global scale, including at subtelomeric regions. Increased events of telomeric sister chromatid exchanges—a hallmark of ALT-positive cells[113,114]—occur when DNA methylation is lost by DNMT deficiency.[91] Additional ALT cell features—heterogeneous telomere length and ALT-associated APBs[83]—are displayed in these DNMT-deficient cells, showing that loss of DNA methylation occurs together with elevated telomeric recombination.[91] While subtelomeric hypomethylation is suggested to permit ALT activity,[91] it is not mandatory that all subtelomeric regions be hypomethylated for ALT recombination to occur.[115]

Although a hypomethylated subtelomere appears to elicit characteristics observed in ALT-positive cells,[91] telomerase-positive cells have hypermethylated subtelomeric regions.[115] Although the extent of subtelomeric CpG methylation in healthy cells is not known, it appears that the epigenetic status of the subtelomere is altered in both ALT- and telomerase-positive cells. That increase in telomere length—caused by *DNMT* knockdown leading

to hypomethylated subtelomeres—occurred while other telomeric heterochromatic marks such as histone methylation were unchanged suggests that DNA methylation exerts higher order control of the telomere length.[91] As the subtelomeric assembly of each chromosome arm is variable, with subtelomeric repeat sequences ranging from <10 kb to >300 kb,[64] the number of CpG and, hence, the extent of subtelomeric methylation is likely to be different among human chromosomes. Currently, subtelomeric methylation is determined by methylation-specific PCR;[116] however, this method is limited in that the amplicon size is very small (< 200 bp), and so the result reflects the methylation status of few cytosine residues in the possible 500 kb subtelomeric region.[64] The conception of optimal methods that would allow for the definitive subtelomeric methylation status across each chromosome arm, and comparison of this status with chromosome arm–specific telomere length[117] remain important goals.

It was initially believed that telomeric sequences were transcriptionally silent; however, telomeres encode telomeric repeat-containing RNA (TERRA)[118] known to localize at the telomere.[118,119] Noncoding TERRA contains telomeric and subtelomeric sequences,[120] and, recently, TERRA transcription was shown to be negatively regulated by cytosine methylation of its promoter, housed in the subtelomere.[115,121] Increased methylation of the subtelomere, a notable feature of telomerase-expressing cells, results in silencing of subtelomeric/telomeric transcription of TERRA, hence suggesting telomerase is inhibited by TERRA, and that this transcriptional silencing may be selected in cancer cells.[115] Whether the inhibition of telomerase by TERRA occurs primarily *in situ* or *in trans* is unknown,[115] and although TERRA transcription has been shown to be higher in ALT-positive cells than telomerase-positive cells, this is likely due to an increased TERRA signal by the generally longer telomeres characteristic of heterogeneous ALT cells.[115] Despite the importance of folate as a methyl donor, there are no published studies on the relationship of folate status with subtelomere methylation and/or TERRA expression.

Telomeric chromatin and histone modifications

The human genetic code is organized within the cell as chromatin in the form of DNA packages of

146 bp wound around a nucleosome comprising pairs of each histone, H2A, H2B, H3, and H4.[122] DNA methylation at CpG dinucleotides, along with histone acetylation, induces reversible changes on chromatin structure. Condensed and transcriptionally silent chromatin or heterochromatin largely contains methylated cytosine residues and histones that are deacetylated. Histone modifications typical of heterochromatic telomeres include increased trimethylation of histones H3 (lysine 9) and H4 (lysine 20) and lowered acetylation of histones H3 and H4.[123] Other modifications at H3 and H4 tails include phosphorylation, ubiquitination, and methylation.[122] The observation that induced changes in telomeric heterochromatin, via histone methyltransferase (HMTase) knockdown, imparted abnormal elongation of telomeric sequence, suggests involvement of histone modifications in telomere length control.[124] Another exemplar of histone modification affecting telomere function includes heterochromatin protein 1 (HP1) that is involved in telomere capping and telomeric function.[125] HP1 functions to cap the telomere by binding directly to the telomeric sequence, while telomere elongation and transcriptional regression of the telomere by HP1 can occur via interaction with histone H3 methylated at lysine 9.[126,127]

Telomere length, diet, and folate

It is generally recognized firsthand that those who have a healthy lifestyle appear to live longer. Since an *in vitro* study showed that vitamin C enrichment slows telomere attrition in a human endothelial cell line,[128] various *in vivo* studies have investigated the effect of dietary components on the telomere length in humans. These associative studies have shown that vitamin D[129] and vitamin E intake,[130] multivitamin use,[131] dietary fiber consumption,[132] and intake of marine omega-3 fatty acid[133] were correlated with longer telomeres; whereas processed meat consumption,[134] increased alcohol intake,[135] and low fruit and vegetable intake, as well as increased meat intake[136] were dietary patterns that were negatively associated with telomere length. The potential effects of additional nutrients on telomere mechanics have recently been published.[137]

Plasma homocysteine concentration—which increases when folate and B12 are deficient—has been shown to be inversely associated with telomere length in human cross-sectional studies comprising up to 1319 subjects.[138–140] The attrition of telomeric sequence induced by elevated homocysteine is possibly mediated by increased oxidative stress or inflammation,[138,140] or the increased demand for proliferation of certain cell types, in these cases hematopoietic stem cells.[140] This negative effect of homocysteine on the telomere length is purported to also be the effect of folate deficiency on the telomere, as the amino acid and vitamin are inversely correlated, and as such it is suggested that the effect would be mitigated by increased folate intake.[138,140] To date, constituents of the folate pathway have not been adequately studied for their effect on telomere length in humans. As yet, B$_{12}$ has been reported to have no effect on the telomere length[7,138] even though plasma B$_{12}$ is considered an important factor in folate and homocysteine metabolism and should be considered in statistical analyses involving these measures. The effect of folate on the telomere length appears to be complex, on the basis of the few studies that have explored the relationship. In one study, low levels of plasma folate were correlated with the shorter telomere length in the older male cohort, though no such effect was observed in corresponding older female participants or in younger adults.[138] Perplexingly, in another study, plasma folate was inversely correlated with the longer telomere length when folate levels were below the cohort median, yet once plasma levels were above this level, the relationship with the telomere length was positive.[7] In a recent review, it has been suggested that folate deficiency might induce telomere attrition and/or dysfunction by molecular mechanisms, including (1) the excision of increased uracil in the telomeric hexamer repeat that is known to generate abasic sites and DNA breaks; (2) the aberrant epigenetic state of the subtelomeric DNA; and (3) inefficient binding of the shelterin proteins to the telomeric DNA due to reduced affinity to uracil and/or abasic sites, resulting from excision repair of uracil in the telomere sequence.[47] Under conditions of folate deficiency, incorporation of uracil instead of thymine in DNA is increased.[4,141] Uracil might also arise in the telomeric hexamer repeat due to spontaneous deamination of cytosine. Excision repair of uracil in DNA has a range of molecular consequences, including generation of abasic sites through base excision repair pathways, which can cause single- or double-stranded DNA breaks and chromosomal aberrations.[4,142,143] A lowered

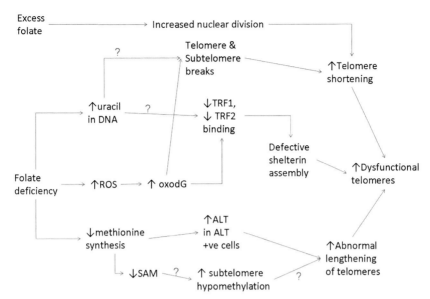

Figure 4. Possible mechanisms by which folate deficiency or excess may influence telomere structure and function: indentifies plausible but untested mechanisms.

synthesis of dTTP from dUMP has been suggested to accelerate telomere shortening,[143] while successive uracil misincorporation within the telomere could result in shorter telomeres as single-stranded breaks of the G-rich strand may not be repairable or cause degradation of the complementary C-rich strand.[143] However, continued investigation, both *in vitro* and *in vivo*, is required in order to validate or repudiate these plausible mechanisms and to better undstand the biological impact of folate deficiency on telomere function.

Knowledge gaps and conclusion

It is evident that dietary deficiency of micronutrients, including folate, may have an effect on the telomere length and function in humans. The development of a nutrient profile for optimal telomere function and maintenance in the general population is a clear goal in this field. Doing so on an individual level by employing principles of nutritional genomics and genetics, while arduous, could be a cost-effective approach to prevention of those chronic disease conditions that are often exacerbated by genomic disturbances caused by nutritional deficiencies.[47,144] In the case of folate, it is still unclear whether (1) deficiency causes increased uracil in the telomere and if, as a result, base excision and attempted repair causes telomere breaks and shortening; (2) low levels induce subtelomeric

hypomethylation and whether the degree of this epigenetic modification can affect the length and function of the telomere; and (3) whether decreased levels of folate cause nucleoplasmic bridges or chromosome fusions that specifically involve telomeric and/or subtelomeric sequences. The effect of genetic polymorphisms that alter the activity of enzymes required in folate uptake, transport, and metabolism on the telomere length and function remains unexplored and should be thoroughly investigated for interactive effects with folate status.

It is apparent that there is not one distinct test for telomere integrity and function. Instead there are a suite of assays that individually measure, for example, telomere length (both absolute[145,146] and chromosome arm specific),[117,147] subtelomeric methylation[115,116] and TERRA RNA expression,[119] telomere dysfunction,[148] ALT mechanism presence,[149] and telomerase activity.[150] Despite the likely importance of telomere base sequence mutation, there do not appear to be any published methods that can detect DNA base damage within the telomere hexamer repeat. It has been shown that DNA damage repair within the telomeric region is less efficacious than repair to regions of the coding sequence,[151–153] with both the rate and degree of telomeric repair declining with age.[152] To be able to detect base damage within the telomeric sequence would be valuable, as the telomere is rich in guanine and thymine residues, and, as such, it may be particularly vulnerable to guanine oxidation and increased incorporation of uracil under oxidative stress and folate deficiency conditions, respectively. In conclusion, as summarized in Figure 4, there are several potential mechanisms by which folate deficiency or excess may adversely affect telomere length, dynamics, and function. Several of these possible mechanisms need to be rigorously tested to obtain a deeper understanding of these fundamental processes that may be instrumental in refining decisions on folate requirements for maintenance of chromosomal stability.

Acknowledgment

Caroline Bull kindly proofread the manuscript and provided constructive suggestions to improve the content of this review.

Conflicts of interest

The authors declare no conflicts of interest.

References

1. Appling, D.R. 1991. Compartmentation of folate-mediated one-carbon metabolism in eukaryotes. *FASEB J.* **5:** 2645–2651.

2. Benesh, F.C. & G.F. Carl. 1978. Methyl biogenesis. *Biol. Psychiatr.* **13:** 465–480.

3. Bailey, L.B. & J.F. Gregory, 3rd. 1999. Folate metabolism and requirements. *J. Nutr.* **129:** 779–782.

4. Blount, B.C. *et al.* 1997. Folate deficiency causes uracil misincorporation into human DNA and chromosome breakage: implications for cancer and neuronal damage. *Proc. Natl. Acad. Sci. USA* **94:** 3290–3295.

5. Koutmos, M. *et al.* 2008. Metal active site elasticity linked to activation of homocysteine in methionine synthases. *Proc. Natl. Acad. Sci. USA* **105:** 3286–3291.

6. Matthews, R.G. & C.W. Goulding. 1997. Enzyme-catalyzed methyl transfers to thiols: the role of zinc. *Curr. Opin. Chem. Biol.* **1:** 332–339.

7. Paul, L. *et al.* 2009. Telomere length in peripheral blood mononuclear cells is associated with folate status in men. *J. Nutr.* **139:** 1273–1278.

8. Smith, A.D., Y.I. Kim & H. Refsum. 2008. Is folic acid good for everyone? *Am. J. Clin. Nutr.* **87:** 517–533.

9. Shammas, N.W. *et al.* 2008. Elevated levels of homocysteine predict cardiovascular death, nonfatal myocardial infarction, and symptomatic bypass graft disease at 2-year follow-up following coronary artery bypass surgery. *Prev. Cardiol.* **11:** 95–99.

10. Picerno, I. *et al.* 2007. Homocysteine induces DNA damage and alterations in proliferative capacity of T-lymphocytes: a model for immunosenescence? *Biogerontology* **8:** 111–119.

11. Smithells, R.W. *et al.* 1981. Apparent prevention of neural tube defects by periconceptional vitamin supplementation. *Arch. Dis. Child* **56:** 911–918.

12. MRC Vitamin Study Research Group. 1991. Prevention of neural tube defects: results of the Medical Research Council Vitamin Study. *Lancet* **338:** 131–137.

13. Bhutta, Z.A. & B. Hasan. 2002. Periconceptional supplementation with folate and/or multivitamins for preventing neural tube defects: RHL commentary. The WHO Reproductive Health Library 2002 last revised 7 January 2002; Retrieved March 2011 from: http://apps.who.int/rhl/pregnancy_childbirth/antenatal_care/nutrition/bhcom/en/index.html.

14. Ames, B.N. & P. Wakimoto. 2002. Are vitamin and mineral deficiencies a major cancer risk? *Nat. Rev. Cancer* **2:** 694–704.

15. Jang, H., J.B. Mason & S.W. Choi. 2005. Genetic and epigenetic interactions between folate and aging in carcinogenesis. *J. Nutr.* **135:** 2967S–2971S.

16. Olovnikov, A.M. 1971. Principle of marginotomy in template synthesis of polynucleotides. *Dokl. Akad. Nauk. SSSR* **201:** 1496–1499.

17. Olovnikov, A.M. 1973. A theory of marginotomy. The incomplete copying of template margin in enzymic synthesis of polynucleotides and biological significance of the phenomenon. *J. Theor. Biol.* **41:** 181–190.

18. Watson, J.D. 1972. Origin of concatemeric T7 DNA. *Nat. N. Biol.* **239:** 197–201.

19. Sitte, N., G. Saretzki & T. von Zglinicki. 1998. Accelerated telomere shortening in fibroblasts after extended periods of confluency. *Free Radic. Biol. Med.* **24:** 885–893.

20. Lindsey, J. *et al.* 1991. In vivo loss of telomeric repeats with age in humans. *Mutat. Res.* **256:** 45–48.

21. Vaziri, H. *et al.* 1993. Loss of telomeric DNA during aging of normal and trisomy 21 human lymphocytes. *Am. J. Hum. Genet.* **52:** 661–667.

22. Allsopp, R.C. *et al.* 1992. Telomere length predicts replicative capacity of human fibroblasts. *Proc. Natl. Acad. Sci. USA* **89:** 10114–10118.

23. Harley, C.B., A.B. Futcher & C.W. Greider. 1990. Telomeres shorten during ageing of human fibroblasts. *Nature* **345:** 458–460.

24. Harley, C.B. *et al.* 1992. The telomere hypothesis of cellular aging. *Exp. Gerontol.* **27:** 375–382.

25. Lundblad, V. & J.W. Szostak. 1989. A mutant with a defect in telomere elongation leads to senescence in yeast. *Cell* **57:** 633–643.

26. Donate, L.E. & M.A. Blasco. 2011. Telomeres in cancer and ageing. *Philos. Trans. R. Soc. Lond. B. Biol. Sci.* **366:** 76–84.

27. Epel, E.S. *et al.* 2004. Accelerated telomere shortening in response to life stress. *Proc. Natl. Acad. Sci. USA* **101:** 17312–17315.

28. McGrath, M. *et al.* 2007. Telomere length, cigarette smoking, and bladder cancer risk in men and women. *Cancer Epidemiol. Biomarkers Prev.* **16:** 815–819.

29. Panossian, L.A. *et al.* 2003. Telomere shortening in T cells correlates with Alzheimer's disease status. *Neurobiol. Aging* **24:** 77–84.

30. Guan, J.Z. *et al.* 2008. A percentage analysis of the telomere length in Parkinson's disease patients. *J. Gerontol. A. Biol. Sci. Med. Sci.* **63:** 467–473.

31. Steer, S.E. *et al.* 2007. Reduced telomere length in rheumatoid arthritis is independent of disease activity and duration. *Ann. Rheum. Dis.* **66:** 476–480.

32. Fitzpatrick, A.L. *et al.* 2007. Leukocyte telomere length and cardiovascular disease in the cardiovascular health study. *Am. J. Epidemiol.* **165:** 14–21.

33. Wiemann, S.U. *et al.* 2002. Hepatocyte telomere shortening and senescence are general markers of human liver cirrhosis. *FASEB J.* **16:** 935–942.

34. Svenson, U. *et al.* 2008. Breast cancer survival is associated with telomere length in peripheral blood cells. *Cancer Res.* **68:** 3618–3623.

35. De Meyer, T. *et al.* 2007. Paternal age at birth is an important determinant of offspring telomere length. *Hum. Mol. Genet.* **16:** 3097–3102.

36. Kimura, M. *et al.* 2008. Offspring's leukocyte telomere length, paternal age, and telomere elongation in sperm. *PLoS Genet.* **4:** 1–9.

37. Njajou, O.T. *et al.* 2007. Telomere length is paternally inherited and is associated with parental lifespan. *Proc. Natl. Acad. Sci. USA* **104:** 12135–12139.

38. Unryn, B.M., L.S. Cook & K.T. Riabowol. 2005. Paternal age is positively linked to telomere length of children. *Aging Cell* **4:** 97–101.

39. Lu, Y. *et al.* 2010. Parents' ages at birth and risk of adult-onset hematologic malignancies among female teachers in California. *Am. J. Epidemiol.* **171:** 1262–1269.

40. Choi, J.Y. *et al.* 2005. Association of paternal age at birth and the risk of breast cancer in offspring: a case control study. *BMC Cancer* **5:** 143–152.

41. Hodgson, M.E., B. Newman & R.C. Millikan. 2004. Birthweight, parental age, birth order and breast cancer risk in African-American and white women: a population-based case-control study. *Breast Cancer Res.* **6:** R656–R667.

42. Xue, F. *et al.* 2007. Parental age at delivery and incidence of breast cancer: a prospective cohort study. *Breast Cancer Res. Treat.* **104:** 331–340.

43. Zhang, Y. *et al.* 1999. Parental age at child's birth and son's risk of prostate cancer. The Framingham Study. *Am. J. Epidemiol.* **150:** 1208–1212.

44. Griffith, J.D. *et al.* 1999. Mammalian telomeres end in a large duplex loop. *Cell* **97:** 503–514.

45. Greider, C.W. 1999. Telomeres do D-loop-T-loop. *Cell* **97:** 419–422.

46. Karlseder, J. *et al.* 1999. p53- and ATM-dependent apoptosis induced by telomeres lacking TRF2. *Science* **283:** 1321–1325.

47. Bull, C. & M. Fenech. 2008. Genome-health nutrigenomics and nutrigenetics: nutritional requirements or 'nutriomes' for chromosomal stability and telomere maintenance at the individual level. *Proc. Nutr. Soc.* **67:** 146–156.

48. Keefe, D.L. and L. Liu. 2009. Telomeres and reproductive aging. *Reprod. Fertil. Dev.* **21:** 10–14.

49. de Lange, T. 2005. Shelterin: the protein complex that shapes and safeguards human telomeres. *Genes Dev.* **19:** 2100–2110.

50. Xin, H., D. Liu & Z. Songyang. 2008. The telosome/shelterin complex and its functions. *Genome. Biol.* **9:** 232–239.

51. Palm, W. & T. de Lange. 2008. How shelterin protects mammalian telomeres. *Annu. Rev. Genet.* **42:** 301–334.

52. Jennings, B.J., S.E. Ozanne & C.N. Hales. 2000. Nutrition, oxidative damage, telomere shortening, and cellular senescence: individual or connected agents of aging? *Mol. Genet. Metab.* **71:** 32–42.

53. Songyang, Z. & D. Liu. 2006. Inside the mammalian telomere interactome: regulation and regulatory activities of telomeres. *Crit. Rev. Eukaryot. Gene Expr.* **16:** 103–118.

54. Verdun, R.E. & J. Karlseder. 2007. Replication and protection of telomeres. *Nature* **447:** 924–931.

55. Verdun, R.E. & J. Karlseder. 2006. The DNA damage machinery and homologous recombination pathway act consecutively to protect human telomeres. *Cell* **127:** 709–720.

56. Chuang, T.C. *et al.* 2004. The three-dimensional organization of telomeres in the nucleus of mammalian cells. *BMC Biol.* **2:** 12–20.

57. Sukenik-Halevy, R. *et al.* 2009. Telomere aggregate formation in placenta specimens of pregnancies complicated with pre-eclampsia. *Cancer Genet. Cytogenet.* **195:** 27–30.

58. Caporali, A. *et al.* 2007. Telomeric aggregates and end-to-end chromosomal fusions require Myc box II. *Oncogene* **26:** 1398–1406.

59. Crott, J.W. *et al.* 2001. The effect of folic acid deficiency and MTHFR C677T polymorphism on chromosome damage in human lymphocytes in vitro. *Cancer Epidemiol. Biomarkers Prev.* **10:** 1089–1096.

60. James, S.J. *et al.* 1994. The effect of folic-acid and/or methionine deficiency on deoxyribonucleotide pools and cell-cycle distribution in mitogen-stimulated rat lymphocytes. *Cell Proliferation* **27:** 395–406.

61. Fenech, M. *et al.* 2011. Molecular mechanisms of micronucleus, nucleoplasmic bridge and nuclear bud formation in mammalian and human cells. *Mutagenesis* **26:** 125–132.

62. Mitchell, T.R. *et al.* 2009. Arginine methylation regulates telomere length and stability. *Mol. Cell Biol.* **29:** 4918–4934.

63. Zhu, X.D. *et al.* 2003. ERCC1/XPF removes the 3′ overhang from uncapped telomeres and represses formation of telomeric DNA-containing double minute chromosomes. *Mol. Cell* **12:** 1489–1498.

64. Riethman, H., A. Ambrosini & S. Paul. 2005. Human subtelomere structure and variation. *Chromosome Res.* **13:** 505–515.

65. Hayflick, L. & P.S. Moorhead. 1961. The serial cultivation of human diploid cell strains. *Exp. Cell Res.* **25:** 585–621.

66. Awaya, N. *et al.* 2002. Telomere shortening in hematopoietic stem cell transplantation: a potential mechanism for late graft failure? *Biol. Blood Marrow Transplant.* **8:** 597–600.

67. Biroccio, A. *et al.* 2003. Inhibition of c-Myc oncoprotein limits the growth of human melanoma cells by inducing cellular crisis. *J. Biol. Chem.* **278:** 35693–35701.

68. Wright, W.E. & J.W. Shay. 1992. The two-stage mechanism controlling cellular senescence and immortalization. *Exp. Gerontol.* **27:** 383–389.

69. Counter, C.M. *et al.* 1992. Telomere shortening associated with chromosome instability is arrested in immortal cells which express telomerase activity. *EMBO J.* **11:** 1921–1929.

70. Londono-Vallejo, J.A. *et al.* 2004. Alternative lengthening of telomeres is characterized by high rates of telomeric exchange. *Cancer Res.* **64:** 2324–2327.

71. Harley, C.B. 1991. Telomere loss: mitotic clock or genetic time bomb? *Mutat. Res.* **256:** 271–282.

72. Martens, U.M. *et al.* 1998. Short telomeres on human chromosome 17p. *Nat. Genet.* **18:** 76–80.

73. Beghelli, S. *et al.* 1998. Pancreatic endocrine tumours: evidence for a tumour suppressor pathogenesis and for a tumour suppressor gene on chromosome 17p. *J. Pathol.* **186:** 41–50.

74. Cornelis, R.S. *et al.* 1994. Evidence for a gene on 17p13.3, distal to TP53, as a target for allele loss in breast tumors without p53 mutations. *Cancer Res.* **54:** 4200–4206.

75. Stocklein, H. *et al.* 2008. Detailed mapping of chromosome 17p deletions reveals HIC1 as a novel tumor suppressor gene candidate telomeric to TP53 in diffuse large B-cell lymphoma. *Oncogene* **27:** 2613–2625.

76. White, G.R. *et al.* 1996. High levels of loss at the 17p telomere suggest the close proximity of a tumour suppressor. *Br. J. Cancer* **74:** 863–870.

77. Chopin, V. & D. Leprince. 2006. [Chromosome arm 17p13.3: could HIC1 be the one ?]. *Med. Sci.* **22:** 54–61.

78. Kimura, M. *et al.* 2004. Methylenetetrahydrofolate reductase C677T polymorphism, folic acid and riboflavin are important determinants of genome stability in cultured human lymphocytes. *J. Nutr.* **134:** 48–56.

79. Morin, G.B. 1989. The human telomere terminal transferase enzyme is a ribonucleoprotein that synthesizes TTAGGG repeats. *Cell* **59:** 521–529.

80. Teixeira, M.T. *et al.* 2004. Telomere length homeostasis is achieved via a switch between telomerase- extendible and -nonextendible states. *Cell* **117:** 323–335.

81. Bryan, T.M. *et al.* 1997. Evidence for an alternative mechanism for maintaining telomere length in human tumors and tumor-derived cell lines. *Nat. Med.* **3:** 1271–1274.

82. Bryan, T.M. *et al.* 1995. Telomere elongation in immortal human cells without detectable telomerase activity. *EMBO J.* **14:** 4240–4248.

83. Muntoni, A. & R.R. Reddel. 2005. The first molecular details of ALT in human tumor cells. *Hum. Mol Genet.* **14 Spec No. 2:** R191–R196.

84. Powers, H.J. 2005. Interaction among folate, riboflavin, genotype, and cancer, with reference to colorectal and cervical cancer. *J. Nutr.* **135:** 2960S–2966S.

85. Berger, S.H., D.L. Pittman & M.D. Wyatt. 2008. Uracil in DNA: consequences for carcinogenesis and chemotherapy. *Biochem. Pharmacol.* **76:** 697–706.

86. Jiang, W.Q. *et al.* 2007. Identification of candidate alternative lengthening of telomeres genes by methionine restriction and RNA interference. *Oncogene* **26:** 4635–4647.

87. Murnane, J.P. 2006. Telomeres and chromosome instability. *DNA Repair* **5:** 1082–1092.

88. Albertson, D.G. 2006. Gene amplification in cancer. *Trends Genet.* **22:** 447–455.

89. Fenech, M. & J.W. Crott. 2002. Micronuclei, nucleoplasmic bridges and nuclear buds induced in folic acid deficient human lymphocytes-evidence for breakage-fusion-bridge cycles in the cytokinesis-block micronucleus assay. *Mutat. Res.* **504:** 131–136.

90. Thomas, P., K. Umegaki & M. Fenech. 2003. Nucleoplasmic bridges are a sensitive measure of chromosome rearrangement in the cytokinesis-block micronucleus assay. *Mutagenesis* **18:** 187–194.

91. Gonzalo, S. *et al.* 2006. DNA methyltransferases control telomere length and telomere recombination in mammalian cells. *Nat. Cell Biol.* **8:** 416–424.

92. Blasco, M.A. 2004. Carcinogenesis Young Investigator Award. Telomere epigenetics: a higher-order control of telomere length in mammalian cells. *Carcinogenesis* **25:** 1083–1087.

93. Gonzalo, S. & M.A. Blasco. 2005. Role of Rb family in the epigenetic definition of chromatin. *Cell. Cycle* **4:** 752–755.

94. Maeda, T. *et al.* 2009. Aging-related alterations of subtelomeric methylation in sarcoidosis patients. *J. Gerontol. A. Biol. Sci. Med. Sci.* **64:** 752–760.

95. Maeda, T. *et al.* 2009. Age-related changes in subtelomeric methylation in the normal Japanese population. *J. Gerontol. A. Biol. Sci. Med. Sci.* **64:** 426–434.

96. Maeda, T. *et al.* 2009. Aging-associated alteration of subtelomeric methylation in Parkinson's disease. *J. Gerontol. A. Biol. Sci. Med. Sci.* **64:** 949–955.

97. Goldberg, A.D., C.D. Allis & E. Bernstein. 2007. Epigenetics: a landscape takes shape. *Cell* **128:** 635–638.

98. Ambros, V. 2004. The functions of animal microRNAs. *Nature* **431:** 350–355.

99. Okano, M., S. Xie & E. Li. 1998. Dnmt2 is not required for de novo and maintenance methylation of viral DNA in embryonic stem cells. *Nucl. Acids Res.* **26:** 2536–2540.

100. Yoder, J.A., C.P. Walsh & T.H. Bestor. 1997. Cytosine methylation and the ecology of intragenomic parasites. *Trends Genet.* **13:** 335–340.

101. Iguchi-Ariga, S.M. & W. Schaffner. 1989. CpG methylation of the cAMP-responsive enhancer/promoter sequence TGACGTCA abolishes specific factor binding as well as transcriptional activation. *Genes Dev.* **3:** 612–619.

102. Choi, S.W. *et al.* 2005. Folate supplementation increases genomic DNA methylation in the liver of elder rats. *Br. J. Nutr.* **93:** 31–35.

103. Friso, S. & S.W. Choi. 2002. Gene-nutrient interactions and DNA methylation. *J. Nutr.* **132:** 2382S–2387S.

104. de Lange, T. *et al.* 1990. Structure and variability of human chromosome ends. *Mol. Cell Biol.* **10:** 518–527.

105. Murray, A.W. & J.W. Szostak. 1986. Construction and behavior of circularly permuted and telocentric chromosomes in *Saccharomyces cerevisiae*. *Mol. Cell Biol.* **6:** 3166–3172.

106. Riethman, H. 2008. Human subtelomeric copy number variations. *Cytogenet. Genome Res.* **123:** 244–252.

107. Riethman, H. *et al.* 2004. Mapping and initial analysis of human subtelomeric sequence assemblies. *Genome Res.* **14:** 18–28.

108. Lander, E.S. *et al.* 2001. Initial sequencing and analysis of the human genome. *Nature* **409:** 860–921.

109. Riethman, H. *et al.* 2003. Human subtelomeric DNA. *Cold Spring Harb. Symp. Quant. Biol.* **68:** 39–47.

110. Brock, G.J., J. Charlton & A. Bird. 1999. Densely methylated sequences that are preferentially localized at telomere-proximal regions of human chromosomes. *Gene* **240:** 269–277.

111. Steinert, S., J.W. Shay & W.E. Wright. 2004. Modification of subtelomeric DNA. *Mol. Cell Biol.* **24:** 4571–4580.

112. Stover, P.J. 2009. One-carbon metabolism-genome interactions in folate-associated pathologies. *J. Nutr.* **139:** 2402–2405.

113. Bailey, S.M., M.A. Brenneman E.H. Goodwin. 2004. Frequent recombination in telomeric DNA may extend the proliferative life of telomerase-negative cells. *Nucl. Acids Res.* **32:** 3743–3751.

114. Bechter, O.E. *et al.* 2004. Telomeric recombination in mismatch repair deficient human colon cancer cells after telomerase inhibition. *Cancer Res.* **64:** 3444–3451.

115. Ng, L.J. *et al.* 2009. Telomerase activity is associated with an increase in DNA methylation at the proximal subtelomere and a reduction in telomeric transcription. *Nucl. Acids Res.* **37:** 1152–1159.

116. Lee, M.E. *et al.* 2009. Subtelomeric DNA methylation and telomere length in human cancer cells. *Cancer Lett.* **281:** 82–91.

117. Baird, D.M. *et al.* 2003. Extensive allelic variation and ultrashort telomeres in senescent human cells. *Nat. Genet.* **33:** 203–207.

118. Azzalin, C.M. *et al.* 2007. Telomeric repeat containing RNA and RNA surveillance factors at mammalian chromosome ends. *Science* **318:** 798–801.

119. Schoeftner, S. & M.A. Blasco. 2008. Developmentally regulated transcription of mammalian telomeres by DNA-dependent RNA polymerase II. *Nat. Cell Biol.* **10:** 228–236.

120. Luke, B. and J. Lingner 2009. TERRA: telomeric repeat-containing RNA. *EMBO J.* **28:** 2503–2510.

121. Nergadze, S.G. *et al.* 2009. CpG-island promoters drive transcription of human telomeres. *RNA* **15:** 2186–2194.

122. Geiman, T.M. & K.D. Robertson. 2002. Chromatin remodeling, histone modifications, and DNA methylation-how does it all fit together? *J. Cell. Biochem.* **87:** 117–125.

123. Yehezkel, S. *et al.* 2008. Hypomethylation of subtelomeric regions in ICF syndrome is associated with abnormally short telomeres and enhanced transcription from telomeric regions. *Hum. Mol. Genet.* **17:** 2776–2789.

124. Garcia-Cao, M. *et al.* 2004. Epigenetic regulation of telomere length in mammalian cells by the Suv39h1 and Suv39h2 histone methyltransferases. *Nat. Genet.* **36:** 94–99.

125. Fanti, L. *et al.* 1998. The heterochromatin protein 1 prevents telomere fusions in Drosophila. *Mol. Cell* **2:** 527–538.

126. Perrini, B. *et al.* 2004. HP1 controls telomere capping, telomere elongation, and telomere silencing by two different mechanisms in Drosophila. *Mol. Cell* **15:** 467–476.

127. Savitsky, M. *et al.* 2002. Heterochromatin protein 1 is involved in control of telomere elongation in Drosophila melanogaster. *Mol. Cell Biol.* **22:** 3204–3218.

128. Furumoto, K. *et al.* 1998. Age-dependent telomere shortening is slowed down by enrichment of intracellular vitamin C via suppression of oxidative stress. *Life Sci.* **63:** 935–948.

129. Richards, J.B. *et al.* 2007. Higher serum vitamin D concentrations are associated with longer leukocyte telomere length in women. *Am. J. Clin. Nutr.* **86:** 1420–1425.

130. Tanaka, Y., Y. Moritoh & N. Miwa. 2007. Age-dependent telomere-shortening is repressed by phosphorylated alpha-tocopherol together with cellular longevity and intracellular oxidative-stress reduction in human brain microvascular endotheliocytes. *J. Cell. Biochem.* **102:** 689–703.

131. Xu, Q. *et al.* 2009. Multivitamin use and telomere length in women. *Am. J. Clin. Nutr.* **89:** 1857–1863.

132. Cassidy, A. *et al.* 2010. Associations between diet, lifestyle factors, and telomere length in women. *Am. J. Clin. Nutr.* **91:** 1273–1280.

133. Farzaneh-Far, R. *et al.* 2010. Association of marine omega-3 fatty acid levels with telomeric aging in patients with coronary heart disease. *JAMA* **303:** 250–257.

134. Nettleton, J.A. *et al.* 2008. Dietary patterns, food groups, and telomere length in the Multi-Ethnic Study of Atherosclerosis (MESA). *Am. J. Clin. Nutr.* **88:** 1405–1412.

135. Pavanello, S. *et al.* 2011. Shortened telomeres in individuals with abuse in alcohol consumption. *Int. J. Cancer.* doi:10.1002/ijc.25999.

136. Diaz, V.A. *et al.* 2010. Effect of healthy lifestyle behaviors on the association between leukocyte telomere length and coronary artery calcium. *Am. J. Cardiol.* **106:** 659–663.

137. Paul, L. 2011. Diet, nutrition and telomere length. *J. Nutr. Biochem.* [Epub ahead of print].

138. Bull, C.F. *et al.* 2009. Telomere length in lymphocytes of older South Australian men may be inversely associated with plasma homocysteine. *Rejuvenation Res.* **12:** 341–349.

139. Panayiotou, A.G. *et al.* 2010. Leukocyte telomere length is associated with measures of subclinical atherosclerosis. *Atherosclerosis* **211:** 176–181.

140. Richards, J.B. *et al.* 2008. Homocysteine levels and leukocyte telomere length. *Atherosclerosis* **200:** 271–277.

141. Duthie, S.J. & A. Hawdon. 1998. DNA instability (strand breakage, uracil misincorporation, and defective repair) is increased by folic acid depletion in human lymphocytes in vitro. *FASEB J.* **12:** 1491–1497.

142. Ahmad, S.I., S.H. Kirk & A. Eisenstark. 1998. Thymine metabolism and thymineless death in prokaryotes and eukaryotes. *Annu. Rev. Microbiol.* **52:** 591–625.

143. Toussaint, M., I. Dionne & R.J. Wellinger. 2005. Limited TTP supply affects telomere length regulation in a telomerase-independent fashion. *Nucl. Acids Res.* **33:** 704–713.

144. Fenech, M.F. 2010. Dietary reference values of individual micronutrients and nutriomes for genome damage prevention: current status and a road map to the future. *Am. J. Clin. Nutr.* **91:** 1438S–1454S.

145. O'Callaghan, N. *et al.* 2008. A quantitative real-time PCR method for absolute telomere length. *Biotechniques* **44:** 807–809.

146. O'Callaghan, N.J. & M. Fenech. 2011. A quantitative PCR method for measuring absolute telomere length. *Biol. Proced. Online* **13:** 3.

147. Britt-Compton, B. *et al.* 2006. Structural stability and chromosome-specific telomere length is governed by cis-acting determinants in humans. *Hum. Mol. Genet.* **15:** 725–733.

148. Gisselsson, D. *et al.* 2002. Centrosomal abnormalities, multipolar mitoses, and chromosomal instability in head and neck tumours with dysfunctional telomeres. *Br. J. Cancer* **87:** 202–207.

149. Henson, J.D. *et al.* 2009. DNA C-circles are specific and quantifiable markers of alternative-lengthening-of-telomeres activity. *Nat. Biotechnol.* **27:** 1181–1185.

150. Kim, N.W. *et al.* 1994. Specific association of human telomerase activity with immortal cells and cancer. *Science* **266:** 2011–2015.

151. Petersen, S., G. Saretzki & T. von Zglinicki. 1998. Preferential accumulation of single-stranded regions in telomeres of human fibroblasts. *Exp. Cell Res.* **239:** 152–160.

152. Kruk, P.A., N.J. Rampino & V.A. Bohr. 1995. DNA damage and repair in telomeres: relation to aging. *Proc. Natl. Acad. Sci. USA* **92:** 258–262.

153. von Zglinicki, T., R. Pilger & N. Sitte. 2000. Accumulation of single-strand breaks is the major cause of telomere shortening in human fibroblasts. *Free Radic. Biol. Med.* **28:** 64–74.

154. Blasco, M.A. 2005. Telomeres and human disease: ageing, cancer and beyond. *Nat. Rev. Genet.* **6:** 611–622.

Ann. N.Y. Acad. Sci. ISSN 0077-8923

ANNALS OF THE NEW YORK ACADEMY OF SCIENCES

Issue: *Nutrition and Physical Activity in Aging, Obesity, and Cancer*

Stem cell engineering: limitation, alternatives, and insight

Jeong Mook Lim,[1,2] Myungook Lee,[1] Eun Ju Lee,[3] Seung Pyo Gong,[4] and Seung Tae Lee[5]

[1]WCU Biomodulation and Department of Agricultural Biotechnology, Seoul National University, Seoul, Korea. [2]Cancer Research Institute, Seoul National University Hospital, Seoul, Korea. [3]Medical Research Center, Seoul National University Hospital, Seoul, Korea. [4]Department of Marine Biomaterials and Aquaculture, Pukyong National University, Busan, Korea. [5]Department of Animal Biotechnology, Kangwon National University, Chunchon, Korea

Address for correspondence: Jeong Mook Lim, Laboratory of Stem Cell and Biomodulation, WCU Biomodulation, Seoul National University, Seoul 151-742, Korea. limjm@snu.ac.kr

The 21st century will see improvements in the quality of human life. The development of new therapeutic technologies will prevent prevalent diseases and enable recovery from currently incurable diseases. The development of cell and tissue replacement therapies using stem cells and their progenitors will accelerate the development of causative treatments. The effort expended thus far in developing cell therapies has revealed many technical limitations. Thus, we must explore conceptual changes in the feasibility of stem cell therapy. This paper introduces the current limitations to stem cell engineering and ways to overcome these limitations, which will provide new insight into their clinical application.

Keywords: stem cells; limitation; tissue-derived; cell niche; cell transformation model

Introduction

Following the first report of the establishment of pluripotent embryonic stem cell (ESC) lines in humans,[1] the development of tissue regeneration therapy was anticipated. People suffering from various incurable diseases were enthusiastic at the news, and many biologists and clinicians anticipated the clinical application of stem cells. Tremendous effort has been made to develop an efficient means of differentiating stem cells into target cells to replace dysfunctional cells in patients. However, scientists soon learned that it is extremely difficult to control the fate and differentiation of pluripotent stem cells. A prerequisite for developing stem cell therapy is to secure immune specificity (i.e., immune tolerance), and it is difficult to establish pluripotent stem cell lines because of technical and ethical obstacles. There has been intense debate over the use of ESC lines for clinical purposes, as the establishment of stem cells requires the sacrifice of viable embryos. There is still room for improvement in the regulation of stem cell self-renewal without cellular and genetic transforma-

tion *in vitro*. The randomized or spontaneous differentiation of stem cells into target cells is another obstacle; it is necessary to know which stem cell stage (e.g., undifferentiated, differentiating, or differentiated) is the best for optimizing cell migration, homing, and regaining tissue function after transplantation. All of these limitations and questions should be addressed at the preclinical and clinical levels.

This paper briefly reviews how scientists have developed alternative methodologies for stem cell manipulation to overcome the current limitations to stem cell engineering. It focuses on the introduction of alternatives for securing immune-specific stem cells and summarizes how scientists have coped with current issues in human cloning by replacing the techniques used to establish ESCs. Scientific progress in establishing induced pluripotent stem (iPS) cells and enriching tissue-specific stem cells from various tissues is also introduced. Finally, we suggest how stem cell fate can be regulated using an artificial environment and discuss alternative uses of stem cells or iPS cells, instead of direct clinical applications.

doi: 10.1111/j.1749-6632.2011.06093.x

Strategies for overcoming current limitations to stem cell engineering

Alternatives to the ethical problems with therapeutic cloning

The establishment of human ESCs (hESCs) led people to anticipate ways to overcome various incurable diseases caused by genetic disorders and organ malfunction.[2] However, research on the clinical application of hESCs inevitably involves the sacrifice of human oocytes and embryos, which has invoked an ethical debate among scientists and ethicists. Problems related to human cloning were increased by the generation of cloned embryos to establish "patient-specific" hESCs. This forced the development of the new concept of "therapeutic cloning," in contrast to "reproductive cloning."[3] In therapeutic cloning, nonimplantable embryos are used to establish ESCs through the nuclear transfer of somatic cells; in comparison, the knockout of implantation-related genes has been suggested as a method of reproductive cloning.[4] Unfortunately, therapeutic cloning cannot avoid the use of the somatic cell cloning technology, which has been used for reproductive cloning. In addition, the influence of the deletion or inactivation of implantation-related genes on stem cell survival and function is unknown. As an alternative, the use of interspecies embryos for deriving hESCs was suggested.[5,6] The generation of interspecies blastocysts via the nuclear transfer of human cord cells into bovine enucleated oocytes was successful. However, this technique was not developed further because the interspecies embryos had severe genetic and cellular abnormalities and showed developmental retardation. Somatic cell nuclear transfer (SCNT) technology itself has room for improvement, and the elucidation of the mechanisms underlying epigenetic cell reprogramming and phenotypes or mitochondrial inheritance is necessary to establish immune-specific stem cells that are functionally normal. No existing alternative to SCNT technology completely avoids the need for human cloning because the generation of viable embryos is essential for the efficient establishment of hESCs.

For obvious ethical reasons, the United Nations banned human cloning (i.e., "reproductive cloning" via SCNT) and the use of hESCs.[7,8] Nevertheless, there is ongoing debate on this topic, and permission has been granted for "therapeutic cloning." In several countries, ethical, legal, and social investi-gations are prerequisite for government funding of stem cell research, and the ethical guidelines regarding stem cell biotechnology have been strengthened in several countries.

Alternatives to the use of human embryos

To avoid the use of human embryos as a source of pluripotent stem cells, SCNT technology must be replaced with an alternative methodology that does not generate viable embryos. The derivation of embryonic or extraembryonic stem cells by culturing a single blastomere retrieved via a noninvasive embryonic biopsy has been attempted.[9] Such techniques can eliminate the use of viable embryos and SCNT, but they enable only the generation of stem cells with immune specificity for the donor embryo, not adult patients. The fusion of a terminally differentiated cell with an ESC has also been suggested, but patient-specific immunogenicity and chromosome stability cannot be guaranteed.[10]

The existence of adult stem cells in various tissues and organs has been reported. However, it is extremely difficult to find these cells in adult tissues. Finding mitosis-activated, pluripotent cells in the blood and the use of cord blood or umbilical cord cells as a stem cell source have also been considered.[11–13] Tissue-specific stem cells have been found in the intestine,[14] hair follicles,[15] mammary glands,[16] dental pulp, and kidneys.[17,18] Stem cells of different types have been derived from both male and female reproductive tissues. Germline stem cell lines have been established by culturing male and female gonadal tissues and developing gametes.[19–21] Tissue-specific stem cells or stem cell-like cells have also been derived from ovarian stromal tissue of nongermline origin.[22]

In 2006, several research groups derived stem cells without performing SCNT.[23] They reported that terminally differentiated fibroblasts could be transformed into pluripotent stem cells by over-expressing key stemness-related genes, including *Klf-4, c-Myc, Oct-4,* and *Sox-2.*[23] Their pluripotency was confirmed, giving rise to the term *iPS cells.* Since then, iPS cell lines have been established from various tissues, and patient-specific iPS cell lines were subsequently established in humans.[24,25] Theoretically and practically, iPS cell technology entirely eliminates the requirement for therapeutic cloning technology to establish patient-specific stem cells. Nevertheless, despite their apparent pluripotent nature, the properties of iPS cells differ from those of ESCs. Among iPS cell lines with different tissue origins, aberrant patterns of the expression of stemness-related or cell cycle-related genes have been detected.[26] There are even differences in the properties of iPS cells among cell lines of different origins,[27] which reduce the efficiency of iPS cell establishment and differentiation potential.[28] Understanding these differences may provide details on the biological role of cell transformation and dedifferentiation. From a different viewpoint, there are strict limitations to the use iPS cell lines for clinical trials because of the genetic manipulation required to establish iPS cells.

Reducing the immunogenicity of stem cells

The acquisition of immune specificity or immune tolerance during the establishment of stem cells is the first priority in developing clinically feasible stem cell engineering. There are two ways to acquire immune specificity: establishing stem cells using either SCNT or iPS cell technology. Unfortunately, neither method can guarantee the acquisition of immune specificity due to the difficulty in regulating extrachromosomal inheritance and the use of gene manipulation, respectively. The establishment of somatic cell-derived adult stem cells is a good alternative; however, a technique for cell enrichment should be developed. A determination was made, based on this concept, that the parthenogenesis of viable oocytes can be used to establish immune-specific stem cells. The potential of parthenogenetic ESC lines has been reported in human[29] and animal[30] models. The difference in gene expression triggered by parthenogenesis is less than that triggered by strain changes. However, no viable offspring derived from parthenogenesis have been delivered to date, and this is essential for deriving clinically useful stem cells. Regardless, viable embryos derived from parthenogenetic activation could be used for human cloning.

As another alternative, a combination of *in vitro* folliculogenesis for the derivation of viable oocytes and parthenogenetic activation for acquiring immune specificity has been suggested. This methodology is based on the consideration that less than 1% of preantral follicles proceed to the final growth stage to give rise to developmentally competent oocytes, while the remaining immature follicles degenerate. If researchers could mobilize the follicles

fated to degenerate to establish stem cells, it would greatly enhance the efficiency of stem cell engineering without using ovulated oocytes. Accordingly, an attempt has been made to derive patient-specific stem cells by using a combined protocol. Several reports have demonstrated the feasibility of follicle growth-oocyte parthenogenesis in an animal model;[31] however, no trial has been conducted in humans. The derivation of viable embryos via follicle culture cannot completely avoid the need for cloning, and this technology can also be used in reproductive medicine and stem cell engineering.

Suggestions to increase the clinical feasibility of stem cell engineering

New technologies for using somatic cell-derived stem cells

Since the first proposal on the development of iPS cell technology, the major focus in establishing patient-specific stem cells has been directed at using somatic cells instead of cloned embryos with SCNT techniques. Many scientists anticipate the use of mesenchymal tissue as the source of stem cells or stem cell progenitors, including blood, bone marrow, fibroblasts, dental pulp, and adipose tissues.[11,18,32] These cells were originally characterized as being multipotent, while recent reports and clinical trials demonstrated their ability to transdifferentiate into cells from different lineages. For example, bone marrow-derived stromal cells transdifferentiated into cardiomyocytes after being transplanted into myocardium.[33] There are several reports on the transdifferentiation of mesenchymal stromal cells into endodermal and ectodermal cells.[34,35] These reports demonstrate that mesenchymal tissue–derived stem cells are contained in the stromal cell fraction.

Despite these promising results, the clinical application of transdifferentiation technology will be delayed because of difficulty isolating a homogenous stem cell population. An extremely small number of stem cells can be detected in and isolated from the stromal cell fraction in mesenchymal tissue. In fact, pilot studies of the use of mesenchymal stem cells remain at the stage of transplanting the mesenchymal stromal cell fraction, which includes a small fraction of stem cells,[36] and the combined use of stem cell-specific markers may limit the efficient retrieval of stem cells with decreased cell viability.[37] Recently, hematology societies have recommended the use of the term *stromal cell* instead of the term *stem cell of mesenchymal origin* until conclusive results are obtained.

Therefore, the isolation of a homogenous stem cell fraction from a mixed stromal cell population is the most important factor limiting the clinical application of mesenchymal stem cells. Techniques for culturing stem cells should also be optimized. It is extremely difficult to maintain mesenchymal tissue–derived stem cells for more than five subpassages due to their heterogeneity and culture inefficiency.[38] It is necessary to discover new stem cell-specific markers in order to elucidate the nature of the stromal cell fraction isolated from bone marrow,[32] adipose tissue,[32] placenta, amniotic fluid and umbilical cord,[13] blood,[11] and mammalian tissue.[18] Noninvasive technologies must also be developed for the effective isolation of stem cells from a mixed stromal cell population. Finding stem cell progenitors in a mixed population of stromal cells is one alternative for retrieving a homogenous population of tissue-derived stem cells, although no noteworthy results have been obtained. iPS cell technology is one choice for using progenitor cells to obtain homogenous stem cells, and this technology might be modified for clinical applications.

Controlling stem cell fate by creating artificial cell niches

As stated above, dedifferentiated stem cells derived through iPS cell technology have limited potential to be used clinically; they can only be applied clinically as cells to support functional stem cells. Therefore, the original iPS cell technology must be modified to produce clinically useful dedifferentiated somatic cell-derived stem cells. The transformation of terminally differentiated cells into stem cells should be possible without genetic manipulation. Several scientists have tried to establish patient-specific stem cells without genetic manipulation.[39] Immune-specific stem cells are derived from fibroblasts or mesenchymal stromal cells cultured with a stem cell extract.[40] Coculture technology has been used to derive somatic cell-derived stem cells, and our group successfully derived ESC-like stem cells from ovarian tissue cultured with embryonic fibroblasts without genetic manipulation (Figs. 1 and 2).[41] Extensive effort has been expended to establish a standard protocol.

As a more advanced strategy, the use of artificial cell niches for stem cell transformation has been proposed based on the fact that the extracellular matrix (ECM) provides an environment for organizing the cellular architecture and determining cell fate and transformation.[42] In addition to its ability to create a structure-constitution environment, the ECM possesses the capacity to accommodate various biological stimulants that control cellular activity.[43] The ECM, which includes fibronectin, collagen, laminin, vitronectin, and tenascin, can be replaced with synthetic oligopeptides that specifically bind to integrin heterodimers expressed on the cell membrane such as the Arg–Gly–Asp (RGD) peptide sequence, the functional motif of collagen, which induces activation of the integrin $\alpha_5\beta_1$ signal.[44] Several reports have demonstrated that a functional matrix or its conjugate oligopeptides can regulate cell fate, metabolism, and transformation via artificial patterning. Previously, we employed three-dimensional (3D) polyethylene glycol (PEG)-based hydrogel crosslinking with dicysteine-containing peptides and an intervening matrix metalloproteinase-specific cleavage site, and natural ECM matrices that were imitated by the conjugation of adhesion oligopeptides derived from each ECM protein (Figs. 3 and 4).[45] Using this artificial ECM, we attempted to regulate stem cell self-renewal by regulating integrin signaling using integrin-stimulation peptide sequences.[45] Our data clearly showed that mouse ESCs could be maintained successfully using this artificial 3D culture system, and that they maintained their morphology and function.

Novel stem cell models for cell transformation and oncogenesis

Basing our understanding on previous attempts to establish clinically feasible stem cell technologies, we realized that an understanding of cell transformation is needed to develop efficient tools for producing immune-specific stem cells. In fact, cell transformation (or dedifferentiation) into stem cells is similar to stem cell transformation into cancer cells. Most stemness-related genes and mRNAs are also cancer cell specific. We believe that iPS cell technology is a powerful tool for understanding oncogenesis in various tissues and organs. The identification of cancer stem cells in various malignant tumors may provide clues for developing technologies to determine whether cells transform into cancer cells or stem cells. Previously, we

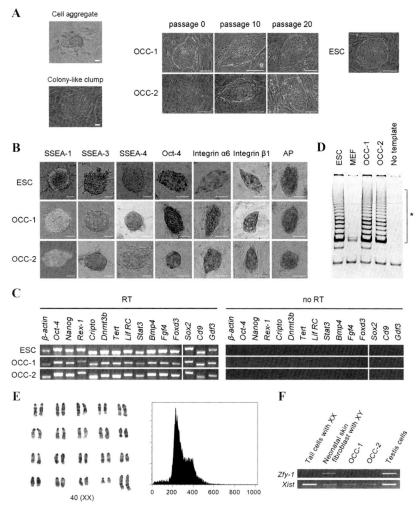

Figure 1. The initial characterization of ovary-derived colony-forming cells (OCCs) derived from the coculture of adult ovarian cells and mouse embryonic fibroblasts (MEF). (A) Cell morphology showing cell aggregates, colony-like clumps, and colony-forming cells on day 7 of primary culture, day 37 after 10 subpassages, and day 67 after 20 subpassages, respectively, with embryonic stem cells (ESCs) as a reference. Scale bar = 50 mm. (B) Antibodies against stage-specific embryonic antigen (SSEA)-1, SSEA-3, and SSEA-4, Oct-4, integrin a_6, integrin b_1, and alkaline phosphatase (AP) were used for cell characterization, with ESCs as a positive control. Similar to the ESCs, the OCCs were positive for SSEA-1, Oct-4, integrin a_6, integrin b_1, and AP. However, both the ESCs and OCCs were negative for SSEA-3 and SSEA-4. Scale bar = 50 mm. (C) Pluripotent cell–specific gene expression by the ESCs and OCCs was monitored by RT-PCR; similar gene expression profiles were detected. (D) Telomerase activity in OCCs as detected by the telomeric repeat amplification protocol assay. A ladder of telomerase products amplified by PCR is shown at six-base increments starting at 50 nucleotides from the location indicated by the asterisk. All lines show high levels of telomerase activity. NC, negative control without added template. (E, F) Karyotyping and sexing of the OCCs. (E) G-banding of air-dried chromosomes in the OCCs was undertaken for exact karyotyping, and the population of diploid cells was estimated using flow cytometry. An image of OCC-B6D2-SNU-1 is shown to represent the established lines; diploidy was detected in the established line. (F) PCR analysis was conducted using the X chromosome–specific primer Xist and Y chromosome–specific primer Zfy. The OCC lines expressed *Xist*, but not *Zfy* (from Gong *et al.*[41]).

determined that the transformation of cells into stem cells without genetic manipulation was possible.[41] However, the specific mechanism of transformation is currently beyond our knowledge of the

regulation of cell function and fate (unpublished data). Further study is necessary to elucidate the mechanism of stem cell transformation, which will greatly contribute to our ability to regulate cell fate

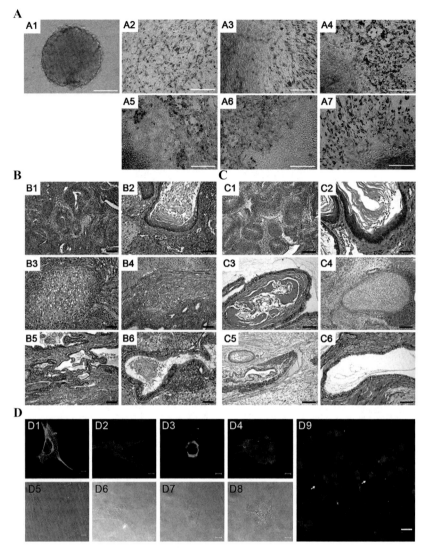

Figure 2. Spontaneous and inducible differentiation of ovary-derived colony-forming cells (OCCs) *in vitro* and *in vivo*. (A) *In vitro* differentiation of OCCs into embryoid bodies on culture in leukemia inhibitory factor (LIF)–free medium. (A1) Embryoid body observed on day 4 of culture. Immunocytochemistry of embryoid bodies was undertaken to detect differentiation along all three germ layers using the specific markers S-100 (A2, ectodermal), nestin (A3, ectodermal), smooth muscle actin (A4, mesodermal), desmin (A5, mesodermal), α-fetoprotein (A6, endodermal), and Troma-1 (A7, endodermal). The results of an analysis of OCC-1 are shown for both established cell lines. Scale bar = 100 mm. (B, C) *In vivo* differentiation of the OCCs following the subcutaneous transplantation of OCC-1 and -2 into NOD-SCID mice. (B) A representative OCC-1–derived teratoma, stained with hematoxylin and eosin, containing (B1) neuroepithelial rosettes, (B2) keratinized stratified squamous epithelial cells, (B3) cartilage, (B4) muscle, (B5) a glandular cuboidal to columnar epithelium, and (B6) ciliated columnar epithelial cells. Scale bar = 50 mm for B1, B4, and B5, and 25 mm for B2 and B3. (C) A representative OCC-2–derived teratoma containing (C1) neuroepithelial rosettes, (C2) keratinized stratified squamous epithelial cells, (C3) an osteoid island showing bony differentiation, (C4) cartilage, (C5) pancreatic tissue, and (C6) ciliated cuboidal epithelial cells. Scale bar = 100 mm for C1 and C5, and 50 mm for C2, C3, C4, and C6. (D) Neuronal cell differentiation of OCCs. (D1) Nestin- and (D2) Tuj1-positive neurons generated 14 days after replating on fibronectin. (D3) O4-positive oligodendrocyte generated eight days and (D4) GFAP-positive astrocytes generated 15 days after replating. (D5-D8) Phase-contrast images of D1–D4. (D9) Merged image of TH- and Tuj1-positive (arrow) neurons generated 19 days after replating on fibronectin. OCCs differentiated in modified N2B27 medium. DAPI (4,6-diamidino-2-phenylindole), blue; TH, green; Tuj1, red. Both established lines exhibited neuronal cell differentiation; the results for OCC-1 are shown for both established cells. Scale bar = 10 mm for D1–D8 and 20 mm for D9 (from Gong *et al.*[41]).

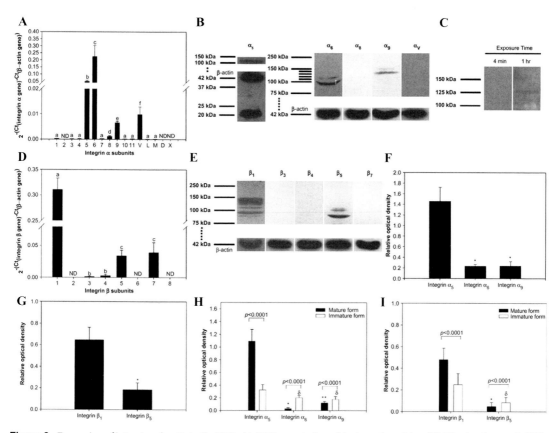

Figure 3. Expression of integrin subunits in the ESCs. (A, D) Transcription of the integrin α (a) and β (d) subunit genes in ESCs. Of the 16 integrin α and eight integrin β subunit genes, real-time PCR showed a significant increase in the transcription of five integrin α and five integrin β subunit genes. (B, C, E) Western blot analysis of integrin α (B, C) and β (E) protein expression in the ESCs. The translation of integrins α_5, α_6, α_9, α_1, and β_5 was identified by immunoblotting and a 4-min film exposure before densitometric analysis. Subsequently, a 1-h exposure was performed for some integrin subunits (α_8, β_3, β_4, β_7, and α_v) that showed no expression using the standard protocol; no expression was detected, except for integrin α_v (C). Both glycosylated mature and non-glycosylated immature forms were observed for integrins α_5, α_6, α_9, β_1, and β_5, and a densitometric analysis of each subunit was performed (F–I). The total amount of each integrin subunit protein expressed (F, G) and the translational levels of mature (with glycosylation) and immature (without glycosylation) protein for each subunit (H, I) are presented as the optical density relative to the level of β-actin expression on the same blot. The greatest total expression of glycosylated mature and nonglycosylated immature proteins was seen for integrins α_5 and β_1, respectively, and significantly more mature than immature integrin α_5 and β_1 was expressed. By contrast, integrins α_6, α_9, and β_5 showed significant decreases in mature relative to immature protein expression. All data shown are the means ± S.D. of five independent experiments. $^{A-F}P < 0.05$; *, **$P < 0.05$; and $^{D}P < 0.05$; ND = not detected (from Lee *et al.*[45]).

and differentiation and to inhibit oncogenesis in various organs.

Conclusions: how far do we go in the future?

Current limitations to the use of stem cells can be summarized as our inability to do the following: (1) harvest immune-specific stem cells; (2) improve the efficiency of stem cell differentiation into target cells; (3) establish transplantation guidelines (optimal stage of transplantation, before or after dif-

ferentiation); (4) establish cell transplantation surgical techniques; (5) improve post-transplantation cell migration without dispersed transplantation, and (6) transplant tissues and organs efficiently and restore their function. The technologies that will be developed to overcome these limitations should meet ethical requirements.

From a clinical viewpoint, there are three major applications of human stem cells of various origins. First, they can be used for cell replacement therapy. Second, human stem cells are a source of

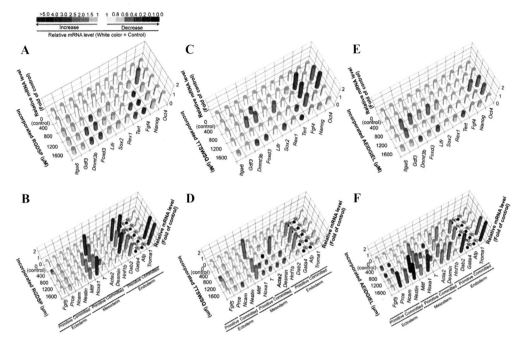

Figure 4. Change in the expression of stemness-related (A, C, E) and differentiation-specific (B, D, F) genes in ESCs after culture in 3D scaffolds containing ECM analog peptides at different concentrations (0, 400, 800, 1200, and 1600 mM). The synthetic adhesion peptides—RGDSP, a ligand for integrins $\alpha_5\beta_1$ and $\alpha_v\beta_5$ (A, B); TTSWSQ, a ligand for integrin $\alpha_6\beta_1$ (C, D); or AEIDGIEL, a ligand for integrin $\alpha_9\beta_1$ (E, F)—were bound to the PEG-based scaffold, and ESCs were subsequently encapsulated within the material. Gene expression was monitored quantitatively by real-time PCR on day 5 of culture in the presence of LIF. In general, stemness-related gene expression was either maintained fully or increased significantly by the addition of 400, 800, and 800 mM RGDSP, TTSWSQ, and AEIDGIEL, respectively. All data shown are the means of four independent experiments. Different colors indicate a significant difference ($P < 0.05$) (from Lee *et al.*[45]).

therapeutic biomaterials. Third, cancer tissue–derived stem cells and stem cells derived through iPS cell technology are an excellent model for cell transformation. To use these applications fully, stem cells must acquire immune specificity or immune tolerance. In terms of quality control and assessment, a homogenous population of stem cells should be secured. Several techniques should be developed, including stem cell culture, stem cell-specific markers, and specific cell niches for stem cell self-renewal and differentiation. An appropriate assessment of stem cell engineering will help establish a better strategy for both basic and clinical research on stem cells.

Acknowledgments

This study was supported by funding from the Stem Cell Research Center of the 21st Century Frontier Research Program (SC-5160) supported by the Ministry of Education, Science, and Technology (MEST), and by the WCU program (R31-10056) through the National Research Foundation of Korea funded by the Ministry of Education, Science, and Technology (MEST). For a certificate, please see:http://www.textcheck.com/certificate/GWTZDS.

Conflicts of interest

The authors declare no conflict of interest.

References

1. Thomson, J.A. 1998. Embryonic stem cell lines derived from human blastocysts. *Science* **282:** 1145–1147.
2. Kehat, I., D. Kenyagin-Karsenti, M. Snir, *et al.* 2002. Human embryonic stem cells can differentiate into myocytes with structural and functional properties of cardiomyocytes. *J. Clin. Invest.* **108:** 407–414.
3. Colman, A. & A. Kind. 2000. Therapeutic cloning: Concepts and practicalities. *Trends Biotechnol.* **18:** 192–196.
4. Meissner, A. & R. Jaenisch. 2006. Generation of nuclear transfer-derived pluripotent ES cells from cloned Cdx2-deficient blastocysts. *Nature* **439:** 212–215.
5. Chang, K.H., J.M. Lim, S.K. Kang, *et al.* 2003. Blastocyst formation, karyotype, and mitochondrial DNA of interspecies embryos derived from nuclear transfer of human cord

fibroblasts into enucleated bovine oocytes. *Fertil. Steril.* **80:** 1380–1387.

6. Chang, K.H., J.M. Lim, S.K. Kang, *et al.* 2004. An optimized protocol of a human-to-cattle interspecies somatic cell nuclear transfer. *Fertil. Steril.* **82:** 960-962.

7. Burley, J. 1999. The ethics of therapeutic and reproductive human cloning. *Semin. Cell Dev. Biol.* **10:** 287–294.

8. United Nations. 2005. International convention against the reproductive cloning of human beings. General Assembly A/59/516/Add.1.

9. Chung, Y., I. Klimanskaya, S. Becker, *et al.* 2008. Human embryonic stem cell lines generated without embryo destruction. *Cell Stem Cell* **2:** 113–117.

10. Tada, M., Y. Takahama, K. Abe, *et al.* 2001. Nuclear reprogramming of somatic cells by in vitro hybridization with ES cells. *Curr. Biol.* **11:** 1553–1558.

11. Zvaifler, N.J., L. Marinova-Mutafchieva, G. Adams, *et al.* 2000. Mesenchymal precursor cells in the blood of normal individuals. *Arthritis Res.* **2:** 477–488.

12. Erices, A., P. Conget, & J.J. Minguell. 2000. Mesenchymal progenitor cells in human umbilical cord blood. *Br. J. Haematol.* **109:** 235–242.

13. Romanov, Y.A., V.A. Svintsitskaya & V.N. Smirnov.2003. Searching for alternative sources of postnatal human mesenchymal stem cells: candidate MSC-like cells from umbilical cord. *Stem Cells* **21:** 105–110.

14. Dekaney, C.M., J.M. Rodriguez, M.C. Graul & S.J. Henning. 2005. Isolation and characterization of a putative intestinal stem cell fraction from mouse jejunum. *Gastroenterology* **129:** 1567–1580.

15. Lyle, S., M. Christofidou-Solomidou, Y. Liu, *et al.* 1998. The C8/144B monoclonal antibody recognizes cytokeratin 15 and defines the location of human hair follicle stem cells. *J. Cell Sci.* **111:** 3179–3188.

16. Welm, B., F. Behbod, M.A. Goodell & J.M. Rosen. 2003. Isolation and characterization of functional mammary gland stem cells. *Cell Prol.* **36**(Suppl.): 17–32.

17. Gronthos, S., M. Mankani, J. Brahim, *et al.* 2000. Postnatal human dental pulp stem cells (DPSCs) *in vitro* and *in vivo*. *Proc. Nat. Acad. Sci. U.S.A.* **97:** 13625–13630.

18. Gupta, S., C. Verfaillie, D. Chmielewski, *et al.* 2006. Isolation and characterization of kidney-derived stem cells. *J. Am. Soc. Nephrol.* **17:** 3028–3040.

19. Hofmann, M.-C., L. Braydich-Stolle & M. Dym. 2005. Isolation of male germ-line stem cells; influence of GDNF. *Dev. Biol.* **279:** 114–124.

20. Johnson, J., J. Canning, T. Kaneko, *et al.* 2004. Germline stem cells and follicular renewal in the postnatal mammalian ovary. *Nature,* **428:** 145–150.

21. Guan, K., K. Nayernia, L.S. Maier, *et al.* 2006. Pluripotency of spermatogonial stem cells from adult mouse testis. *Nature* **440:** 1199–1203.

22. Parrott, J.A. & M.K. Skinner. 2000. Kit ligand actions on ovarian stromal cells: effects on theca cell recruitment and steroid production. *Mol. Reprod. Dev.* **55:** 55–64.

23. Takahashi, K. & S. Yamanaka. 2006. Induction of pluripotent stem cells from mouse embryonic and adult fibroblast cultures by defined factors. *Cell* **126:** 663–676.

24. Yu, J., M.A. Vodyanik, K. Smuga-Otto, *et al.* 2007. Induced pluripotent stem cell lines derived from human somatic cells. *Science* **318:** 1917–1920.

25. Park, I.-H., R. Zhao, J.A. West, *et al.* 2008. Reprogramming of human somatic cells to pluripotency with defined factors. *Nature* **451:** 141–146.

26. Lister, R., M. Pelizzola, R.H. Dowen, *et al.* 2009. Human DNA methylomes at base resolution show widespread epigenomic differences. *Nature* **462:** 315–322.

27. Lister, R., M. Pelizzola, Y.S. Kida, *et al.* 2011. Hotspots of aberrant epigenomic reprogramming in human induced pluripotent stem cells. *Nature* **471:** 68–73.

28. Polo, J.M., S. Liu, M.E. Figueroa, *et al.* 2010. Cell type of origin influences the molecular and functional properties of mouse induced pluripotent stem cells. *Nat. Biotechnol.* **28:** 848–855.

29. Mai, Q., Y. Yu, T. Li, *et al.* 2007. Derivation of human embryonic stem cell lines from parthenogenetic blastocysts. *Cell Res.* **17:** 1008–1019.

30. Cibelli, J.B., K.A. Grant, K.B. Chapman, *et al.* 2002. Parthenogenetic stem cells in nonhuman primates. *Science* **295:** 819.

31. Kim, I.W., S.P. Gong, C.R. Yoo, *et al.* 2009. Derivation of developmentally competent oocytes by the culture of preantral follicles retrieved from adult ovaries: maturation, blastocyst formation, and embryonic stem cell transformation. *Fertil. Steril.* **92:** 1716–1724.

32. Sakaguchi, Y., I. Sekiya, K. Yagishita & T. Muneta. 2005. Comparison of human stem cells derived from various mesenchymal tissues: superiority of synovium as a cell source. *Arthritis Rheum.* **52:** 2521–2529.

33. Kawada, H., J., Fujita, K., Kinjo, *et al.* 2004. Nonhematopoietic mesenchymal stem cells can be mobilized and differentiate into cardiomyocytes after myocardial infarction. *Blood* **104:** 3581–3587.

34. Woodbury, D., K. Reynolds & I.B. Black. 2002. Adult bone marrow stromal stem cells express germline, ectodermal, endodermal, and mesodermal genes prior to neurogenesis. *J. Neurosci. Res.* **69:** 908–917.

35. Jiang, Y., B.N. Jahagirdar, R.L. Reinhardt, *et al.* 2002. Pluripotency of mesenchymal stem cells derived from adult marrow. *Nature,* **418:** 41–49.

36. Pittenger, M.F., A.M. Mackay, S.C. Beck, *et al.* 1999. Multilineage potential of adult human mesenchymal stem cells. *Science* **284:** 143–147.

37. Booth, L.H. & K. O'Halloran 2011. A comparison of biomarker responses in the earthworm *Aporrectodea caliginosa* to the organophosphorus insecticides diazinon and chlorpyrifos. *Environ. Toxicol. Chem.* **20:** 2494–2502.

38. Banfi, A., A. Muraglia, B. Dozin, *et al.* 2000. Proliferation kinetics and differentiation potential of ex vivo expanded human bone marrow stromal cells: implications for their use in cell therapy. *Exp. Hematol.* **28:** 707–715.

39. Kossack, N., J. Meneses, S. Shefi, *et al.* 2009. Isolation and characterization of pluripotent human spermatogonial stem cell-derived cells. *Stem Cells* **27:** 138–149.

40. Taranger, C.K., A. Noer, A.L. Sørensen, *et al.* 2005. Induction of dedifferentiation, genomewide transcriptional programming, and epigenetic reprogramming by extracts of

carcinoma and embryonic stem cells. *Mol. Biol. Cell.* **16:** 5719–5735.

41. Gong, S.P., S.T. Lee, E.J. Lee, *et al.* 2010. Embryonic stem cell-like cells established by culture of adult ovarian cells in mice. *Fertil. Steril.* **93:** 2594–2601.

42. Spradling, A., D. Drummond-Barbosa & T. Kai. 2001. Stem cells find their niche. *Nature* **414:** 98–104.

43. Carey, D.J. 1991. Control of growth and differentiation of vascular cells by extracellular matrix proteins. *Annu. Rev. Physiol.* **53:** 161–177.

44. Rowley, J.A., G. Madlambayan & D.J. Mooney. 1999. Alginate hydrogels as synthetic extracellular matrix materials. *Biomaterials* **20:** 45–53.

45. Lee, S.T., J.I. Yun, Y.S. Jo, *et al.* 2010. Engineering integrin signaling for promoting embryonic stem cell self-renewal in a precisely defined niche. *Biomaterials* **31:** 1219–1226.

Ann. N.Y. Acad. Sci. ISSN 0077-8923

ANNALS OF THE NEW YORK ACADEMY OF SCIENCES

Issue: *Nutrition and Physical Activity in Aging, Obesity, and Cancer*

Inhibitory mechanism of lycopene on cytokine expression in experimental pancreatitis

Hyeyoung Kim

Department of Food and Nutrition, Brain Korea 21 Project, College of Human Ecology, Yonsei University, Seoul, South Korea

Address for correspondence: Hyeyoung Kim, Department of Food and Nutrition, College of Human Ecology, Yonsei University, Seoul 120-749, South Korea. kim626@yonsei.ac.kr

Reactive oxygen species (ROS) are important mediators to induce pancreatitis. Serum levels of antioxidant enzymes and carotenoids including lycopene are lower in patients with pancreatitis than those of healthy subjects. The cholecystokinin (CCK) analog cerulein induces similar pathologic events as shown in human pancreatitis. Recent studies show that high doses of cerulein activate NF-κB and induce the expression of inflammatory cytokines, in pancreatic acinar cells, which is mediated by the activation of NADPH oxidase. Lycopene functions as a very potent antioxidant to suppress the induction of inflammatory cytokines, in pancreatic acinar cells stimulated with cerulein. In this review, the possible beneficial effect of lycopene on experimental pancreatitis shall be discussed based on its antioxidant activity.

Keywords: lycopene; pancreatitis; oxidative stress

Introduction

Increased production of reactive oxygen species (ROS) has been demonstrated in the pathogenesis of pancreatitis. Lower status of carotenoids was reported in patients with chronic pancreatitis than those in healthy subjects.[1] Supplementation of carotenoids reduces the complications of the patients with chronic pancreatitis, even though the absorption of carotenoids is relatively low in patients with pancreatitis. Carotenoids play several biological roles, including antioxidant activity, immune modulation, and regulation of cellular differentiation.[2,3] Supplementation of carotenoids has been suggested for inhibiting the progression of symptoms in patients with cancer and heart disease.[4–6] Lycopene shows potent antioxidant activity among carotenois *in vitro* assay systems.[7,8] Since ROS are produced in pancreatic acinar cells [9] as well as infiltrated neutrophils [10,11] during pancreatitis, lycopene might be beneficial for preventing or reducing inflammatory events in pancreas.

Oxidative stress and pancreatitis

Oxidative stress has been reported as one of the important pathogenic factors in human acute and chronic pancreatitis since serum levels of antioxidants including carotenoids were reduced in the patients with pancreatitis.[1,11–16] Cytokines such as interleukin-1β (IL-1β), interleukin-6 (IL-6), and tumor necrosis factor-α (TNF-α) mediate pancreatic inflammation.[17–19] IL-1β and TNF-α are released from activated macrophage and aggravate pancreatic inflammation with the action of IL-6.[20–24] Cytokine expression is mainly regulated by nuclear factor-κB (NF-κB).[25,26] Cytokines and ROS are known stimulators for NF-κB activation in various cells.[27]

Cerulein pancreatitis as an experimental model

Cerulein is a cholecystokinin (CCK) analog that induces similar physiological and biochemical changes shown in human acute pancreatitis. The pathological events include dysregulation of secretion of amylase and lipase and infiltration of neutrophils into pancreas.[28–32] CCK has two receptors, CCK_1 (CCK_A) and CCK_2 (CCK_B) receptors,[33] that mediate G-protein–coupled receptor-initiated inflammatory signaling (Fig. 1). Binding of cerulein to the CCK receptor initiates transient increase in

doi: 10.1111/j.1749-6632.2011.06107.x

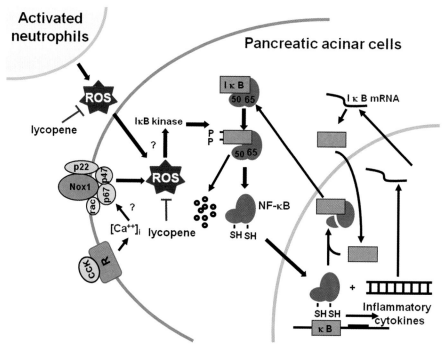

Figure 1. Inhibition by lycopene on cerulein-induced activation of NF-κB and cytokine expression in pancreatic acinar cells. Cerulein binds the CCK receptor (R), which is a G-protein–coupled receptor. Ligand receptor binding initiates a transient increase in intracellular Ca^{2+}. Ca^{2+} may activate NADPH oxidase by stimulating tanslocation of cytosolic subunits ($p47^{phox}$, $p67^{phox}$) to the membrane and activating small G protein rac in pancreatic acinar cells. ROS, produced by an NADPH oxidase, induce the activation of IκB kinase, which in turn phosphorylates IκB in the cytosol. IκB is an inhibitory subunit bound to NF-κB, a p65/p50 heterodimer in the cytosol. Phosphorylated IκB is ubiquitinated and degraded in a proteasome-dependent manner. NF-κB translocates to the nucleus and regulates cytokine expression. NF-κB is recycled after binding to κB in the nucleus and transported to the cytosol. ROS are produced in pancreatic acinar cells or infiltrated neutrophils. Scavenging ROS by lycopene inhibits activation of the oxidant-sensitive transcription factor NF-κB and thus suppresses cytokine expression in pancreatic acinar cells. 50, NF-κB subunit p50; 65, NF-κB subunit p65; CCK, cholecystokinin; p22, $p22^{phox}$; p67, $p67^{phox}$; p47, $p47^{phox}$. This figure is adapted and modified from our previous paper.[34]

intracellular Ca^{2+}. Ca^{2+} may activate NADPH oxidase by stimulating tanslocation of cytosolic subunits ($p47^{phox}$, $p67^{phox}$) to the membrane and activating small G protein rac to produce ROS in pancreatic acinar cells.[34] ROS are considered the major pathogenic factors in pancreatitis.[35,36] NF-κB activation and cytokine expression are mediated by ROS in cerulein-stimulated pancreatic acinar cells.[9] It has been reported that ROS induce the expression to IL-1β, IL-6, and TNF-α in the development of pancreatitis.[37,38] We previously prepared an *in vitro* model of pancreatitis using freshly isolated pancreatic acinar cells cocultured with freshly isolated neutrophils primed with 4β-phorbol 12β-myristate 13α-acetate (PMA).[39] The PMA-primed neutrophils activated acinar cells to induce the expression of inflammatory cytokines. Therefore, ROS

may be produced in both infiltrated neutrophils and pancreatic acinar cells during pancreatitis. Antioxidants that scavenge ROS or inhibitors that suppress the production of ROS may prevent the development of pancreatitis by inhibiting the upstream signaling for inflammation in pancreas.

Antioxidant and anti-inflammatory activities of lycopene

Lycopene contributes to the red color of tomatoes. It is an effective antioxidant as well as a singlet oxygen quencher.[40,41] Recently, we showed that lycopene inhibited NF-κB activation and IL-6 expression in pancreatic acinar cells.[42] Lycopene reduced peroxynitrite- or oxidative stress–induced DNA damage in Chinese hamster lung fibroblasts[43,44] and Hep3B cells in a dose-dependent manner.[45] Lycopene reduced the levels of cytokines such as IL-6 in older women[46] and prostate cancer cell cultures,[47] while it suppressed the expression of intracellular adhesion molecule-1 (ICAM-1) by inhibiting NF-κB activation in human umbilical endothelial cells.[48] Lycopene inhibited activation of NF-κB and mitogen-activated protein kinases in murine dendritic cells.[49] Therefore, lycopene could inhibit the induction of inflammatory cytokines by suppressing NF-κB activation through its antioxidant action in pancreatic acinar cells (Fig. 1). The antioxidant activity of lycopene is closely related to its anti-inflammatory activity.

The intake of lycopene reduced serum levels of oxidative stress indices such as lipid peroxides.[50] Malnutrition leads to carotenoid deficiency, and simple dietary supplementation improves lycopene status, even in patients with malabsorption.[51] In this aspect, dietary supplementation of carotenoids may be beneficial for preventing the development of pancreatitis, especially for people in the state of malnutrition due to smoking or alcohol consumption. The consumption of naturally occurring lycopene-rich fruits and vegetables is recommended for the prevention of oxidative stress–associated inflammatory diseases, including pancreatitis.

Acknowledgments

This study was supported by the Basic Science Research Program through the National Research Foundation of Korea (NRF), funded by the Ministry of Education, Science and Technology (2011–0001177). H.K. is grateful to the Brain Korea 21 Project, College of Human Ecology, Yonsei University.

Conflicts of interest

The author declares no conflicts of interest.

References

1. Quilliot, D. *et al*. 2011. Carotenoid deficiency in chronic pancreatitis: the effect of an increase in tomato consumption. *Eur. J. Clin. Nutr.* **65:** 262–268.
2. Bendich, A. & J.A. Olson. 1989. Biological actions of carotenoids. *FASEB J.* **3:** 1927–1932.
3. Russell, R. 2006. The multifunctional carotenoids: insights into their behavior. *J. Nutr.* **136:** 1690S–2692S.
4. Rao, A.V. & S. Agarwal. 2000. Role of antioxidant lycopene in cancer and heart disease. *J. Am. Coll. Nutr.* **19:** 563–569.
5. Rao, A.V. 2002. Lycopene, tomatoes, and the prevention of coronary heart disease. *Exp. Biol. Med.* **227:** 908–913.
6. Canene-Adams, K. *et al*. 2005. The tomato as a functional food. *J. Nutr.* **135:** 1226–1230.
7. Di Mascio, P., S. Kaiser & H. Sies. 1989. Lycopene as the most efficient biological carotenoid singlet oxygen quencher. *Arch. Biochem. Biophys.* **274:** 532–538.
8. Stahl, W. *et al*. 1998. Carotenoid mixtures protect multilamellar liposomes against oxidative damage: synergistic effects of lycopene and lutein. *FEBS Lett.* **427:** 305–308.
9. Yu, J.H. *et al*. 2002. Suppression of cerulein-induced cytokine expression by antioxidants in pancreatic acinar cells. *Lab. Invest.* **10:** 1359–1368.
10. Schoenberg, M.H. *et al*. 1990. Oxygen free radicals in acute pancreatitis of the rat. *Gut* **10:** 1138–1143.
11. Park, B.K. *et al*. Role of oxygen free radicals in patients with acute pancreatitis. *World J. Gastroenterol.* **10:** 2266–2269.
12. Scott, P. *et al*. 1993. Vitamin C status in patients with acute pancreatitis. *Br. J. Surg.* **80:** 750–754.
13. Schoenberg, M.H., D. Birk & H.G. Beger. 1995. Oxidative stress in acute and chronic pancreatitis. *Am. J. Clin. Nutri.* **62:** 1306S–1314S.
14. Braganza, J.M. *et al*. 1993. Micronutrient antioxidant status in tropical compared with temperate-zone chronic pancreatitis. *Scand. J. Gastroenterol.* **28:** 1098–1104.
15. Van Gossum, A. *et al*. 1996. Deficiency in antioxidant factors in patients with alcohol-related chronic pancreatitis. *Dig. Dis. Sci.* **41:** 1225–1231.
16. Mathew, P. *et al*. 1996. Antioxidants in hereditary pancreatitis. *Am. J. Gastroenterol.* **91:** 1558–1562.
17. Viedma, J.A. *et al*. 1992. Role of interleukin-6 in acute pancreatitis. Comparison with C-reactive protein and phospholipase A. *Gut* **33:** 1264–1267.
18. Heath, D.I. *et al*. 1993. Role of interleukin-6 in mediating the acute phase protein response and potential as an early means of severity assessment in acute pancreatitis. *Gut* **34:** 41–45.
19. Sameshima, H. *et al*. 1993. The role of tumor necrosis factor-alpha in the aggravation of cerulein-induced pancreatitis in rats. *Int. J. Pancreatol.* **14:** 107–115.
20. McKay, C.J. *et al*. 1996. Increased monocyte cytokine production in association with systemic complications in acute pancreatitis. *Br. J. Surg.* **83:** 919–923.
21. Tracey, K.J. & A. Cerami. 1992. Tumor necrosis factor and regulation of metabolism in infection: role of systemic versus tissue levels. *Proc. Soc. Exp. Biol. Med.* **200:** 233–239.
22. Zamir, O. *et al*. 1992. Evidence that tumor necrosis factor participates in the regulation of muscle proteolysis during sepsis. *Arch. Surg.* **127:** 170–174.
23. Schirmer, W.J., J.M. Schirmer & D.E. Fry. 1989. Recombinant human tumor necrosis factor produces hemodynamic changes characteristic of sepsis and endotoxemia. *Arch. Surg.* **124:** 445–448.
24. Kishimoto, T., T. Taga & S. Akira. 1997. Cytokine signal transduction. *Cell* **76:** 253–262.
25. Barnes, P.J. & M. Karin. 1997. Nuclear factor-κB: a pivotal transcription factor in chronic inflammatory diseases. *N. Engl. J. Med.* **336:** 1066–1071.
26. Wulczyn, F.G., D. Krappmann & C. Scheidereit. 1996. The NF-κB/Rel and IκB gene families: mediators of immune response and inflammation. *J. Mol. Med.* **74:** 749–769.

27. Meyer, M., R. Schreck & P.A. Baeuerle. 1993. Hydrogen peroxide and antioxidants have opposite effects on activation of NF-κB and AP-1 in intact cells: AP-1 as secondary antioxidant-responsive factor. *EMBO J.* **12:** 2005–2015.

28. Go, V.W. *et al.* 1993. *The Pancreas: Biology, Pathobiology, and Disease.* 2nd ed. Raven Press. New York.

29. Willemer, S., H.P. Elsasser & G. Adler. 1992. Hormone-induced pancreatitis. *Eur. Surg. Res.* **24**(S1): 29–39.

30. Jensen, R.T. *et al.* 1989. Interaction of CCK with pancreatic acinar cells. *Trends. Pharmacol. Sci.* **10:** 418–423.

31. Sato, S. *et al.* Receptor occupation, calcium mobilization, and amylase release in pancreatic acini: effect of CCK-JMV-180. 1989. *Am. J. Physiol.* **257**(Gastrointest Liver Physiol 20): G202–G209.

32. Lerch, M.M. & G. Adler. 1994. Experimental animal models of acute pancreatitis. *Int. J. Pancreatol.* **15:** 159–170.

33. Alexander, S.D.H., A. Mathie & J.A Peters. 2001. Nomenclature supplement. *Trends Pharmacol. Sci.* **22:** S1–S145.

34. Okumura, N., A. Sakakibara & T. Hayakawa. 1982. Pancreatic endocrine function in experimental pancreatolithiasis in dogs. *Am. J. Gastroenterol.* **77:** 392–396.

35. Aho, H.J., T.J. Nevalainen & V.T. Havia. 1982. Human acute pancreatitis. A light and electron microscopic study. *Acta Pathol. Microbiol. Immunol. Scand. Section A.* **90:** 367–373.

36. Uys, C.J., S. Bank & I.N. Marks. 1973. The pathology of chronic pancreatitis in Cape Town. *Digestion* **9:** 454–468.

37. Heath, D.L., D.H. Cruickshank & M. Gudgeon. 1993. Role of interleukin-6 in mediating the acute phase protein response and potential as an early means of severity assessment in acute pancreatitis. *Gut* **66:** 41–45.

38. Norman, J., M. Franz & A. Riker. 1994. Rapid elevation of systemic cytokines during acute pancreatitis and their origination within the pancreas. *Surg. Forum.* **45:** 148–150.

39. Seo, J.Y. *et al.* 2002. Oxidative stress-induced cytokine production in isolated rat pancreatic acinar cells: effects of small molecule antioxidants. *Pharmacology* **64:** 63–70.

40. Di Mascio, P., S. Kaiser & H. Sies. 1989. Lycopene as the most efficient biological carotenoid singlet oxygen quencher. *Arch. Biochem. Biophys.* **274:** 532–538.

41. Stahl, W. *et al.* 1998. Carotenoid mixtures protect multilamellar liposomes against oxidative damage: synergistic effects of lycopene and lutein. *FEBS Lett.* **427:** 305–308.

42. Kang, M., K.S. Park & H. Kim. 2011. Lycopene inhibits IL-6 expression in cerulein-stimulated pancreatic acinar cells. *Gene Nutr.* **6:** 117–123.

43. Muzandu K. *et al.* 2006. Effect of lycopene and beta-carotene on peroxynitrite-mediated cellular modifications. *Toxicol. Appl. Pharmacol.* **215:** 330–340.

44. Muzandu, K. *et al.* 2005. Lycopene and beta-carotene ameliorate catechol estrogen-mediated DNA damage. *Jpn. J. Vet. Res.* **52:** 173–184.

45. Park, Y.O., E.S. Hwang & T.W. Moon. 2005. The effect of lycopene on cell growth and oxidative DNA damage of Hep3B human hepatoma cells. *Biofactors* **23:** 129–139.

46. Walston. J. *et al.* 2006. Serum antioxidants, inflammation, and total mortality in older women. *Am. J. Epidemiol.* **163:** 18–26.

47. Feng, D., W.H. Ling & R.D. Duan. 2010. Lycopene suppresses LPS-induced NO and IL-6 production by inhibiting the activation of ERK, p38MAPK, and NF-κB in macrophages. *Inflamm. Res.* **59:** 115–121.

48. Hung, C.F. *et al.* 2008. Lycopene inhibits TNF-α-induced endothelial ICAM-1 expression and monocyte-endothelial adhesion. *Eur. J. Pharmacol.* **586:** 275–282.

49. Kim, G.Y. *et al.* 2004. Lycopene suppresses the lipopolysaccharide-induced phenotypic and functional maturation of murine dendritic cells through inhibition of mitogen-activated protein kinases and nuclear factor-κB. *Immunology* **113:** 203–211.

50. Rao, A.V. & S. Agarwal. 1998. Bioavailability and *in vivo* antioxidant properties of lycopene from tomato products and their possible role in the prevention of cancer. *Nutr. Cancer* **31:** 199–203.

51. Quilliot, D. *et al.* 2011. Carotenoid deficiency in chronic pancreatitis: the effect of an increase in tomato consumption. *Eur. J. Clin. Nutr.* **65:** 262–268.

Ann. N.Y. Acad. Sci. ISSN 0077-8923

ANNALS OF THE NEW YORK ACADEMY OF SCIENCES

Issue: *Nutrition and Physical Activity in Aging, Obesity, and Cancer*

Genomic biomarkers and clinical outcomes of physical activity

Alberto Izzotti

Department of Health Sciences, Faculty of Medicine, University of Genoa, Genoa, Italy

Address for correspondence: Alberto Izzotti, Department of Health Sciences, University of Genoa, Via A. Pastore 1, I-16132, Genoa, Italy. izzotti@unige.it

Clinical and experimental studies in humans provide evidence that moderate physical activity significantly decreases artery oxidative damage to nuclear DNA, DNA-adducts related to age and dyslipedemia, and mitochondrial DNA damage. Maintenance of adequate mitochondrial function is crucial for preventing lipid accumulation and peroxidation occurring in atherosclerosis. Studies performed on human muscle biopsies analyzing gene expression in living humans reveal that physically active subjects improve the expression of genes involved in mitochondrial function and of related microRNAs. The attenuation of oxidative damage to nuclear and mitochondrial DNA by physical activity resulted in beneficial effects due to polymorphisms of glutathione S-transferases genes. Subjects bearing null *GSTM1/T1* polymorphisms have poor life expectancy in the case of being sedentary, which was increased 2.6-fold in case they performed physical activity. These findings indicate that the preventive effect of physical activity undergoes interindividual variation affected by genetic polymorphisms.

Keywords: physical activity; molecular biomarkers; DNA damage; gene expression; gene polymorphisms

Introduction

Chronic degenerative diseases, including cancer and atherosclerosis, arise from the long-term accumulation of molecular alterations inside of the cells comprising the target tissue. In turn, these molecular alterations involve DNA damage, as well as changes in genes, microRNA, and protein expression, resulting in the transformation of genetic damage into phenotypic and functional decrements that determine disease occurrence. Based on this premise, risk factors contribute to the accumulation of these detrimental molecular changes, whereas protective factors hamper these molecular events.

Physical activity is currently recognized as a potent tool for the prevention of chronic degenerative diseases, including cardiovascular diseases and common cancers such as those affecting the colon, breast, prostate, and endometrium. This preventive effect occurs through specific mechanisms that act before the onset of disease in healthy organisms; thus, physical activity is a fundamental tool for primary disease prevention. To understand the mechanism by which physical activity exerts its potent action, this article reviews the effect of physical activity on molecular biomarkers associated with chronic degenerative diseases. This issue is crucial to provide biological plausibility for the preventive effects of physical activity and to clarify the eventual occurrence of interindividual variability in receiving these preventive benefits. To examine this issue, we refer to interventional preventive studies performed on subjects at high risk for cardiovascular diseases. This review article primarily analyzes a series of molecular epidemiology studies.[1–4] In these studies, a cohort of 107 subjects (96 males and 11 females; age 70 ± 0.83 years, mean $\pm$ SE) were divided into two groups according to their physical activity levels. Of the 107 subjects, 51 (48%) were physically active, performing at least 45 min of walking per day at least five days per week. The remaining 56 (52%) subjects were sedentary. The subjects were followed for up to 15 years, between 1992 and 2007. During this period, all of the subjects

doi: 10.1111/j.1749-6632.2011.06091.x

underwent surgical intervention for the removal of aortic atherosclerotic lesions for therapeutic purposes. All patients were active smokers. Details of these patients have been reported previously.[1] All subjects received the same standard medical therapy (antihypertensives and anti-aggregants) at the same hospital. A battery of molecular biomarkers was analyzed in the smooth muscle cells from the medium layer of the 107 aorta specimens, including DNA alterations (e.g., 8-hydroxy-2′-deoxyguanosin [8-oxo-dG], bulky DNA adducts, and the common 4977 bp deletion of mitochondrial DNA) and genetic polymorphisms (e.g., GSTM1, GSTT1, NAT1, NAT2, MTHFR, prothrombin, and factor V Leiden). Clinical outcomes were recorded in terms of morbidity and mortality.

The findings of these studies have been analyzed with a focus on the effect of physical activity on specific molecular biomarkers and clinical outcomes. The results obtained are discussed with reference to the current literature regarding the molecular effects of physical exercise in an effort to understand the mechanisms by which physical activity modulates molecular biomarkers and improves clinical outcomes.

DNA biomarkers and cardiovascular diseases

Bulky DNA adducts were consistently detected by ^{32}P-postlabeling in aorta samples, and their number was related to risk factors such as age, cigarette smoking, hypertension, and high blood lipid level, as previously reported.[3] Compared to inactive subjects, the number of DNA adducts related to age and triglycerides in physically active subjects were significantly ($P < 0.05$) lower by 77% and 34%, respectively (Fig. 1). Mitochondria play a major role in determining the levels of these molecular lesions. Indeed, these organelles are the main endogenous source of intracellular reactive oxygen species accumulating during aging[5] as well as the intracellular location where the lipid catabolism occurs through the beta-oxidation pathway. Accordingly, it is conceivable that the observed decreased in age- and triglyceride-related DNA adducts in physically active subjects is amenable to the improved mitochondrial function consequent to physical exercise, as reported below.

The antioxidant effect in the aorta exerted by physical activity was confirmed by measuring 8-oxo-dG to analyze oxidative DNA lesions. We found that 8-oxo-dG was present at very high levels in the aortas of the examined subjects, with particular reference to the cells contained in the inner layer of the vessel.

In the 107 subjects, a robust correlation between 8-oxo-dG levels in the aorta and blood triglycerides was detected ($r = 0.888$, $P < 0.001$). This finding further supports the hypothesis that the strict relationship occurring between oxidative DNA alterations and defective lipid catabolism and overload in the artery is likely related to the failure of mitochondrion function (see below).

Compared to sedentary subjects, physically active subjects exhibited significantly lower levels of 8-oxo-dG (2.8-fold difference; $P < 0.01$). The levels of 8-oxo-dG were 187.09 ± 94.92 and 66.64 ± 40.18 (mean $\pm$ SE) 8-oxo-dG/10^5 dG in sedentary subjects and active subjects, respectively (Fig. 2, left panel). As reported, this finding may partially be amenable to the improvement of mitochondrial function induced by physical activity. It is known, however, that a variety of other mechanisms contribute to the antioxidant effect of low-endurance physical activity. It has been demonstrated that ultraendurance exercise increases blood antioxidant capacity through elevating hydrophilic antioxidants (uric acid, bilirubin, and vitamin C) and decreases lipophilic antioxidants (carotenoids and g-tocopherol),[6] thus resulting in a general trend toward an increased formation of oxidative DNA alterations.[7] Thus, there is convincing evidence that submaximal resistance exercise increases plasma antioxidants; however, this increase in plasma antioxidants is not efficient for inhibiting lipid oxidation in the case of ultraendurance exercise.[8] This effect depends on the training status as demonstrated by the finding that lipid peroxidation products in blood (i.e., conjugated dienes) after short-term resistance exercise increase only in nonresistance-trained subjects, whereas no increase was observed in trained subjects.[9] Results obtained from 107 elderly subjects undergoing constant low endurance physical activity demonstrate the direct antioxidant effect of this type of exercise on the human artery.[1]

Mitochondrial biomarkers and cardiovascular diseases

Mitochondrial DNA (mtDNA) is very sensitive to alterations induced by both exogenous and

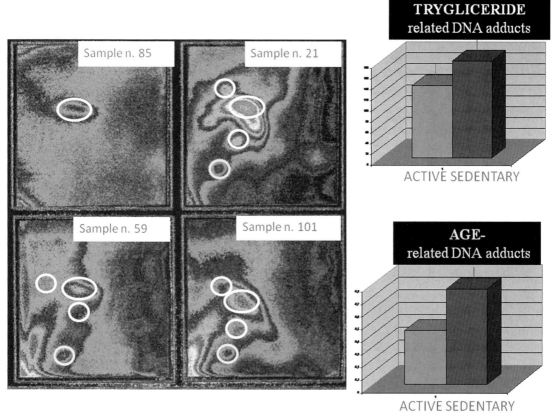

Figure 1. Physical activity decreases formation of bulky DNA adducts as detected by ^{32}P-postlabeling in human aorta (left boxes). DNA adducts are reported as adducts/10^8 normal nucleotides for the 51 physically active subjects (blue) and 56 sedentary subjects (red) (right histograms). White circles in ^{32}P-autoradiograms (left boxes) indicate adducts related with blood triglycerides, whereas yellow circles indicate adducts related with age. Both triglycerides- and age-related adducts are specifically decreased by physical activity.

endogenous genotoxic sources due to a variety of factors, including its nonnucleosomal structure, the lack of effective DNA repair, and a lack of mutation silencing based on triplet codon redundance.[10] MtDNA possesses specific fragile sites, rendering it highly susceptible to deletions resulting from oxidative damage. This damage typically induces a common mtDNA deletion that causes a loss of 4,977 nucleotides up to a total of 16,569 bp, which is the total length of the mitochondrial genome. These lesions are transmitted to mitochondrial progeny, which accumulate in cells over time.[10] The level of the mtDNA 4977 common deletion is remarkably high in human atherosclerotic arteries, especially in subjects older than 75 years.[4] Furthermore, this molecular alteration is the most potent molecu-

lar marker for predicting survival of atherosclerotic patients. Subjects presenting with a high level of this lesion have a 54% decrease in life expectancy compared to other patients.[1] The level of mtDNA 4977 deletion in the artery was highly correlated with those of 8-oxo-dG in the same tissue ($r = 0.829$, $P < 0.05$), a finding related to the endogenous oxidative origin of this mitochondrial molecular lesion. Physical activity resulted in 2.2-fold decrease in the amount of the mtDNA 4977 deletion ($13.0 \pm 0.07\%$ vs. $5.8 \pm 0.04\%$ in sedentary and physically active subjects, respectively; $P < 0.05$) (Fig. 2). The occurrence of this molecular lesion results in a loss of mitochondrial gene domains involved in oxidative phosphorylation (i.e., cytochrome oxidases, ATP synthase, NADH

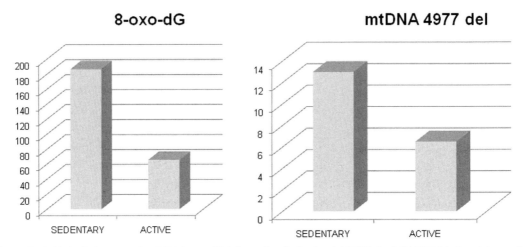

Figure 2. Oxidative lesions to nuclear DNA (8-oxo-dG, left panel) and mitochondrial DNA (mtDNA4977 deletion, right panel) in the aorta of 107 human subjects. The level of these molecular alterations is significantly higher in sedentary than physically active subjects.

dehydrogenase, and cytochrome b) and fatty acid beta-oxidation (i.e., acyl CoA-dehydrogenase). Accordingly, cells bearing the mtDNA 4977 deletion undergo defective oxidative phosphorylation, resulting in an increased endogenous production of reactive oxygen species. Furthermore, mitochondria bearing the mtDNA 4977 deletion cannot perform efficient lipid catabolism through the betaoxidation pathway, as this molecular lesion leads to the main pathogenic step contributing to the intracellular accumulation of lipids. This situation typically occurs in atherosclerosis, in which the hallmark is represented by the transformation of smooth muscle cells into foamy cells. In foamy cells, the cytoplasm is filled with noncatabolized cholesterol and lipid vacuoles (Fig. 3). Thus, the finding that physical activity decreases the occurrence of the mtDNA deletion indicates that this preventive intervention exerts its protective effects through the maintenance of adequate mitochondrial function. This beneficial effect contributes to decreasing oxidative DNA damage, as demonstrated in physically active subjects by the decrease in 8-oxo-dG and age-related DNA adducts. Furthermore, the maintenance of mitochondrial function improves lipid catabolism and lipid-related DNA damage, as demonstrated by the decrease in triglyceride-related DNA adducts in physically active subjects. These mitochondria-related mechanistic issues are supported by the experimental data obtained from the analysis of gene expression at the postgenomic level.

Postgenomic biomarkers and mitochondria

Several studies have examined the influence of physical activity on gene expression in target tissues by collecting muscle biopsies directly from human volunteers. Gene expression in skeletal muscle was compared between sedentary and sprint-trained or endurance athletes by collecting *vastus medialis* muscle biopsies from the thighs and evaluating gene expression by cDNA microarray.[11] The obtained findings demonstrated that oxidative phosphorylation-related mitochondrial genes were significantly upregulated in the trained compared to the sedentary subjects and in the endurance- versus sprint-trained subjects. The expression of these mitochondrial gene clusters involved in fat and carbohydrate oxidation was correlated with O_2 peak consumption.[11]

Using a similar approach, the gene expression profiles of young (21 years) and elderly (70 years) subjects were compared, and 596 genes were found to be differentially expressed. Gene expression was also evaluated in elderly subjects before and after a 6-month resistance exercise-training program. Prior to the exercise training, the transcriptome profile showed a dramatic enrichment of genes associated with mitochondrial function and age (e.g., cytochrome c oxidase). Following exercise training, the transcriptional signature of aging was markedly reversed back to that of younger levels for most

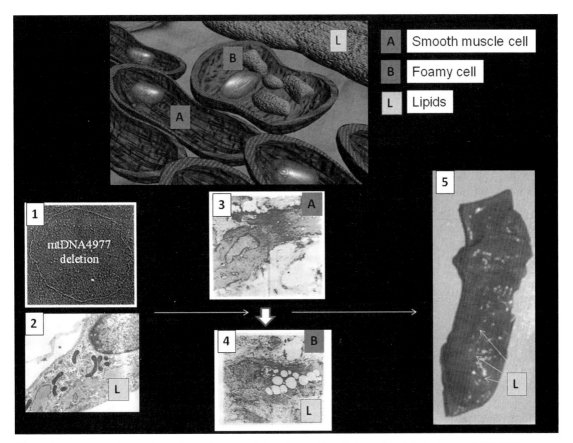

Figure 3. Phenotypic change of smooth muscle artery cells into foamy cells and atherosclerosis. Mitochondrial DNA 4977 common deletion (panel 1) resulting from oxidative stress causes loss of mitochondrial genes involved in mitochondria lipid catabolism (panel 2), thus inducing in cytoplasm lipids accumulation and transforming smooth muscle cells (panel 3) into foamy cells (panel 4). This step is fundamental for the accumulation of lipid material into the atherosclerotic plaque (panel 5).

genes that were affected by both age and exercise. Before exercise training, older adults were 59% weaker than younger subjects, but after 6 months of training in the older adults, strength improved significantly such that they were only 38% weaker than the younger adults. It was concluded that healthy older adults show evidence of mitochondrial impairment and muscle weakness, which can be partially reversed at the phenotypic level and substantially reversed at the transcriptome level following six months of resistance exercise training.[12] These findings indicate that physical activity reverses aging in human skeletal muscle, which is mainly due to an altered expression of mitochondrial genes.

Given that physical exercise is fundamental for maintaining the physiological expression of mitochondrial genes, it has also been demonstrated that

inactivity is a potent factor for altering the expression of the same genes. Gene expression was analyzed in the soleus muscle of the calf in the same 12 subjects before and after 5 weeks of physical inactivity.[13] A remarkable (up to threefold) significant decrease in the expression of mitochondrial genes involved in oxidative phosphorylation (e.g., citrate synthase, pyruvate dehydrogenase, cytochrome c oxidase, succinate dehydrogenase, cytochrome b, and NADH dehydrogenase), aerobic response (nuclear respiratory factor 1), mitochondrial biogenesis (peroxisome proliferator-activated receptor gamma coactivator 1-alpha and -beta and DNA polymerase γ), mitochondrial gene transcription (mitochondrial RNA polymerase; mtDNA helicase; and mitochondrial transcription factor A, B1, and B2), glucose delivery (glucose transporter 4), and carnitine activity (carnitine palmitoyl transferase) was detected.[13] Similar results have been obtained by studying cardiac muscle cells in rats, demonstrating that physical exercise exerts beneficial effects on the expression of genes involved in energy production, mitochondrial function, lipid catabolism, angiogenesis, and antioxidant response.[14]

Together, these studies provide evidence that physical activity is absolutely required for maintaining at the physiological level mitochondrial function.

MicroRNA and physical activity

MicroRNAs represent the master post-transcriptional regulators of gene expression. It has been demonstrated that microRNA expression is dramatically altered, not only under pathological conditions including cancer, but also in healthy organisms undergoing exposure to genotoxic agents such as cigarette smoke.[15] A recent study examined the role of physical exercise on microRNAs in healthy mice.[16] C57BL/6 mice were divided into physically active (4 weeks of exercise) and an inactive control group (cast limb). Microarray analysis was performed by cDNA microarray of calf gastrocnemius muscle. MiR-696 was revealed as the most sensitive microRNA undergoing activity-related alterations in expression. In particular, miR-696 was downregulated following physical exercise and upregulated following immobilization. Peroxisome proliferator-activated receptor-gamma coactivator 1-alpha (PPAR-g), which is a pivotal regulator of mitochondrial biogenesis, was found to be the master target gene regulated by miR-696. Based on the inhibitory role of microRNAs for selectively silencing the expression of their target genes, the expression of both PPAR-g mRNA and protein were upregulated following physical activity, thus being inversely related to miR-696 expression. This mechanistic link between physical activity and mitochondrial biogenesis and function was confirmed by *in vitro* transfection of miR-696 into cultured myocytes, demonstrating a 30% decrease in mitochondria DNA copy number in transfected cells as evaluated by qPCR that was paralleled by a remarkable decrease of mitochondrial function as evaluated by mitotracker.[16] These results provide evidence at the miRNome level that physical activity is fundamental for maintaining a physiological level of mitochondrial function in muscle cells.

Relationship of biomarkers modulated by physical activity and clinical outcomes

Based on the reported findings, there is convincing evidence that physical activity is fundamental for maintaining physiological mitochondrial function in muscle cells, including smooth muscle cells composing the medium layer of human arteries. We previously reported that high levels of mitochondrial failure associated with the accumulation of the mtDNA 4977 deletion in these cells results in a dramatic decrease in atherosclerotic patient survival.[1] In the same study, we analyzed the effects of protective factors on increasing the survival rate, demonstrating that the most potent protective factor is physical activity. We found that the survival rate was significantly ($P < 0.05$) increased by 34% in physically active subjects whose life expectancy, over a 15-year follow-up, was 2.4 years longer than those of sedentary subjects. Furthermore, physical activity decreased the incidence of not only mortality but also morbidity. The number of hospitalizations per year per single patient was 0.76 in sedentary subjects versus 0.28 in physically active subjects, showing a significant 2.7-fold difference. These findings are consistent with the established beneficial effects of physical activity on cardiovascular diseases.[17] Our study,[1] however, revealed that these benefits of physical activity are subject to remarkable interindividual variation. Accordingly, we have evaluated the influence of gene polymorphisms.

Influence of gene polymorphisms on the preventive effects of physical exercise

In our previous studies,[1,2] we evaluated a variety of gene polymorphisms for their influence on biomarkers modulated by physical activity and on clinical outcomes. The gene polymorphisms included polymorphic genes involved in thrombosis (*factor II* prothrombin and *factor V* Leiden), metabolism (*MTHFR*, *NAT1/2*), DNA repair (*OGG1*), and antioxidant defense (*GSTM1/T1*). Among these genetic polymorphisms, only those involved in antioxidant defense exerted a significant influence on both molecular biomarkers and clinical outcomes. In particular, the *GSTM1/T1* genes undergo a homozygous deletion polymorphism that results in a lack of gene activity referred to as a "null" polymorphism. Such an occurrence, i.e., the

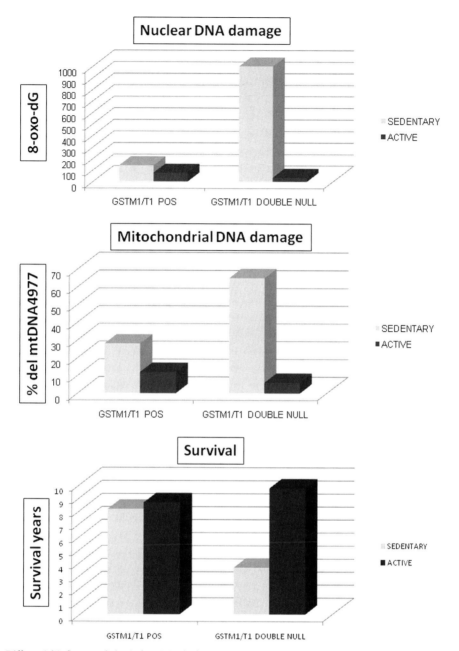

Figure 4. Differential influence of physical activity (sedentary vs. active) on aorta oxidative-DNA damage (upper panel), aorta mitochondrial-DNA damage (middle panel), and survival time (lower panel) as related to *GSTM1/T1* gene polymorphisms. Preventive effects of physical activity are mainly exerted in *GSTM1/T1* double null subjects.

double *GSTM1/T1* null polymorphism, occurred in 22% of the 107 subjects examined. Both oxidative DNA alterations (8-oxo-dG) and the mtDNA 4977 deletion in arterial smooth muscle cells were significantly higher in subjects bearing the homozygous double null deletion compared to wild-type carriers. We found that this phenomenon was strongly influenced by physical activity. No significant difference was observed between the wild-type and double null genotype carriers at the level of these

Table 1. Examples of polymorphic genes supposed to play a role in sport performance and clinical outcomes of physical exercise

Polymorphic gene	Chromosome location	Function	Effects on physical activity outcomes	Reference
Angiotensin-converting enzyme (ACE)	17q.23.3	Renin-angiotensin converting enzyme	I variant allele gives rise to lower enzyme activity and is associated with enhanced endurance performance and an anabolic response to intense exercise training. This effect may be related to an increase in slow-twitch rather than fast-twitch muscle fibers. The lower ACE enzyme activity associated with the II genotype raises nitric oxide, which in turn improve the efficiency of mitochondrial respiration and hence muscle function.	19–22
Alpha-actinin-3 (ACTN3)	11q31.1	Encodes a Z-disc structural protein that is found only in fast glycolytic type 2 muscle fibers. Anchors actin to myosin type 1 aerobic slow fibers	Nonmutant version associated with sprint performance, mutant version associated with endurance (in elite athletes only)	23
Heme oxygenase 1 (HO1)	22q12.3	Catalyzes the degradation of heme antioxidant; regulates cardiovascular function and its adaptive response through carbon monoxide production activating adaptive responses such as vasodilatation	Individuals with a CC genotype presented better cardiac adaptation than their CT and TT counterparts after endurance training	24
Hypoxia-inducible factor-1alpha (HIF1a)	14q23.2	Under hypoxic conditions activates the transcription of over 40 genes (e.g., erythropoietin, glucose transporters, glycolytic enzymes, vascular endothelial growth factor, etc.) increasing oxygen delivery and facilitating metabolic adaptation to hypoxia	HIF1A Pro582Ser (rs11549465) genotype distributions more frequent in elite endurance athletes than in controls	25

Continued

Table 1. *Continued*

Polymorphic gene	Chromosome location	Function	Effects on physical activity outcomes	Reference
Insulin-like growth factor 1 (IGF1)	12q23.2	Glucose homeostasis and cell proliferation. Mediate their intracellular actions through the PI 3-K and RAS/RAF/MAPK signaling pathways and downstream effectors include mTOR, p70 S6 kinase, ERK, and JNK	Synergistic effect between IGF1 polymorphisms and myostatin on the left ventricular mass in male athletes	26
Mitochondrial DNA haplotypes	mtDNA	Mutations in mitochondrial genes have been related to impaired cardiac function and exercise intolerance	Haplogroup T 13368A negatively associated with the status of elite endurance athlete. This mitochondrial variant could be related with a lower capacity to respond to endurance training, probably involved in a lower adaptability to endurance training, thus determining a lower chance to reach the condition of elite endurance athlete	27
Nuclear respiratory factor 2 (NRF2)	2q31	Activates peroxisome proliferator-activated receptor-gamma coactivator 1-alpha triggering mitochondrial biogenesis	A/C rs12594956 and C/T rs8031031 SNPs are associated with elite endurance athletes	28
Nitric oxide oxigenase 3 (NOS 3)	7q36.1	Catalyzes the generation of nitric oxide and L-citrulline from L-arginine and molecular oxygen. Critical mediator of cardiovascular homeostasis through regulation of the diameter of blood vessels	T/C (T) rs2070744 polymorphism associated with elite performance in power-oriented athletic events (throwing, jumping, sprinting)	29

oxidative biomarkers (8-oxo-dG and mtDNA 4977 deletion) in physically active subjects, whereas a remarkable difference was recorded for sedentary subjects (Fig. 4), This finding indicates that subjects lacking antioxidant defenses due to their adverse genetic polymorphism, i.e., the double null carriers, receive the greatest benefit of physical activity in terms of antioxidant effects, thereby replacing the lack of endogenous antioxidant defenses due to their genetic profile. This feature is reflected in the clinical outcomes. The survival rate was quite similar between the wild-type and double null

Table 2. Molecular biomarkers and related phenotypic outcomes on which physical activity induced a significant protective effect in *in vivo* studies.

DNA damage	Messenger RNA	Micro RNA	Protein	Related phenotypic outcome	Analyzed tissue	Organism	Reference
DNA adducts					Smooth muscle cells aorta	107 humans	1
8-oxo-dG				Morbidity mortality	Smooth muscle cells aorta	107 humans	1
Mitochondrial-DNA deletion				Morbidity mortality	Smooth muscle cells aorta	107 humans	1
Cytogenetic-damage (micronuclei, DNA-fragmentation)					Blood lymphocytes	Metanalysis	7
	Genes involved in carbohydrate oxidative phosphorylation and lipid beta-oxidation			O$_2$ peak consumption	Skeletal muscle	20 humans	11
	Cytochrome c oxidase, age-related gene expression signature			Strength increase	Skeletal muscle	51 humans	12
	Oxidative phosphorylation, mitochondria biogenesis and function				Skeletal muscle	12 humans	13
	Energy production, mitochondrial function, lipid catabolism, angiogenesis, antioxidant response				Cardiac muscle	Sprague–Dawley rats	14
		miR-696	PPAR-gamma; mitochondrial biogenesis and function		Skeletal muscle	C57BL/6 mice	16

carriers, with no significant influence of their activity level (Fig. 4, left-lower panel). Conversely, the difference in survival rate between the wild-type and double null carriers was maximized in sedentary subjects (Fig. 4, right-lower panel), in which the mean survival period during the 15-year follow-up was only 3.6 years for sedentary subjects versus 9.7 years (i.e., 2.7-fold longer) in physically active subjects. These results indicate that there is remarkable interindividual variation in response to the preventive benefits of physical activity and that selected subcategories are highly sensitive to these beneficial effects. The concept that genetic polymorphisms influence the outcomes of physical activity, mainly in terms of athletic performance, was explored by a recent review that took into account the most important studies performed.[18] A total of 239 gene polymorphisms have been found to be related to physical activity outcomes, mainly in terms of athletic performance. Of the 239 polymorphisms, 214 are located in autosomal genes, 7 on the X chromosome, and 18 in mitochondrial genes. Most studies to date, however, were based on small sample sizes and thus cannot provide definitive evidence that DNA sequence variants in a given gene are reliably associated with human variation in fitness and performance traits. Furthermore, unlike the data described here, the reviewed studies did not use any molecular biomarkers to support the causality of the purported association. The polymorphic genes found to be more strictly associated with physical activity outcomes, mainly in terms of athletic performance, are reported in Table 1.

Conclusions

Evidence showing that physical activity is required for maintaining muscle cell function as related to adequate mitochondrial function, thus avoiding or delaying tissue aging, exists at both the genomic, and postgenomic levels. Genomic evidence includes the attenuation of oxidative DNA damage to nuclear DNA in terms of 8-oxo-dG and to mitochondrial DNA in terms of the mtDNA 4977 deletion. Postgenomic evidence includes improved gene and microRNA expression profiles paralleled by phenotypic findings, such as increases in proteins involved in mitochondrial function and increases in biogenesis and muscle strength. A summary of these findings reviewed in this paper is reported in Table 2. Taken together, these findings provide evidence of the preventive beneficial effects exerted by physical activity at the molecular level. These benefits mainly focus on maintaining the physiological function of the mitochondria, thus avoiding their age-related decay and reflecting on the biology of the whole cell and tissue. This mechanism bears relevance not only to skeletal muscle cells, but also for cardiac muscle cells and vascular smooth muscle cells, thus affecting athletic performance as well as the occurrence and prevention of cardiovascular diseases.

In conclusion, there is currently adequate experimental evidence at both the genomic and postgenomic levels that physical activity of moderate intensity is able, through the activation of specific molecular mechanisms, to (1) prevent molecular damage and mitochondrial alterations induced by aging, (2) decrease morbidity and mortality as related to cardiovascular diseases and cancer, and (3) exert protective effects, primarily in subjects with poor antioxidant defenses due to their genetic profiles. Conversely, the lack of physical activity is the main factor responsible for increasing age-related physical decay in muscle cells and the occurrence of chronic degenerative diseases such as cancer and atherosclerosis.

Acknowledgments

This study was supported by the Italian Association for Cancer Research grant no. 8909.

Conflicts of Interests

The author declares no conflicts of interest.

References

1. Izzotti, A. *et al.* 2007. Survival of atherosclerotic patients as related to oxidative stress and gene polymorphisms. *Mutat. Res.* **621:** 119–128.
2. Izzotti, A. *et al.* 2001. Increased DNA alterations in atherosclerotic lesions of individuals lacking the *GSTM1* genotype. *FASEB J.* **15:** 752–757.
3. De Flora, S. *et al.* 1997. Molecular epidemiology of atherosclerosis. *FASEB J.* **11:** 1021–1031.
4. Bogliolo, M. *et al.* 1999. Detection of the "4977 bp" mitochondrial DNA deletion in human atherosclerotic lesions. *Mutagenesis* **14:** 77–82.
5. Izzotti, A. *et al.* 1999. Age-related increases of 8-hydroxy-2'-deoxyguanosine and DNA protein cross-link in mouse organs. *Mutat. Res.* **446:** 215–223.
6. Neubauer, O. *et al.* 2010. Antioxidant responses to an acute ultra-endurance exercise: impact on DNA stability and indications for an increased need for nutritive antioxidants in the early recovery phase. *Br. J. Nutr.* **104:** 1129–1138.
7. Reichhold, S. *et al.* 2009. Endurance exercise and DNA stability: is there a link to duration and intensity? *Mutat. Res. Rev.* **682:** 28–38.
8. Ramel, A. *et al.* 2004. Correlations between plasma noradrenaline concentrations, antioxidants, and neutrophil counts after submaximal resistance exercise in men. *Br. J. Sports Med.* **38:** E22.
9. Ramel, A. *et al.* 2004. Plasma antioxidants and lipid oxidation after submaximal resistance exercise in men. *Eur. J. Nutr.* **43:** 2–6.
10. Izzotti, A. 2009. Gene environment interactions in non-cancer degenerative diseases. *Mutat. Res.* **667:** 1–3.

11. Stepto, N.K. *et al.* 2009. Global gene expression in skeletal muscle from well-trained strength and endurance athletes. *Med. Sci. Sports Exerc.* **41:** 546–565.

12. Melov, S. *et al.* 2007. Resistance exercise reverses aging in human skeletal muscle. *PLoS One* **23:** e465.

13. Timmons, J.A. *et al.* 2006. Expression profiling following local muscle inactivity in humans provides new perspective on diabetes-related genes. *Genomics* **87:** 165–172.

14. Simonsen, M.L. *et al.* 2010. Acute physical activity effects on cardiac gene expression. *Exp. Physiol.* **95:** 1071–1080.

15. Izzotti, A. *et al.* 2009. Downregulation of microRNA expression in the lung of rats exposed to cigarette smoke. *FASEB J.* **23:** 806–812.

16. Aoi, W. *et al.* 2010. The microRNA miR-696 regulates PGC-1{alpha} in mouse skeletal muscle in response to physical activity. *Am. J. Physiol. Endocrinol. Metab.* **298:** 799–806.

17. Shiroma, E.J. *et al.* 2010. Physical activity and cardiovascular health: lessons learned from epidemiological studies across age, gender, and race/ethnicity. *Circulation* **122:** 743–752.

18. Bray, M.S. *et al.* 2009. The human gene map for performance and health-related fitness phenotypes: the 2006–2007 update. *Med. Sci. Sports Exerc.* **41:** 35–73.

19. Myerson, S. *et al.* 1999. Human angiotensin I-converting enzyme gene and endurance performance. *J. Appl. Physiol.* **87:** 1313–1316.

20. Williams, A.G. *et al.* 2000. The ACE gene and muscle performance. *Nature* **403:** 614.

21. Alvarez, R. *et al.* 2000. Genetic variation in the renin–angiotensin system and athletic performance. *Eur. J. Appl. Physiol.* **82:** 117–120.

22. Folland, J. *et al.* 2000. Angiotensin-converting enzyme genotype affects the response of human skeletal muscle to functional overload. *Exp. Physiol.* **85:** 575–579.

23. Druzhevskaya, A.M. *et al.* 2008. Association of the ACTN3 R577X polymorphism with power athlete status in Russians. *Eur. J. Appl. Physiol.* **103:** 631–634.

24. He, Z. *et al.* 2008. Association between HMOX-1 genotype and cardiac function during exercise. *Appl. Physiol. Nutr. Metab.* **33:** 450–460.

25. Döring, F. *et al.* 2010. A common haplotype and the Pro582Ser polymorphism of the hypoxia-inducible factor-1alpha (HIF1A) gene in elite endurance athletes. *J. Appl. Physiol.* **108:** 1497–1500.

26. Karlowatz, R.J. *et al.* 2011. Polymorphisms in the IGF1 signalling pathway including the myostatin gene are associated with left ventricular mass in male athletes. *Br. J. Sports Med.* **45:** 36–41.

27. Castro, M.G. *et al.* 2007. Mitochondrial haplogroup T is negatively associated with the status of elite endurance athlete. *Mitochondrion* **7:** 354–357.

28. Eynon, N. *et al.* 2010. Interaction between SNPs in the NRF2 gene and elite endurance performance. *Physiol. Genomics.* **42:** 78–81.

29. Gómez-Gallego, F. *et al.* 2009. The -786 T/C polymorphism of the NOS3 gene is associated with elite performance in power sports. *Eur. J. Appl. Physiol.* **107:** 565–569.

Ann. N.Y. Acad. Sci. ISSN 0077-8923

Impact of endurance and ultraendurance exercise on DNA damage

Karl-Heinz Wagner,[1,2] Stefanie Reichhold,[1] and Oliver Neubauer[1,2]

[1]Department of Nutritional Sciences, Emerging Field "Oxidative Stress and DNA Stability," University of Vienna, Vienna, Austria [2]School of Medical Sciences and School of Public Health, Griffith University (Gold Coast Campus), Australia

Address for correspondence: Karl-Heinz Wagner, Department of Nutritional Science, Emerging Field "Oxidative Stress and DNA Stability," Althanstraße 14, 1090 Vienna, Austria. karl-heinz.wagner@univie.ac.at

Regular moderate physical activity reduces the risk of several noncommunicable diseases. At the same time, evidence exists for oxidative stress resulting from acute and strenuous exercise by enhanced formation of reactive oxygen and nitrogen species, which may lead to oxidatively modified lipids, proteins, and possibly negative effects on DNA stability. The limited data on ultraendurance events such as an Ironman triathlon show no persistent DNA damage after the events. However, when considering the effects of endurance exercise comparable to a (half) marathon or a short triathlon distance, no clear conclusions could be drawn. In order to clarify which components of exercise participation, such as duration, intensity, frequency, or training status of the subjects, have an impact on DNA stability, more information is clearly needed that combines the measurement of DNA damage, gene expression, and DNA repair mechanisms before, during, and after exercise of differing intensities and durations.

Keywords: ultraendurance exercise; endurance exercise; physical activity; DNA damage; training status

Oxidative stress–induced DNA damage and insufficient DNA repair have been discussed to play a significant role in processes that lead to chronic diseases, such as cancer, diabetes, and arteriosclerosis.[1] It is well documented that regular moderate physical activity is associated with various health benefits, including decreased risk of the mentioned diseases;[2–4] however, acute, but not regular, strenuous exercise may induce oxidative stress via enhanced formation of reactive oxygen (ROS) and nitrogen species (RNS).[5,6] The potential mechanisms involved in this formation are increased oxygen consumption, autoxidation of catecholamines, activation of inflammatory cells due to muscle tissue damage, and ischemia and/or hypoxia/reoxygenation damage.[7]

ROS formation results in oxidative modifications of lipids, proteins, and nucleic acids.[7–9] Since oxidative modifications of DNA can lead to mutations[10] and exceptionally high volumes of exercise are also associated with a substantial oxidative stress, concerns have arisen about the health effects of competing in endurance and ultraendurance exercise events, particularly when participants are not optimally trained.[11] Based on the U-shaped relationship between exercise and health in general, much has to be learned on exercise of different durations, intensities, and types on oxidative stress responses and DNA stability. The current work of our group is focusing on the effects of ultraendurance exercise on oxidative stress and DNA stability.

Methods commonly used to evaluate DNA damage linked to exercise

Comprehensive reviews have been published on the various methods that quantify genotoxicity in human studies[12] and therefore are not the subject of this paper.

Very briefly, the most commonly applied methodologies to describe changes in DNA stability during or after physical activity are the micronucleus (MN) assay; its more developed test, the cytokinesis-block micronucleus cytome (CBMN Cyt) assay; the single cell gel electrophoresis (SCGE or COMET) assay; the DNA base oxidation product 8-hydroxy-2′-deoxyguanosine (8-OHdG); and, rare also, the sister chromatid exchange (SCE) assay.[13]

doi: 10.1111/j.1749-6632.2011.06106.x
 © 2011 New York Academy of Sciences. **115**

The CBMN Cyt assay detects genome instability, including chromosome breakage, loss, and rearrangement, in addition to gene amplification and nondisjunction. Micronuclei (MNi), nucleoplasmic bridges (NPBs), and nuclear buds (Nbuds) are measured as end points of this assay. Nucleoplasmic bridges originate from dicentric chromosomes resulting from misrepaired DNA breaks or telomere end fusion. Nuclear buds are formed as a consequence of gene amplification.[14–16]

The SCGE assay, under alkaline conditions (standard version), is a simple, rapid, and sensitive method that detects DNA strand breaks and alkali-labile sites. The key principle of the method is based on the migration of damaged DNA in an electric field, forming comet-shaped images.[17] The relative amount of DNA in the tail represents the frequency of DNA strand breaks. In order to detect oxidized pyrimidines and purines, isolated nuclei are treated with the lesion-specific enzymes endonuclease (ENDO) III and formamidopyrimidine glycosylase (FPG).[18]

8-OHdG, which is formed after the oxidation of guanine, is mainly determined in urine and white blood cells.[1] For 8-OHdG, the analytical aspect is of high importance since it can be measured with more- and less-reliable methods. An overview on this specific topic can be found elsewhere.[12,19]

SCEs arise during DNA replication as a consequence of breakage and rejoining of sister chromatids.[20]

The questions that now arise are whether endurance exercise at all, and particularly ultraendurance exercise, might induce DNA damage and if there are some further interactions influencing the link, such as training performance or frequency.

The studies summarized in Tables 1–3 have applied one or more of these methods for the evaluation of DNA stability before, during, and after exercise and refer to exercise that was specifically done in the field, but not under laboratory conditions (e.g., on a cycle ergometer or a treadmill run). All the details describing the studies and the circumstances such as the type of physical activity conducted, the number of subjects, their training status, and much more are given in the table as far as it has been described in the original work.

Field studies of endurance exercise

Thus far, relatively few studies have examined the effect of competitive half or full marathons or short-distance triathlons on DNA damage.

The first event investigated for its DNA-damaging potential was a half marathon. Around 80% of the 12 subjects tested showed an increase in DNA migration (SCGE assay) 24 h after the race. Blood was only sampled pre- and 24 h postexercise, which precludes further conclusions concerning the time-course of DNA damage thereafter.[21] Similar results were reported by Hartmann *et al.*,[22] who studied six athletes participating in a short-distance triathlon (2.5 h duration). Blood was sampled seven times over a period of five days, with the first sample collected prerace. Their results show that DNA migration remained elevated compared to prerace, until five days postrace in the basic SCGE assay. No changes were observed in FPG-sensitive sites in the SCGE assay, urinary 8-OHdG, and MNi frequencies, so it was concluded that the detected events were not due to oxidation of DNA bases and do not lead to chromosome damage. One main limitation of both studies is the few number of subjects investigated. Partly consistent with these findings, elevated levels of DNA single-strand breaks found in the SCGE assay 24 h, and 7 and 14 days after a marathon occurred.[23] FPG-sensitive sites were also increased immediately after the marathon, reaching a maximum one day after the race. Furthermore, oxidative effects on pyrimidines, detected with the lesion-specific ENDO III as well as urinary 8-OHdG, were significantly elevated immediately after the marathon until seven days later. In contrast, Brivita *et al.* found no change in the levels of endogenous DNA strand breaks and FPG-sensitive sites immediately after a half marathon and a marathon race in 10 subjects.[24] However, pyrimidine oxidation was significantly increased, and the *ex vivo* resistance to DNA damage induced by hydrogen peroxide was decreased after the event. In the latter studies, only two time points, 10 days before and immediately after the race, were investigated.

Based on the findings reviewed above, a clear conclusion of the effects of competitive endurance exercise lasting less than four hours on DNA stability remains elusive. Although the majority of studies have found increased levels of DNA strand breaks 24 hours after competitive endurance exercise, the

Table 1. Studies investigating the effects of competitive endurance exercise on markers of DNA damage

Reference	Experimental protocol[a]	Subjects[b] (trained/ untrained/VO$_2$max)	Method[c]	End point[d]	Sample matrix[e]	Summary of results[f]
21	Half marathon	12 MT (45 ± 25 km/w running)	COMET	SBs, AP	leu	↑ 24 h after half marathon in 10 subjects
22	Short-distance triathlon (1.5 km swimming, 40 km cycling, 10 km running)	6 T	COMET	SBs, AP	leu	↑ 24 h until 5 d after race
			+FPG	FPG-ss .	leu	↔ immediately after race
			HPLC-ECD	8- OHdG	urine; 24 h	↔ 1 d until 4 d after race
			MN	Mni	lymph	↔ 2 d and 4 d after race
23	Marathon	14 runners	COMET	SBs, AP	PBMC	↑ 24 h after marathon; still ↑ 14 d after race
		20 control	+FPG	FPG-s s.	PBMC	↑ immediately until 24 h after marathon
			+ENDO III	ENDO III-s s	PBMC	↑ immediately after race; still ↑ 14 d after race
			ELISA	8-OHdG	urine; 8 h	↑ immediately after race; still ↑ 14d after race
24	Half marathon and marathon	10 WT half marathon	COMET	SBs, AP	lymph	↔ immediately after races
		(4.2 h running/w; 5 m, 5 f)	+FPG	FPG-s s	lymph	↔ immediately after races
		12 WT marathon	+ ENDO III	ENDO III-s s	lymph	↑ after both races
		(3.5 h running/w; 10 m, 2 f)	+ H$_2$O$_2$	*ex vivo* SSB Induction	lymph	↑ immediately after races

Studies listed by their type and duration of exercise. h = hour; w = week; d = day.

[a]Experimental protocols showing the type of exercise that was performed. Duration and intensity of exercise are indicated in parentheses.

[b]Number of subjects indicated as untrained (UT), trained (T; do their regular training), moderately trained (MT), well-trained (WT), males (m), and females (f).Training status (VO$_2$max, training per week or month) is given in parentheses.

[c]Analytical methods: high performance liquid chromatography with electrochemical detection (HPLC-ECD), single cell gel electrophoresis assay (COMET), single cell gel electrophoresis assay with formamidopyrimidine glycosylase treatment (+FPG), single cell gel electrophoresis assay with endonuclease III treatment (+ENDO III), single cell gel electrophoresis assay with H$_2$O$_2$ treatment, sister chromatid exchange assay (SCE), micronucleus assay (MN), micronucleus assay including X-ray irradiation (MN+X-ray), and enzyme linked immuno assay (ELISA).

[d]The end points are outlined as 8-hydroxy-2′-deoxyguanosine (8-OHdG), 8-oxo-7,8-dihydro-2′-deoxyguanosine (8-oxodG), strand breaks (SBs), apurinic/apyrimidinic sites (AP), micronuclei (MNi), formamidopyrimidine glycosylase-sensitive sites (FPG-s s), endonuclease III-sensitive sites (ENDO III-s s), single strand breaks (SSB), nucleoplasmic bridges (NPB), and nuclear buds (Nbuds).

[e]Samples included lymphocytes (lymph), leucocytes (leu), urine and its collection period, white blood cells (WBC), peripheral blood mononuclear cells (PBMC), and plasma.

[f]Effects are described as no significant change (↔), significant increase (↑), and significant decrease (↓).

Table 2. Studies investigating the effects of competitive ultraendurance exercise on markers of DNA damage

Reference	Experimental protocol[a]	Subjects[b] (trained/ untrained/ VO$_2$max)	Method[c]	End point[d]	Sample matrix[e]	Summary of results[f]
28	8–11 h vigorous exercise/day for 30 d	23 T	HPLC-ECD	8-oxodG	urine; spot	↑ after 30 d period
29	Ultramarathon (2 d) (40 km, 90 km)	79 m (272 km running/month) 16 f (219 km running/month)	HPLC-ECD	8 -O HdG	urine; spot	↑ after 1 run; back to initial levels after 2 runs
30	4 d supramarathon (93 km, 120 km, 56 km, 59 km; road running)	5 WT	ELISA	8-OHdG	urine; 12 h	↑ after 24 h; back to initial levels on day 4
25	Ultramarathon (50 km)	11 f (VO$_2$max: ∼55.0 mL/kg/min) 11 m (VO$_2$max: ∼60.0 mL/kg/min) divided in to supplement/placebo group	COMET	SBs, AP	leu	↑ at midrace; back to initial levels 2 h after race
26	Ironman triathlon (3.8 km swimming, 180 km cycling, 42 km running)	28 WT (VO$_2$max: 5 8.9 mL/kg/min)	COMET	SBs, AP	lymph	↑1 d after race; back to initial levels 5 d after race
			+FPG	FPG-s s	lymph	↔
			+ENDO III	ENDO III-s s	lymph	↑ 5 d after race compared to 1 d after race; back to initial levels 19 d after race
27	Ironman triathlon (3.8 km swimming, 180 km cycling, 42 km running)	20 WT (VO$_2$max: 60.8 mL/kg/min)	MN	Mni	lymph	↓ immediately and further 19 d after race
			MN	Nbuds	lymph	↑ 5 d after race; back to initial levels 19 d after race
			MN	NPB	lymph	↓ 19 d after race

[a–f] See Table 1.

Table 3. Studies investigating the effects of noncompetitive endurance exercise and periods of intensified training on markers of DNA damage

Reference	Experimental protocol[a]	Subjects[b] (trained/ untrained/ VO$_2$max)	Method[c]	Endpoint[d]	Sample matrix[e]	Summary of results[f]
31	Road running (30 ± 6 km/d) for 8 d	10 long-distance runners	HPLC-ECD	8-OHdG	urine; 24 h	↑ during 8 d period
32	14 d of winter training	15 T supplement group 15 T placebo group	ELISA	8-OHdG	urine; 24 h	↑ 7 d after start of training
33	90 min swimming (1500 m) or 70 min running (15 km)	9 T swimmers 9 T runners	HPLC-ECD HPLC-ECD	8 -O HdG 8-OHdG	lymph urine; spot	↓ after swimming; ↔ after running ↔ after swimming; ↔ after running
34	Running (20 km)	11 T distance runners (VO$_2$max: 57.5 mL/kg/mm)	HPLC-ECD	8-OHdG	urine; 24 h	↔ 1 d until 3 d after the test
35	Long-distance road running (8–110 km/w)	32 T long-distance runners 32 control	HPLC-ECD	8-OHdG	urine; 24 h urine; spot	↔; no differences between groups
36	Road running (10 km at 7 5% heart rate max)	8 UT	ELISA	8 -OHdG	plasma	↓ immediately after run; 24 h back to initial levels
38	4 w of overload training (referring to program of long-distance triathletes)	9 WT triathletes (VO$_2$max: 66.0 mL/kg/min) 6 N T (VO$_2$max: 42.8 mL/kg/min	COMET	SBs, AP	leu	↔ immediately after overload training
39	4 w of overload training (referring to program of long-distance triathletes)	7 WT supplement group 10 WT placebo group	COMET	SBs, AP	leu	↑ immediately after overload training in both groups

[a–f] See Table 1.

results are not consistent due to different experimental designs, differences in the size of study groups, and differences in the training status of the subjects. With respect to the observation periods, it is important to emphasize that monitoring DNA stability ≤24 hours after exercise is too short be-cause major alterations in DNA repair mechanisms seem to occur thereafter.[23,25–27]

Field studies of ultraendurance exercise

The effect of prolonged vigorous exercise on the formation of urinary 8-oxodG has been investigated by Poulsen *et al.*[28] Their trained participants underwent a 30-day training program, including 8–11 hours of vigorous exercise per six days per week in the Danish Army; oxidative DNA modifications increased thereby by 33%. Two studies with a repeated day's running performance showed an increase in DNA repair systems, leading to adaptation and normalization of oxidative DNA damage.[29,30]

In a two-day marathon, urinary 8-OHdG was assessed in hobby athletes. Oxidized bases increased after a 6-h run at day one. At day two, after 13 hours of running, a reduction was observed that was discussed to be due to an acceleration of the DNA repair system.[29] Similar results were seen after a super marathon (four-day race), where urinary 8-OHdG levels were increased at the first days, but declined to baseline at the fourth and last day of running.[30]

Completing an ultramarathon with an average duration of seven hours, a significantly higher proportion of damaged cells (10%) midrace was found compared to that prerace.[25] However, within two hours the values had returned to baseline. Almost one week after the event, the number of damaged cells significantly decreased to lower levels than at prerace, suggesting that DNA damage was not persistent due to DNA repair. Data from our working group in Ironman triathletes supported this finding.[26] The number of DNA strand breaks significantly decreased one day after an Ironman triathlon, returned to baseline values five days postrace, and significantly declined further below baseline values 19 days after the race. Although no changes in the FPG-sensitive sites were observed, ENDO III–sensitive sites increased five days after the race and declined to baseline values three weeks postrace. Surprisingly, the number of MNi decreased significantly after the race, remained at a low level until five days postrace, and was significantly lower than at baseline after 19 days postrace.[27] NPBs and Nbuds remained unchanged. These data suggest that duration and intensity, based on an Ironman triathlon race, do not lead to chromosomal alterations.

Concluding the results, which examined the effects of competitive ultraendurance exercise on various markers of DNA damage, no persistent DNA damage was observed. It seems plausible that extensive training for ultraendurance events results in adaptation and increased activity of DNA repair systems.

Noncompetitive field studies with endurance exercise and periods of intensified training

Contrary to field studies, less is known on periods of prolonged training. In a competition-simulating experiment, long-distance runners completed 20 km in 79.2 ± 2.4 minutes in a noncompetitive environment.[31] No change in urinary 8-OHdG was assessed, either three days before, or three days after, the test. When long-distance runners were compared with nonactive controls, no differences in the urinary 8-OHdG levels were found at rest; however, no data on the subjects' training statuses were shown.[32] In contrast, decreased levels of plasma 8-OHdG (measured with ELISA) was found immediately after a 10-km run (1 ± 0.2-h duration), which returned to baseline 24 hours after exercise.[33]

Urinary 8-OHdG was increased in long-distance runners during an eight-day running camp, with an average running distance of 30 ± 6 km/day. However, it decreased to pretraining levels on the day after the camp was concluded.[34] During two weeks of winter training at an altitude of more than 2,500 m, urinary 8-OHdG (quantified with ELISA), increased in the placebo and antioxidant supplementation group (for details see, Table 1), one week after the start of the training.[35] Unfortunately, potential training adaptations on exercise-induced effects could not be estimated due to missing data on the training schedule. 8-OHdG in urine and lymphocytes was measured in nine trained swimmers and runners before and within 15 min after 90 min of swimming (1.5 km) or 70 min of running (15 km).[36] 8-OHdG content of lymphocyte DNA decreased immediately after swimming, but not after running. Urinary 8-OHdG did not change significantly. Interestingly, the preexercise levels of 8-OHdG in the DNA of lymphocytes were reported to be higher in swimmers compared to runners; however, due to missing data on the training status, the reasons can only be speculated upon, such as the intensity of an individual's training. Palazzetti *et al.* investigated the effects of an intense training period on DNA stability (SCGE assay) in a group of male well-trained triathletes. No changes were found in the first study,[37] but in another,[38] an increase regarding the levels of DNA strand breaks was observed immediately after four weeks of overloaded training. Based on the published data, it can be concluded that the effects of exercise on DNA is influenced by the duration of exercise (acute or chronic intervention) and DNA repair enzyme activity.

The studies that investigated the effects of noncompetitive endurance exercise on DNA are inconsistent in their outcomes due to the use of different experimental designs, missing trainings data, and various methods for the detection of DNA damage.

Impact of adaptation and lifestyle data on published papers

Based on the available data on this issue, no clear differences appear between DNA stability/damage on the one hand, and exercise durations and intensities on the other.[39] However, some important points can be concluded.

DNA damage after competitive ultraendurance exercise in well-trained subjects does not appear to be persistent. Although levels of DNA strand breaks increase 24 hours after competitive endurance exercise, the evidence of exercise-induced effects on sustained DNA damage is limited, due to the short monitoring periods. It is particularly noticeable that most of the studies lack follow-up observations during recovery; additionally, the study groups are generally small, reducing the likelihood of detecting significant effects.

Thus, there is need for larger cohorts of subjects to be tested in order to obtain statistically stronger results (especially to clarify the effect of different training status on the DNA/training-induced effects). Further, in many studies information on lifestyle, smoking habits, alcohol consumption, medication, and diet is missing, although it is needed for the assessment of DNA modulation/stability.[14] Moreover, very often, an indication of the subjects' training statuses and the used exercise protocols are weakly reported.

The outcomes also lead to the conclusion that adaptive effects of regular exercise play an essential role on antioxidant defences and can also account for improved resistance of trained athletes to DNA damage.[8,40–42] In this context, the concept of hormesis, which is characterized as a dose–response phenomenon where a low dose of a substance or environmental factor stimulates adaptation, whereas a high dose tends to inhibit adaptation, provides a tempting hypothesis to explain the protective effects of exercise.[43] During exercise, low levels of ROS formation can stimulate adaptive mechanisms, that is,

expression of antioxidant enzymes and upregulation of DNA repair enzyme activity, which can lead to decreased oxidative damage or apoptosis.[39–41,44,45]

An additional physiological response after exercise is increased plasma antioxidant capacity[26,46,47] caused by the intake of antioxidants such as vitamin C and alpha-tocopherol during the race, tissue mobilization of these vitamins,[46,48–50] and/or because of increased endogenous synthesis of the hydrophilic antioxidant uric acid via the metabolism of purines, by xanthine oxidase, during intense exercise.[46,47]

Conclusion and future aspects

The exact mechanism by which physical exercise influences DNA stability requires further investigation. Based on the presented publications, no clear direction can be pointed out, since major determinants are missing in many papers. Future investigations should combine DNA damage parameters with DNA repair mechanisms and should also look at gene level before, during, and after exercise in order to add knowledge to the mechanisms that maintain DNA stability in response to vigorous exercise.

Acknowledgment

Parts of the studies described in the paper were supported by the Austrian Science Fund, Vienna, Austria.

Conflicts of interest

The authors declare no conflicts of interest.

References

1. Wu, L.L., C.C. Chiou, P.Y. Chang & J.T. Wu. 2004. Urinary 8-OHdG: a marker of oxidative stress to DNA and a risk factor for cancer, atherosclerosis and diabetics. *Clin. Chim. Acta.* **339:** 1–9.
2. Blair, S., H. Kohl III, C. Barlow, *et al.* 1995. Changes in physical fitness and all-cause mortality: a prospective study of healthy and unhealthy men. *J. Am. Med. Assoc.* **273:** 1093–1098.
3. Kruk, J. & H. Aboul-Enein. 2007. Physical activity and cancer prevention: updating the evidence. The role of oxidative stress in carcinogenesis. *Curr. Cancer Ther. Rev.* **3:** 81–95.
4. Hamman, R.F., R.R. Wing, S.L. Edelstein, *et al.* 2006. Effect of weight loss with lifestyle intervention on risk of diabetes. *Diabetes Care* **29:** 2102–2107.
5. Packer, L., E. Cadenas & K.J.A. Davies. 2008. Free radicals and exercise: an introduction. *Free Radic. Biol. Med.* **44:** 123–125.
6. Halliwell, B. 2007. Oxidative stress and cancer: have we moved forward? *Biochem. J.* **401:** 1–11.

7. König, D., K-H. Wagner, I. Elmadfa & A. Berg. 2001. Exercise and oxidative stress: significance of antioxidants with reference to inflammatory, muscular, and systemic stress. *Exerc. Immunol. Rev.* **7:** 108–133.

8. Sachdev, S.S. & K.J.A. Davies. 2008. Production, detection, and adaptive responses to free radicals in exercise. *Free Radic. Biol. Med.* **44:** 215–223.

9. König, D, O. Neubauer, L. Nics, *et al.* 2007. Biomarkers of exercise-induced myocardial stress in relation to inflammatory and oxidative stress. *Exerc. Immunol. Rev.* **13:** 15–36.

10. Poulsen, H. 2005. Oxidative DNA modifications. *Exp. Toxicol. Pathol.* **57:** 161–169.

11. Knez, W., J. Coombes & D. Jenkins. 2006. Ultra-endurance exercise and oxidative damage: implications for cardiovascular health. *Sports Med.* **36:** 429–441.

12. Knasmüller, S., A. Nersesyan, M. Misík, *et al.* 2008. Use of conventional and -omics based methods for health claims of dietary antioxidants: a critical overview. *Br. J. Nutr.* **99:** ES3–52.

13. Wagner, K-H., S. Reichhold, C. Hölzl, *et al.* 2010. Well-trained, healthy triathletes experience no adverse health risks regarding oxidative stress and DNA damage by participating in an ultra-endurance event. *Toxicology.* **278:** 211–216.

14. Fenech, M. 2007. Cytokinesis-block micronucleus cytome assay. *Nat. Protoc.* **2:** 1084–1104.

15. Thomas, P., K. Umegaki & M. Fenech. 2003. Nucleoplasmic bridges are a sensitive measure of chromosome rearrangement in the cytokinesis-block micronucleus assay. *Mutagenesis* **18:** 187–194.

16. Bonassi S. A. Znaor, M. Ceppi, *et al.* 2007. An increased micronucleus frequency in peripheral blood lymphocytes predicts the risk of cancer in humans. *Carcinogenesis* **28:** 625–631.

17. Dusinská, M. & A. Collins. 2008. The comet assay in human biomonitoring: gene-environment interactions. *Mutagenesis* **23:** 1–15.

18. Collins, A.R., S.J. Duthie & V.L. Dobson. 1993. Direct enzymic detection of endogenous oxidative base damage in human lymphocyte DNA. *Carcinogenesis* **14:** 1733–1735.

19. Cooke, M.S., R. Olinski & S. Loft. 2008. Measurement and meaning of oxidatively modified DNA lesions in urine. *Cancer Epidemiol. Biomark. Prev.* **17:** 3–14.

20. Wilson D.M. III & L.H. Thompson. 2007. Molecular mechanisms of sister-chromatid exchange. *Mutat. Res.- Fundam. Mol. Mech. Mutagen.* **616:** 11–23.

21. Niess, A., M. Baumann, K. Roecker, *et al.* 1998. Effects of intensive endurance exercise on DNA damage in leucocytes. *J. Sports Med. Phys. Fit.* **38:** 111–115.

22. Hartmann, A., S. Pfuhler, C. Dennog, *et al.* 1998. Exercise-induced DNA effects in human leukocytes are not accompanied by increased formation of 8-hydroxy-2′-deoxyguanosine or induction of micronuclei. *Free Radic. Biol. Med.* **24:** 245–251.

23. Tsai, K., T.G. Hsu, K.M. Hsu, *et al.* 2001. Oxidative DNA damage in human peripheral leukocytes induced by massive aerobic exercise. *Free Radic. Biol. Med.* **31:** 1465–1472.

24. Briviba, K., B. Watzl, K. Nickel, *et al.* 2005. A half-marathon and a marathon run induce oxidative DNA damage, reduce antioxidant capacity to protect DNA against damage and modify immune function in hobby runners. *Redox Rep.* **10:** 325–331.

25. Mastaloudis, A., T.W. Yu, R.P. O'Donnell, *et al.* Endurance exercise results in DNA damage as detected by the comet assay. *Free Radic. Biol. Med.* **36:** 966–975.

26. Reichhold, S., O. Neubauer, C. Hoelzl, *et al.* 2009. DNA damage in response to an Ironman triathlon. *Free Rad. Res.* **43:** 753–760.

27. Reichhold, S., O. Neubauer, V. Ehrlich, *et al.* 2008. No acute and persistent DNA damage after an Ironman triathlon. *Cancer Epidemiol. Biomarkers Prev.* **17:** 1913–1919.

28. Poulsen, H.E., S. Loft & K. Vistisen. 1996. Extreme exercise and oxidative DNA modification. *J. Sports Sci.* **14:** 343–346.

29. Miyata, M., H. Kasai, K. Kawai, *et al.* 2008. Changes of urinary 8-hydroxydeoxyguanosine levels during a two-day ultramarathon race period in Japanese non-professional runners. *Int. J. Sports Med.* **29:** 27–33.

30. Radak, Z., J. Pucsuk, S. Boros, *et al.* 2000. Changes in urine 8-hydroxydeoxyguanosine levels of super-marathon runners during a four-day race period. *Life Sci.* **66:** 1763–1767.

31. Sumida, S., K. Okamura, T. Doi, *et al.* 1997. No influence of a single bout of exercise on urinary excretion of 8-hydroxy-deoxyguanosine in humans. *Biochem. Mol. Biol. Int.* **42:** 601–609.

32. Pilger, A., D. Germadnik, D. Formanek, *et al.* 1997. Habitual long-distance running does not enhance urinary excretion of 8-hydroxydeoxyguanosine. *Eur. J. Appl. Physiol. Occup. Physiol.* **75:** 467–469.

33. Itoh, H., T. Ohkuwa, Y. Yamazaki, *et al.* 2006. Influence of endurance running on plasma 8-hydroxy-deoxyguanosine levels in humans. *Jpn. J. Phys. Fit. Sports Med.* **55:** 241–245.

34. Okamura, K., T. Doi, K. Hamada, *et al.* 1997. Effect of repeated exercise on urinary 8-hydroxy-deoxyguanosine excretion in humans. *Free Radic. Res.* **26:** 507–514.

35. Pfeiffer, J., E. Askew, D. Roberts, *et al.* 1999. Effect of antioxidant supplementation on urine and blood markers of oxidative stress during extended moderate-altitude training. *Wildern. Environ. Med.* **10:** 66–74.

36. Inoue, T., Z. Mu, K. Sumikawa, *et al.* 1993. Effect of physical exercise on the content of 8-hydroxydeoxyguanosine in nuclear DNA prepared from human lymphocytes. *Cancer Sci.* **84:** 720–725.

37. Palazzetti, S., M. Richard, A. Favier & I. Margaritis. 2003. Overloaded training increases exercise-induced oxidative stress and damage. *Can. J. Appl. Physiol.* **28:** 588–604.

38. Palazzetti, S., A.S. Rousseau, M.J. Richard, *et al.* 2004. Antioxidant supplementation preserves antioxidant response in physical training and low antioxidant intake. *Br. J. Nutr.* **91:** 91–100.

39. Reichhold, S., O. Neubauer, A.C. Bulmer, *et al.* 2009. Endurance exercise and DNA stability: is there a link to duration and intensity? *Mutat. Res. Rev.* **682:** 28–38.

40. Radak, Z., H.Y. Chung & S. Goto. 2008. Systemic adaptation to oxidative challenge induced by regular exercise. *Free Radic. Biol. Med.* **44:** 153–159.

41. Ji, J.J. 2008. Modulation of skeletal muscle antioxidant defense by exercise: role of redox signalling. *Free Radic. Biol. Med.* **44:** 142–152.

42. Ji, L.L., M.-C. Gomez-Cabrera & J. Vina. 2006. Exercise and hormesis: activation of cellular antioxidant signaling pathway. *Ann. N.Y. Acad. Sci.* **1067:** 425–435.

43. Mattson M.P. 2008. Hormesis defined. *Ageing Res. Rev.* **7:** 1–7.

44. Gomez-Cabrera, M.-C., E. Domenech & J. Vina. 2008. Moderate exercise is an antioxidant: upregulation of antioxidant genes by training. *Free Radic. Biol. Med.* **44:** 126–131.

45. Mooren, F., A. Lechtermann & K. Völker. 2004. Exercise-induced apoptosis of lymphocytes depends on training status. *Med. Sci. Sports Exerc.* **36:** 1476–1483.

46. Neubauer, O., D. König, N. Kern, *et al.* 2008. No indications of persistent oxidative stress in response to an Ironman triathlon. *Med. Sci. Sports Exerc.* **40:** 2119–2128.

47. Liu, M.-L., R. Bergholm, S. Makimattila, *et al.* 1999. A marathon run increases the susceptibility of LDL to oxidation in vitro and modifies plasma antioxidants. *Am. J. Physiol.- Endocrinol. Metab.* **276:** E1083–1091.

48. Poulsen, H., A. Weimann & S. Loft. 1999. Methods to detect DNA damage by free radicals: relation to exercise. *Proc. Nutr. Soc.* **58:** 1007–1014.

49. Neubauer O, S. Reichhold, L. Nics, *et al.* 2010. Antioxidant responses to an acute ultra-endurance exercise: impact on DNA stability and indications for an increased need for nutritive antioxidants in the early recovery phase. *Br. J. Nutr.* **104:** 1129–1138.

50. Mastaloudis, A., J.D. Morrow, D.W. Hopkins, *et al.* 2004. Antioxidant supplementation prevents exercise-induced lipid peroxidation, but not inflammation, in ultramarathon runners. *Free Radic. Biol. Med.* **36:** 1329–1341.

Ann. N.Y. Acad. Sci. ISSN 0077-8923

ANNALS OF THE NEW YORK ACADEMY OF SCIENCES

Issue: *Nutrition and Physical Activity in Aging, Obesity, and Cancer*

Myricetin is a potent chemopreventive phytochemical in skin carcinogenesis

Nam Joo Kang,[1] Sung Keun Jung,[2] Ki Won Lee,[3,5,6,*] and Hyong Joo Lee[4,5]

[1]School of Food Science and Biotechnology, Kyungpook National University, Daegu, Republic of Korea. [2]Hormel Institute, University of Minnesota, Austin, Minnesota, USA. [3]Food Science and Biotechnology Program, Department of Agricultural Biotechnology, [4]WCU Biomodulation Program, Department of Agricultural Biotechnology, [5]Center for Agricultural Biomaterials, Seoul National University, Seoul, Republic of Korea. [6]Advanced Institutes of Convergence Technology, Suwon-si, Gyeonggi-do, Republic of Korea

Address for correspondence: Hyong Joo Lee, Department of Agricultural Biotechnology, Seoul National University, Seoul 151-921, Republic of Korea. leehyjo@snu.ac.kr; Ki Won Lee, Department of Agricultural Biotechnology, Seoul National University, Seoul 151–921, Republic of Korea, kiwon@snu.ac.kr

Myricetin is a widely distributed flavonol that is found in many plants, including tea, berries, fruits, vegetables, and medicinal herbs. Abundant sources provide interesting insights into the multiple mechanisms by which myricetin mediates chemopreventive effects on skin cancer. Myricetin strongly inhibited tumor promoter–induced neoplastic cell transformation by inhibiting MEK, JAK1, Akt, and MKK4 kinase activity directly. In a mouse skin model, myricetin attenuated the ultraviolet B (UVB)–induced COX-2 expression and skin tumor formation by regulating Fyn. Myricetin-mediated inactivation of Akt in the UVB response plays a role in regulating UVB-induced carcinogenesis. Recently, myricetin was found to inhibit UVB-induced angiogenesis by targeting PI3-K in an SKH-1 hairless mouse skin tumorigenesis model. Raf kinase is a critical target for myricetin in inhibiting the UVB-induced formation of wrinkles and suppression of type I procollagen and collagen levels in mouse skin. Accumulated data suggest that myricetin acts as a promising agent for the chemoprevention of skin cancer.

Keywords: myricetin; skin carcinogenesis; chemoprevention; signaling pathway

Introduction

Myricetin (3,3′,4′,5,5′,7-hexahydroxyflavone, Fig. 1) is a flavonol and a polyphenol. It is found in many plants, including tea, berries, fruits, vegetables, and medicinal herbs.[1] In berries, vegetables, and fruits, myricetin occurs mostly in the form of glycosides,[2] rather than free aglycones, and high levels of myricetin are found in the skins of many fruits, such as red grapes.[3] Myricetin is commonly consumed in our diet in vegetables, in fruits, and in beverages such as tea and wine.[4] Some of the consumed myricetin is absorbed by the gastrointestinal tract, whereas the remainder is metabolized by the gastrointestinal microflora.[5] The liver is largely responsible for the metabolism of the absorbed myricetin, and the intestinal wall and kidney are secondary sites. The major metabolite of myricetin is 3,5-dihydroxyphenylacetic acid, which is excreted in the urine.[5] The structure of myricetin is similar to that of quercetin. The hydroxylation of quercetin at position 5′ in the B ring leads to the formation of myricetin.[3] However, few studies have evaluated the biological activities of myricetin, although it is similar to quercetin and is abundant in plants and foods. Myricetin has greater antiradical activity than other flavonoids, and it scavenges oxygen radicals and inhibits lipid peroxidation.[6] The anticarcinogenic effects of myricetin have been attributed to various mechanisms, including their antioxidative activity, the inhibition of enzymes that activate carcinogens, the modification of signal transduction pathways, and interactions with other proteins. This review discusses the antiskin carcinogenic mechanisms of myricetin, focusing on its interactions with cellular protein kinase and the modification of signal

doi: 10.1111/j.1749-6632.2011.06122.x

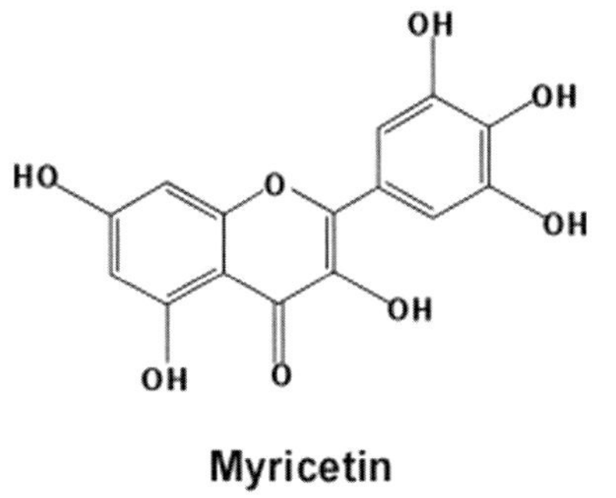

Figure 1. Chemical structure of myricetin.

transduction pathways as potential targets for the chemopreventive effects of myricetin in skin cancer.

Target proteins regulating the signaling pathway for skin carcinogenesis

Skin cancer is currently the most common type of human cancer.[7,8] Although substantial progress has been made in developing new skin cancer therapies, skin cancer is still a global health problem. When ultraviolet (UV) irradiation, the primary ecological carcinogen in the development of skin cancer, stimulates clonal expansion of aberrant skin cells, resulting in skin carcinogenesis, multiple cellular signaling pathways are involved (Fig. 2).[9] One or more molecules may strongly direct these signaling pathways toward the development of carcinogenesis. Such molecules may be targets for the chemoprevention of skin cancer. In particular, published evidence reports that enzymes and proteins are critical signal regulators in skin carcinogenesis.[9]

Src family tyrosine kinases
The Src family kinases (SFKs), 60-kDa nonreceptor tyrosine kinases, comprise nine very similar tyrosine kinases: Src, Lck, Hck, Fyn, Blk, Lyn, Fgr, Yes, and Yrk. Increased SFK activity is related to cellular events, including cell differentiation, proliferation, migration, and survival.[10] A study showed that UV radiation induces the activation of Src,[11] and c-Src kinase activity in skin tumors is elevated by 4- to 20-fold, compared to normal skin.[12] The activation of Fyn, another member of the Src family, plays a critical role in the development of skin cancer.[10,13] A recent *in vivo* study showed that in 14-Fyn (K14) transgenic mice, increased epidermal Fyn levels activated p44/42 MAP kinases, STAT3, and PDK-1.[14] The epidermal growth factor receptor (EGFR) and

Src cooperate in several functions, including regulating cell proliferation and apoptosis.[15]

The MAPK pathway
MAPK signaling pathways are commonly upregulated in various cancer cell types,[16] and these pathways are involved in cell proliferation and survival. Among the components of the MAPK pathways, the Raf/MEK/ERK cascade is a core signaling component in cell proliferation, differentiation, and apoptosis, as well as in development, growth, and inflammation via the transmission of signals from cell surface receptors to the nucleus.[17] Raf, named for rapidly accelerated fibrosarcoma, is a serine/threonine kinase that functions in the Ras/Raf/MEK/ERK mitogen-activated protein kinase (MAPK) signaling pathway.[18] The Raf/ERK pathway is the most critical mediator of Ras-dependent carcinogenesis in all cell types. UV irradiation induces Raf activation *in vitro* and *in vivo*.[19,20] One study reported that blocking MEK/ERK activity suppressed UV-induced skin cancer.[21] Using interfering B-Raf RNA, it showed that activated B-Raf is involved in transformed and tumorigenic growth of melanomas[22] and that B-Raf mutation is related to early carcinogenesis events in both melanocytic and nonmelanocytic skin tumors.[23] In addition, Raf is one of the signal molecules in the ultraviolet A (UVA)-induced production of matrix metalloproteinase 1 (MMP-1) in human dermal fibroblasts.[24] MKK4 is a component of stress-activated MAP kinase signaling modules, and it is expressed ubiquitously. It directly phosphorylates and activates the c-Jun N-terminal kinase (JNK) and p38 families of MAP kinases in response to environmental stress, proinflammatory cytokines, and developmental cues.[25] Therefore, this pathway is an attractive target for the development of novel anticancer agents.

The PI3-K/Akt pathway
In recent years, the phosphatidylinositol-3-kinase (PI3-K)/Akt signaling pathway has been identified as a main player in human cancer, including skin cancer.[26] PI3-Ks phosphorylate phosphatidylinositol 4,5-bisphosphate (PIP2) and convert PIP2 into phosphatidylinositol 2,4,5-triphosphate, or PIP3, a critical second messenger that recruits Akt (protein kinase B, PKB) to activate cell growth, proliferation, and survival signaling.[26,27] One study showed that UV irradiation triggers the activation of EGFR

UVB

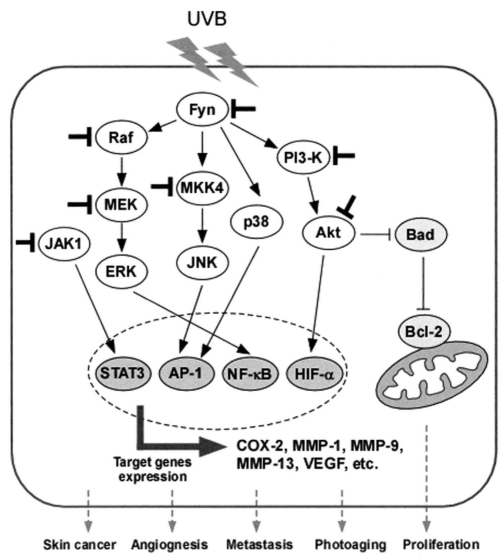

Figure 2. General scheme of signaling cascades in skin carcinogenesis and simplified depiction of the proposed antiskin cancer mechanism of myricetin. If cellular receptors recognize the oncogenic stimuli, Fyn is activated. Activated Fyn phosphorylates MAPK upstream proteins, including Raf and MKKs. The signaling cascades result in MAPKs phosphorylation and activation. MAPK pathways lead to expression of oncogenic proteins. Besides MAPKs, PI3-K is also activated by Fyn. Activated PI3-K leads to activation of Akt, and consequently turns on downstream signals to induce oncogenic gene expression. Akt inactivates several proapoptotic factors, including Bad. Along with MAPK and PI3-K pathways, activated transcription factors go into the nucleus and activate the expression of specific target genes in skin carcinogenesis. In summary, these signaling cascades result in skin cancer, angiogenesis, metastasis, aging, and proliferation.

and subsequently upregulates the phosphorylation of Akt, which is involved in mediating cell survival.[28] Moreover, the Akt level increased throughout this process due to increased PI3-K activity in chemically induced mouse skin carcinogenesis.[29] Activated Akt promotes cell survival by inhibiting apoptosis via the inactivation of several proapoptotic factors, includ-

ing the Bcl-2-associated death promoter (Bad).[30] Studies have also shown that Akt regulates the activation of NF-κB and AP-1, which are pivotal transcription factors involved in neoplastic transformation and the development of cancer.[31,32] Therefore, the PI3-K/Akt pathway is also considered an attractive target for cancer prevention or treatment.

The JAK/STAT3 pathway

The JAK family consists of nonreceptor tyrosine protein kinases and plays a critical role in cell survival, proliferation, differentiation, and apoptosis.[33] JAK kinase is required for the tyrosine phosphorylation of signal transducers and activators of transcription 3 (STAT3), which is activated by cytokines and growth factors. STATs are DNA-binding transcriptional factors,[34] and STAT1, STAT3, and STAT5 are frequently activated in human cancers, with a higher incidence of abnormal STAT3 activation in almost all tumors studied.[35] STAT3 is constitutively activated in a number of human malignancies, including breast cancer, lung cancer, melanoma, brain tumors, prostate cancer, and pancreatic adenocarcinoma.[36] Therefore, the JAK1–STAT3 pathway has been suggested as playing a critical role in cell transformation and carcinogenesis.

Other signaling pathways

Cyclooxygenase (COX), a rate-limiting enzyme for producing prostanoids such as prostaglandins, prostacyclins, and thromboxanes, is involved in skin carcinogenesis. COX has two main isoforms: COX-1 and COX-2. COX-1 is constitutively expressed in most tissues, whereas COX-2 is inducible by a variety of tumor-promoting agents.[37] It has been observed that COX-2 is upregulated after UVB exposure in both human and murine skin cells,[38] and upregulated COX-2 expression in skin epidermis is involved in the development of skin cancer.[39] Celecoxib, a specific COX-2 inhibitor, reduced the risk of skin cancer in mouse skin models.[40] In addition, lack of one allele of COX-2 mice had a 50–65% reduction of tumor multiplicity and a marked decrease in tumor size in a TPA-induced murine tumorigenesis model.[41] Cyclooxygenase-2 expression is critical for chronic UV-induced murine skin carcinogenesis.[41] Thus, developing an agent that can suppress COX-2 expression could be a critical strategy for the chemoprevention of skin cancer.

Angiogenesis is the growth of blood vessels, and blood vessels help tumors to grow by feeding the cancer cells with essential oxygen and nutrients. Skin tumors are highly angiogenic.[42] In the progression of malignant melanoma, the role of angiogenesis is well documented. Many angiogenic factors, including vascular endothelial growth factor (VEGF) and matrix metalloproteinases (MMPs), are upregulated in cutaneous malignant melanoma.[43] In the skin of VEGF transgenic mice, microvascular density and adhesion increased.[44] MMPs are also involved in tumor progression, invasion, and angiogenesis via remodeling of the extracellular matrix (ECM).[45] During the angiogenic processs, several MMPs, including MMP-9, MMP-13, and membrane-type 1 MMP, have been reported to play an important role in the degradation of the basement membrane and perivascular ECM components, modulation of angiogenic factors and production of endogenous angiogenic inhibitors.[46] Hypoxia-inducible factor-1 (HIF-1) is a heterodimeric transcription factor that plays a critical role in the cellular response to hypoxia. HIF-1 regulates the transcription of a broad range of genes that facilitate responses to the hypoxic environment, including genes regulating angiogenesis.[47] Among the HIF-α subunits, HIF-1α is expressed ubiquitously and has a major role in regulating oxygen homeostasis and tumor formation.[48,49] In addition, HIF-1α can be induced in an oxygen-independent manner by various cytokines through the PI3-K/Akt signal transduction pathway.[50]

Antiskin carcinogenic effects of myricetin

Antitumor promoting effects

Carcinogenesis is characterized as a multistage process that includes initiation, promotion, and progression stages. Cancer prevention strategies that involve intervention at the tumor promotion stage, a reversible and long-term process, seem to be more practical than those intervening at the tumor initiation stage, which is an irreversible and short-term process. The neoplastic transformation of cells is one of the major events occurring during carcinogenic processes. Additionally, elevated levels of COX-2 are frequently observed in various types of transformed and cancerous cells.[51] Therefore, inhibiting COX-2 expression and neoplastic transformation could be an effective strategy for delaying carcinogenesis.

Myricetin strongly inhibited the phorbol ester-induced upregulation of COX-2 expression in JB6 P$^+$ mouse epidermal (JB6 P$^+$) cells by targeting the NF-κB pathway.[52] A recent study showed that myricetin strongly inhibited tumor promoter–induced neoplastic cell transformation by inhibiting MEK kinase activity directly.[53] *Ex vivo* binding data showed that myricetin bound directly with MEK1 and a pull-down assay of Sepharose 4B-myricetin-coupled beads with three MEK1 deletion mutants further demonstrated that myricetin bound directly to MEK1 without competing with ATP. Another study demonstrated that myricetin can bind directly to Janus kinase 1/signal transducer and activator of transcription 3 (JAK1/STAT3) molecules, which play a role in cell transformation and carcinogenesis, to inhibit cell transformation in EGF-activated mouse JB6 P$^+$ cells.[54] Direct binding and kinase activity inhibition of Akt by myricetin downregulated downstream molecular events, including 12-*O*-tetradecanoylphorbol-13-acetate (TPA)–induced AP-1 activation, cyclin D1 expression, cell cycle progression, and cell transformation.[55] Other studies of myricetin showed that it can also bind with MKK4 directly and that it attenuated tumor necrosis factor-alpha (TNF-α)–induced JNK and ERK phosphorylation, AP-1 activation, and VEGF expression.[56] Docking data revealed that myricetin fits easily into the ATP-binding site of MKK4, located between the N- and C-lobes of the kinase domain. The surface of the putative myricetin-binding site in MKK4 accommodates the compound without any steric collision, leading to high inhibitory activity of MKK4. It can form hydrogen bonds with the backbone of the hinge region in MKK4, as do other ATP-competitive kinase inhibitors. In addition, myricetin readily docks in the ATP-binding site of Fyn.[57] As a result of binding with Fyn, myricetin attenuated the ultraviolet B (UVB)–induced COX-2 expression in mouse skin. Moreover, pretreatment with myricetin significantly suppressed the incidence of UVB-induced skin tumors in a dose-dependent manner.[57] In light of these results, myricetin constitutes a promising antiskin carcinogenic agent that suppresses the MAPK, Akt, Fyn, and JAK1/STAT3 pathways.

Polycyclic aromatic hydrocarbons (PAHs) are one of the groups of carcinogens to cause skin cancer,[58] and myricetin reduced PAHs-induced skin tumorigenesis in several animal models.[59] Topical application of myricetin prevented skin cancer development in SENCAR mice using 7,12-dimethylbenz(a)anthracene, benzo(a)pyrene and *N*-methyl-*N*-nitrosourea as the initiating agent.[59] Furthermore, myricetin delayed the beginning and development of skin tumors in BALB/c mice induced by PAHs.[59] Myricetin was also found to inhibit the mutagenicity of several bay-region diol-epoxides of PAHs inducing benzo(a)pyrene (BP) in the epidermis of SENCAR mice.[60] An-

other study showed that myricetin inhibited epidermal cytochrome P-450–dependent monooxygenases and BP metabolism.[61] These results suggest that myricetin is capable of inhibiting the carcinogenic effects of PAHs in the skin.

Antiapoptotic effects

Apoptosis is an active suicide mechanism that eliminates unwanted or potentially deleterious cells under a variety of physiological and pathological circumstances in multicellular organisms. It is generally accepted that the induction of apoptosis following UV radiation is an important defensive mechanism to ensure the removal of irreversibly damaged and potentially carcinogenic cells. UVB-induced genomic DNA damage has been suggested to be a crucial event triggering the apoptotic program. Furthermore, the formation of reactive oxygen species (ROS) following UV radiation appears to be an additional factor triggering the apoptotic machinery.[62] Since keratinocytes that are too seriously damaged for DNA repair undergo apoptosis, misregulation of the UVB-induced apoptotic process may have a cardinal effect on inducing skin cancer. Therefore, a specific therapeutic strategy designed to improve or decrease the susceptibility of individual cell types to apoptosis could establish the foundation for treating a variety of human diseases, such as cancer.

One study demonstrated that myricetin inactivates Akt to block Bad phosphorylation, leading to a reduced interaction between Bad and 14-3-3β and the mitochondrial translocation of Bad in UVB-irradiated cells.[63] Considering the important role of Akt in carcinogenesis, this study suggested that myricetin-mediated inactivation of Akt in the UVB response plays a role in regulating UVB-induced carcinogenesis. This is the first report to link the modulation of the Akt signaling axis in UVB-induced cell death to the naturally occurring polyphenolic compound myricetin. These findings reveal that a new regulatory mechanism of UVB-induced apoptosis and myricetin may be useful as a potential template for developing better chemopreventive agents against skin cancer.

Antiangiogenic effects

Angiogenesis, the sprouting of new blood vessels, is a crucial part of cancer development.[64] During the prevascular phase of tumor growth, tumors cannot exceed 1–2 mm in diameter. With angiogenesis, however, tumors are able to grow beyond this size and metastasize to other organs.[65] Therefore, various antiangiogenic strategies are currently being tested in clinical trials and are anticipated to provide promising results in cancer treatment.

Myricetin was recently found to inhibit UVB-induced angiogenesis by regulating PI3-K in an SKH-1 hairless mouse skin tumorigenesis model.[66] Topical treatment with myricetin inhibited repetitive UVB-induced neovascularization and platelet/endothelial cell adhesion molecule-1 expression in SKH-1 hairless mouse skin. Myricetin treatment significantly suppressed the induction of VEGF, MMP-9, MMP-13, and HIF-1α expression by chronic UVB irradiation.[66] The results of a kinase and pull-down assay indicated that myricetin suppressed UVB-induced PI3-K activity directly by binding with PI3-K, and subsequently attenuated the UVB-induced phosphorylation of Akt/p70[S6K] in mouse skin. An X-ray crystallographic study indicated that myricetin inhibits PI3-K activity by fitting into the ATP binding pocket of PI3-K; however, there is no evidence of a direct interaction between myricetin and PI3-K *in vivo*. These results are the first to demonstrate that myricetin inhibits UVB-induced HIF-1α expression and attenuates the UVB-induced phosphorylation of Akt by regulating PI3-K activity *in vivo* in mouse skin.

Antiaging effects

The specific damage produced in skin by repeated exposure to UV light is known as photoaging. Photoaging damage is characterized by histological changes, including damage to collagen fibers, excessive deposition of abnormal elastic fibers, and increased levels of glycosaminoglycans,[67] resulting in a wrinkled, lax, and coarse appearance with uneven pigmentation and brown spots.[68,69] Histological and ultrastructural studies have demonstrated such alterations in the dermal connective tissues of photoaged skin.[67]

Inflammation is also strongly related to skin aging. With age, the immune system becomes less effective and its capacity to manage the inflammatory response is reduced.[70] This leads to increased inflammatory activity. The term *inflammaging* describes this close relationship. Inflammation can become chronic if tissue health is not restored or occurs in response to stable low-grade irritation.[70] In this case, the immune system continues to produce low levels of inflammatory chemicals, including free radicals, leading to persistent inflammation and to continuous damage to the surrounding tissues. An excess of ROS in the skin can chronically activate NF-κB, a proinflammatory transcription factor, leading to the continued release of inflammatory mediators and to chronic inflammation. These ROS can be overgenerated by aging, external stresses (such as UV, pollution, toxins, and chemical irritants), and internal stresses (lifestyle, diet, and lack of sleep). Therefore, chronic inflammation also plays an important role in skin aging.

Flavonoid compounds possess antioxidant properties and could be useful in the prevention of photoaging. In a recent study, myricetin repressed UVA-induced MMP-1 activation in human dermal fibroblasts,[71] suggesting that it might be useful in preventing UV-induced skin aging. The inhibitory effects of flavonoids (myricetin, quercetin, kaempferol, luteolin, apigenin, and chrysin) on the UVA-induced collagenase activities and expression depend on the number of OH groups in these chemical structures. Compared with flavonol, myricetin had a greater inhibitory effect on UVA-induced MMP-1 activity. Another study demonstrated that myricetin protected keratinocytes against UVB-induced keratinocyte death.[72] The protective mechanisms of myricetin in keratinocytes against UVB-induced photodamage involve the inhibition of UVB-induced intracellular hydrogen peroxide production, lipid peroxidation, and JNK activation. Using a chronic UVB irradiation-induced skin aging model, myricetin inhibited UVB-induced photoaging in mouse skin.[73] Furthermore, this antiphotoaging effect of myricetin involved the suppression of MMP-9 expression through the direct inhibition of Raf kinase activity, suggesting that Raf kinase is a critical target for myricetin in inhibiting the UVB-induced formation of wrinkles and suppression of type I procollagen and collagen levels in mouse skin. Computer modeling showed that the hydroxyl groups at positions 3' and 4' of myricetin make H bonds with the backbone carbonyl group of Gly595 and the side chain of Thr598, thereby holding the activation loop of B-Raf in an inactive conformation. These results suggest that myricetin is a potent antiskin aging agent.

Conclusion

Studies clearly demonstrate that myricetin can bind directly to central kinases such as PI3-K, Akt, JAK1, Raf1, MEK1, MKK4, and Fyn, which regulate multiple cell signaling pathways in skin carcinogenesis. Notably, this one natural phytochemical can bind several protein kinases to target multiple pathways. Phytochemicals with multiple targets are ideal agents for treating chronic diseases, such as cancer, because these diseases, especially cancer, always involve changes in multiple cellular signaling pathways. Therefore, the regulation of multiple cell signaling pathways by myricetin may control the behavior of skin cancer cells, as well as other cancer cells, by inhibiting cell growth and inducing apoptosis, both of which are regulated by multiple pathways. Future X-ray crystallography investigations of the myricetin–protein kinase complexes are required to elucidate the exact binding modes.

Acknowledgments

This work was supported by grants from the World Class University Program (R31-2008-00-10056-0) and the National Leap Research Program (No. 2010-0029233) through the National Research Foundation of Korea funded by the Ministry of Education, Science and Technology, Republic of Korea.

Conflicts of interest

The authors declare no conflicts of interest.

References

1. Hertog, M.G. *et al.* 1993. Dietary antioxidant flavonoids and risk of coronary heart disease: the Zutphen Elderly Study. *Lancet* **342:** 1007–1011.
2. Koeppen, B.H. & K. Herrmann. 1977. Flavonoid glycosides and hydroxycinnamic acid esters of blackcurrants (Ribes nigrum). *Phenolics of fruits 9. Z Lebensm Unters Forsch.* **164:** 263–268.
3. Mattivi, F. *et al.* 2006. Metabolite profiling of grape: flavonols and anthocyanins. *J. Agric. Food Chem.* **54:** 7692–7702.
4. Hertog, M.G. *et al.* 1993. Intake of potentially anticarcinogenic flavonoids and their determinants in adults in The Netherlands. *Nutr. Cancer* **20:** 21–29.
5. Griffiths, L.A. & G.E. Smith. 1972. Metabolism of myricetin and related compounds in the rat. Metabolite formation in vivo and by the intestinal microflora in vitro. *Biochem. J.* **130:** 141–151.
6. Formica, J.V. & W. Regelson. 1995. Review of the biology of Quercetin and related bioflavonoids. *Food Chem. Toxicol.* **33:** 1061–1080.
7. Luo, J.L. *et al.* 2001. UV-induced DNA damage and mutations in Hupki (human p53 knock-in) mice recapitulate p53 hotspot alterations in sun-exposed human skin. *Cancer Res.* **61:** 8158–8163.
8. Newell, G.R. *et al.* 1988. Incidence of cutaneous melanoma in the United States by histology with special reference to the face. *Cancer Res.* **48:** 5036–5041.
9. Bode, A.M. & Z. Dong. 2003. Mitogen-activated protein kinase activation in UV-induced signal transduction. *Sci. STKE* **167:** 1–15.
10. Thomas, S.M. & J.S. Brugge. 1997. Cellular functions regulated by Src family kinases. *Annu. Rev. Cell Dev. Biol.* **13:** 513–609.
11. Matsumoto, T. *et al.* 2002. Overexpression of a constitutively active form of c-Src in skin epidermis increases sensitivity to tumor promotion by 12-O-tetradecanoylphorbol-13-acetate. *Mol. Carcinog.* **33:** 146–155.
12. Slaga, T.J. *et al.* 1986. Critical genetic determinants and molecular events in multistage skin carcinogenesis. *Symp. Fundam. Cancer Res.* **39:** 31–44.
13. Ayli, E.E. *et al.* 2008. Activation of Src-family tyrosine kinases in hyperproliferative epidermal disorders. *J. Cutan. Pathol.* **35:** 273–277.
14. Matsumoto, T. *et al.* 2003. Targeted expression of c-Src in epidermal basal cells leads to enhanced skin tumor promotion, malignant progression, and metastasis. *Cancer Res.* **63:** 4819–4828.
15. Calautti, E. *et al.* 1995. Fyn tyrosine kinase is involved in keratinocyte differentiation control. *Genes Dev.* **9:** 2279–2291.
16. Sebolt-Leopold, J.S. & R. Herrera. 2004. Targeting the mitogen-activated protein kinase cascade to treat cancer. *Nat. Rev. Cancer* **4:** 937–947.
17. Cobb, M.H. & E.J. Goldsmith. 1995. How MAP kinases are regulated. *J. Biol. Chem.* **270:** 14843–14846.
18. Sundaram, M. & M. Han. 1995. The C. elegans ksr-1 gene encodes a novel Raf-related kinase involved in Ras-mediated signal transduction. *Cell* **83:** 889–901.
19. Djavaheri-Mergny, M. & L. Dubertret. 2001. UV-A-induced AP-1 activation requires the Raf/ERK pathway in human NCTC 2544 keratinocytes. *Exp. Dermatol.* **10:** 204–210.
20. Rodriguez-Viciana, P., C. Sabatier & F. McCormick. 2004. Signaling specificity by Ras family GTPases is determined by the full spectrum of effectors they regulate. *Mol. Cell Biol.* **24:** 4943–4954.
21. Hoyos, B. *et al.* 2002. Activation of c-Raf kinase by ultraviolet light. Regulation by retinoids. *J. Biol. Chem.* **277:** 23949–23957.
22. Huntington, J.T. *et al.* 2004. Overexpression of collagenase 1 (MMP-1) is mediated by the ERK pathway in invasive melanoma cells: role of BRAF mutation and fibroblast growth factor signaling. *J. Biol. Chem.* **279:** 33168–33176.
23. Rajagopalan, H. *et al.* 2002. Tumorigenesis: RAF/RAS oncogenes and mismatch-repair status. *Nature* **418:** 934.
24. Cho, H.J. *et al.* 2007. Ascofuranone suppresses PMA-mediated matrix metalloproteinase-9 gene activation through the Ras/Raf/MEK/ERK- and Ap1-dependent mechanisms. *Carcinogenesis* **28:** 1104–1110.
25. Whitmarsh, A.J. & R.J. Davis. 2007. Role of mitogen-activated protein kinase kinase 4 in cancer. *Oncogene* **26:** 3172–3184.
26. Cantley, L.C. 2002. The phosphoinositide 3-kinase pathway. *Science* **296:** 1655–1657.

27. Yuan, T.L. & L.C. Cantley. 2008. PI3K pathway alterations in cancer: variations on a theme. *Oncogene* **27:** 5497–5510.

28. Engelman, J.A., J. Luo & L.C. Cantley. 2006. The evolution of phosphatidylinositol 3-kinases as regulators of growth and metabolism. *Nat. Rev. Genet* **7:** 606–619.

29. Samuels, Y. *et al.* 2004. High frequency of mutations of the PIK3CA gene in human cancers. *Science* **304:** 554.

30. Brunet, A. *et al.* 1999. Akt promotes cell survival by phosphorylating and inhibiting a Forkhead transcription factor. *Cell* **96:** 857–868.

31. Los, M. *et al.* 2009. Switching Akt: from survival signaling to deadly response. *Bioessays* **31:** 492–495.

32. Ozes, O.N. *et al.* 1999. NF-kappaB activation by tumour necrosis factor requires the Akt serine-threonine kinase. *Nature* **401:** 82–85.

33. Imada, K. & W.J. Leonard. 2000. The Jak-STAT pathway. *Mol. Immunol.* **37:** 1–11.

34. Rane, S.G. & E.P. Reddy. 2000. Janus kinases: components of multiple signaling pathways. *Oncogene* **19:** 5662–5679.

35. Bowman, T. *et al.* 2000. STATs in oncogenesis. *Oncogene* **19:** 2474–2488.

36. Klampfer, L. 2006. Signal transducers and activators of transcription (STATs): novel targets of chemopreventive and chemotherapeutic drugs. *Curr. Cancer Drug Targets* **6:** 107–121.

37. Smith, W.L., D.L. DeWitt & R.M. Garavito. 2000. Cyclooxygenases: structural, cellular, and molecular biology. *Annu. Rev. Biochem.* **69:** 145–182.

38. Chen, W. *et al.* 2001. Role of p38 MAP kinases and ERK in mediating ultraviolet-B induced cyclooxygenase-2 gene expression in human keratinocytes. *Oncogene* **20:** 3921–3926.

39. Lee, J.L. *et al.* 2003. Cyclooxygenases in the skin: pharmacological and toxicological implications. *Toxicol. Appl. Pharmacol.* **192:** 294–306.

40. Fischer, S.M. *et al.* 1999. Chemopreventive activity of celecoxib, a specific cyclooxygenase-2 inhibitor, and indomethacin against ultraviolet light-induced skin carcinogenesis. *Mol. Carcinog.* **25:** 231–240.

41. Fischer, S.M. *et al.* 2007. Cyclooxygenase-2 expression is critical for chronic UV-induced murine skin carcinogenesis. *Mol. Carcinog.* **46:** 363–371.

42. Hanahan, D. & J. Folkman. 1996. Patterns and emerging mechanisms of the angiogenic switch during tumorigenesis. *Cell* **86:** 353–364.

43. Liekens, S., E. De Clercq & J. Neyts. 2001. Angiogenesis: regulators and clinical applications. *Biochem. Pharmacol.* **61:** 253–270.

44. Detmar, M. *et al.* 1998. Increased microvascular density and enhanced leukocyte rolling and adhesion in the skin of VEGF transgenic mice. *J. Invest. Dermatol.* **111:** 1–6.

45. Surazynski, A. *et al.* 2008. Extracellular matrix and HIF-1 signaling: the role of prolidase. *Int. J. Cancer* **122:** 1435–1440.

46. Handsley, M.M. & D.R. Edwards. 2005. Metalloproteinases and their inhibitors in tumor angiogenesis. *Int. J. Cancer.* **115:** 849–860.

47. Forsythe, J.A. *et al.* 1996. Activation of vascular endothelial growth factor gene transcription by hypoxia-inducible factor 1. *Mol. Cell. Biol.* **16:** 4604–4613.

48. Iyer, N.V. *et al.* 1998. Cellular and developmental control of O2 homeostasis by hypoxia-inducible factor 1 alpha. *Genes Dev.* **12:** 149–162.

49. Ryan, H.E., J. Lo & R.S. Johnson. 1998. HIF-1 alpha is required for solid tumor formation and embryonic vascularization. *EMBO J.* **17:** 3005–3015.

50. Strieter, R.M. 2005. Masters of angiogenesis. *Nat. Med.* **11:** 925–927.

51. Pai, R. *et al.* 2002. Prostaglandin E2 transactivates EGF receptor: a novel mechanism for promoting colon cancer growth and gastrointestinal hypertrophy. *Nat. Med.* **8:** 289–293.

52. Lee, K.M. *et al.* 2007. Myricetin down-regulates phorbol ester-induced cyclooxygenase-2 expression in mouse epidermal cells by blocking activation of nuclear factor kappa B. *J. Agric. Food Chem.* **55:** 9678–9684.

53. Lee, K.W. *et al.* 2007. Myricetin is a novel natural inhibitor of neoplastic cell transformation and MEK1. *Carcinogenesis* **28:** 1918–1927.

54. Kumamoto, T., M. Fujii & D.X. Hou. 2009. Myricetin directly targets JAK1 to inhibit cell transformation. *Cancer Lett.* **275:** 17–26.

55. Kumamoto, T., M. Fujii & D.X. Hou. 2009. Akt is a direct target for myricetin to inhibit cell transformation. *Mol. Cell Biochem.* **332:** 33–41.

56. Kim, J.E. *et al.* 2009. MKK4 is a novel target for the inhibition of tumor necrosis factor-alpha-induced vascular endothelial growth factor expression by myricetin. *Biochem. Pharmacol.* **77:** 412–421.

57. Jung, S.K. *et al.* 2008. Myricetin suppresses UVB-induced skin cancer by targeting Fyn. *Cancer Res.* **68:** 6021–6029.

58. Buening, M.K. *et al.* 1978. Tumorigenicity of the optical enantiomers of the diastereomeric benzo[a]pyrene 7,8-diol-9,10-epoxides in newborn mice: exceptional activity of (+)-7beta,8alpha-dihydroxy-9alpha,10alpha-epoxy-7,8,9,10-tetrahydrobenzo[a]pyrene. *Proc. Natl. Acad. Sci. USA* **75:** 5358–5361.

59. Mukhtar, H. *et al.* 1988. Exceptional activity of tannic acid among naturally occurring plant phenols in protecting against 7,12-dimethylbenz(a)anthracene-, benzo(a)pyrene-, 3-methylcholanthrene-, and *N*-methyl-*N*-nitrosourea-induced skin tumorigenesis in mice. *Cancer Res.* **48:** 2361–2365.

60. Ashurst, S.W. *et al.* 1983. Formation of benzo(a)pyrene/DNA adducts and their relationship to tumor initiation in mouse epidermis. *Cancer Res.* **43:** 1024–1029.

61. Das, M. *et al.* 1987. Inhibition of epidermal xenobiotic metabolism in SENCAR mice by naturally occurring plant phenols. *Cancer Res.* **47:** 760–766.

62. Ichihashi, M. *et al.* 2003. UV-induced skin damage. *Toxicology* **189:** 21–39.

63. Kim, W. *et al.* 2010. Myricetin inhibits Akt survival signaling and induces Bad-mediated apoptosis in a low dose ultraviolet (UV)-B-irradiated HaCaT human immortalized keratinocytes. *J. Radiat. Res.* **51:** 285–296.

64. Bergers, G. & L.E. Benjamin. 2003. Tumorigenesis and the angiogenic switch. *Nat. Rev. Cancer* **3:** 401–410.

65. Carmeliet, P. & R.K. Jain. 2000. Angiogenesis in cancer and other diseases. *Nature* **407:** 249–257.

66. Jung, S.K. *et al.* 2010. Myricetin inhibits UVB-induced angiogenesis by regulating PI-3 kinase in vivo. *Carcinogenesis* **31:** 911–917.

67. Smith, J.G., Jr. *et al.* 1962. Alterations in human dermal connective tissue with age and chronic sun damage. *J. Invest. Dermatol.* **39:** 347–350.

68. Chung, J.H. *et al.* 2001. Modulation of skin collagen metabolism in aged and photoaged human skin in vivo. *J. Invest. Dermatol.* **117:** 1218–1224.

69. Grewe, M. *et al.* 1993. Analysis of the mechanism of ultraviolet (UV) B radiation-induced prostaglandin E2 synthesis by human epidermoid carcinoma cells. *J. Invest. Dermatol.* **101:** 528–531.

70. Alonso-Fernandez, P. & M. De la Fuente. 2011. Role of the immune system in aging and longevity. *Curr. Aging Sci. Epub ahead of print.*

71. Sim, G.S. *et al.* 2007. Structure activity relationship of antioxidative property of flavonoids and inhibitory effect on matrix metalloproteinase activity in UVA-irradiated human dermal fibroblast. *Arch. Pharm. Res.* **30:** 290–298.

72. Huang, J.H. *et al.* 2010. Protective effects of myricetin against ultraviolet-B-induced damage in human keratinocytes. *Toxicol. In Vitro.* **24:** 21–28.

73. Jung, S.K. *et al.* 2010. Myricetin suppresses UVB-induced wrinkle formation and MMP-9 expression by inhibiting Raf. *Biochem. Pharmacol.* **79:** 1455–1461.

Ann. N.Y. Acad. Sci. ISSN 0077-8923

ANNALS OF THE NEW YORK ACADEMY OF SCIENCES
Issue: *Nutrition and Physical Activity in Aging, Obesity, and Cancer*

Culinary plants and their potential impact on metabolic overload

Ji Yeon Kim[1] and Oran Kwon[1,2]

[1] Department of Nutritional Science and Food Management, Ewha Womans University, Seoul, Korea. [2]BioFood Network, Ewha Womans University, Seoul, Korea

Address for correspondence: Oran Kwon, Department of Nutritional Science and Food Management, Ewha Womans University, 11–1 Daehyeon-dong, Seodaemun-gu, Seoul 120-750, Korea. orank@ewha.ac.kr

Contemporary human behavior has led a large proportion of the population to metabolic overload and obesity. Postprandial hyperlipidemia and hyperglycemia evoke redox imbalance in the short term and lead to complex chronic disease in the long term with repeated occurrence. Complex diseases are best prevented with complex components of plants; thus, current nutrition research has begun to focus on the development of plant-based functional foods and dietary supplements for health and well-being. Furthermore, given the wide range of species, parts, and secondary metabolites, culinary plants can contribute significant variety and complexity to the human diet. Although understanding the health benefits of culinary plants has been one of the great challenges in nutritional science due to their inherent complexity, it is an advantageous pursuit. This review will address the challenges and opportunities relating to studies of the health benefits of culinary plants, with an emphasis on obesity attributed to metabolic overload.

Keywords: culinary plants; metabolic overload; multicomponents; multitargets

Introduction

From ancient times to the present, plants have been valued for their nutritional properties and flavor enhancement. In addition, plant use spanned the range between food and medicine.[1,2] The strong historic bond between plants and human health began to unwind in 1897 when synthetic acetyl salicylic acid (aspirin) was first introduced to the world, and throughout the 20th century more attention was paid to synthetic molecules than plant products. Presently, plant use for human health, including their use as functional foods and dietary supplements, is making a comeback.[3]

There are about 250,000 living plant species. Because the definition of plants is not clear in much of the scientific literature, for the purposes of this review we have used the term *culinary plants* to include fruits, vegetables, herbs, spices, and nuts, excluding fungi and lower plants. All culinary plants may contain a small number of primary compounds from the early products of photosynthesis, then produce a large array of secondary metabolites to protect them against a variety of environmental stresses.[4] For instance, various glycosides of bioactive components cause plants to be unpalatable, thereby reducing consumption by animals.[5] Carotenoids play a key role in the process of photoprotection by facilitating the dissipation of excess absorbed energy as heat under conditions of high sun exposure. They also serve the important functions of light collection under conditions of low light.[6] In fact, a variety of species of higher plants have the flexibility to alter the carotenoid composition of leaves in response to shade environment, with a high demand for efficient light collection or fully sun-exposed sites, with a high demand for photoprotection.[6] Table 1 shows an example of a classification framework for plant-produced secondary metabolites and their sources.[2,7,8] Many large-scale epidemiological studies have found that the health benefits of culinary plants could be attributed to these bioactive components in addition to vitamins, minerals, and fiber.[9–11]

doi: 10.1111/j.1749-6632.2011.06090.x

Table 1. Classification framework for bioactive components in culinary plants and examples of their sources

Classification	Major compounds	Major sources
Polyphenols		
Flavonoids		
Flavonols	fisetin, isorhamnetin, kaempferol, myricetin, quercetin	apple, basil, coriander, cumin, dill, fennel, onion, parsley, tarragon, thyme
Flavones	apigenin, luteolin	oregano, parsley, peppermint, rosemary, thyme
Flavanones	eriodictyol, hesperetin, naringenin	peppermint, rosemary
Flavan-3-ols	(+)-catechin, (+)-gallocatechin, (−)-epigallocatechin, (−)-epicatechin, (−)-epicatechin-3-gallate, theaflavin	nutmeg, teas
Anthocyanidins	cyanidin, delphinidin, malvidin, pelargonidin, peonidin, petunidin	black currant, berries, cherry, eggplant, orange, red grape
Isoflavones	daidzein, genistein	red clover, soybean
Phenolic acids		
Hydroxy-benzoic acid derivatives	gallic acid, salicylic acid, vanillic acid	cumin, sage, thyme
Hydroxy-cinnamic acid derivatives	caffeic acid, *p*-coumaric acid	cumin, fennel
Terpenes		
Monoterpenes	geraniol, limonene, terpineol	basil, caraway, celery seed, coriander, cumin, dill, fennel, mint, marjoram, peppermint, rosemary, sage, spearmint, thyme
Sesquiterpenes	farnesenes, farnesol, humulene	coriander, turmeric
Diterpene	cafestol, cembrene, kahweol, phytol, retinoids (retinol, retinal), taxadiene	chili powder, paprika, red pepper
Triterpenes	squalene, saponins (glycyrrhizin)	shark liver oil, licorice
Tetraterpenes	lycopene, alpha, beta, gamma-carotene	coriander, cumin, fennel, mustard, sage
Vanilloids	capsaicin, curcumin, gingerol, paradol	turmeric, ginger, mustard ginger, ginger oleoresin, paprika, red pepper
Sulfur containing compounds		
Disulfides	diallyl disulfide	garlic
Thiols	allicin	onion

In this review, we first discuss obesity attributed to metabolic overload, as this is a major focus of current functional food and dietary supplement development. We will then discuss the use of culinary plants and their bioactive components in obesity prevention. In addition, the challenges presented by the multicomponent nature of culinary plants and disease complexity are discussed.

Metabolic overload

Contemporary human behavior favors excessive intake of energy and limited energy expenditure. The postprandial state is a dynamic and potentially unstable one. In a single day, the systemic stress of hyperlipidemia and hyperglycemia induces a seemingly trivial redox imbalance. However, over time these biological insults can evoke metabolic, oxidative, and immune imbalance, manifesting in cellular dysfunction, disease, and ultimately death.[12]

Postprandial metabolic overload

The term *postprandial* refers to the time after a meal, which is a dynamic period of metabolic trafficking, biosynthesis, and oxidative metabolism of absorbed substrates. During this state, every major biological system, organ, tissue, and cell is responding with compensatory and adaptive mechanisms to manage the short-term disturbance and restore balance/homeostasis.[12] Under optimal conditions, the movement from balance is modest, allowing for rapid system recovery and negligible opportunity for unfavorable stress. However, considering the fact that most people eat several times a day, postprandial period–induced chronic disease can be attributed to exaggerated metabolic, oxidative, and immune imbalance.[13–16]

Early stage of obesity

In normal physiology, binding of insulin to its receptors in skeletal muscle and adipose tissues normally facilitates glucose entry into the cell via glucose transporter type 4 (GLUT-4).[17] After phosphorylation, glucose is either stored as glycogen or oxidized to form CO_2 and H_2O. Any unoxidized surplus is transformed into fatty acid via malonyl CoA. In addition to stimulating the uptake of glucose, insulin upregulates the lipogenic transcription factor sterol regulatory element-binding protein 1c (SREBP-1c),[18] followed by enzymes for *de novo* fat synthesis. Newly synthesized fatty acids and dietary fatty acids are transported as very low-density lipoproteins (VLDL) and stored as triglyceride in adipocytes, resulting in obesity.[19] At early stages of obesity, adipocytes continue to actively store additional triglycerides and begin to function as endocrine cells. Adipokines such as leptin and adiponectin are secreted to enhance the insulin sensitivity of the peripheral tissues. Therefore, β-oxidation in muscle can often be maintained.[20] Specifically, leptin production increases in proportion to the increase in fat accumulation. Hyperleptinemia downregulates SREBP-1c and activates 5' adenosine monophosphate-activated protein kinase (AMPK)-induced fat oxidation, leading to limited intramyocellular and liver triglyceride deposition.[21]

Adipocyte dysfunction and inflammation

The homeostatic capacity of adipose tissue has its limits, as adipocytes reach large dimensions and can easily suffer mechanical rupture.[22] In parallel, adipocytes begin to secrete adipokines that modulate an inflammatory response in adipose tissue. Specifically, monocyte chemoattractant protein-1 (MCP-1) enhances macrophage infiltration into adipose tissue.[23] A major contribution to the inflammatory nature of obesity is the sharp increase in the activity of tumor necrosis factor-α[24,25] and other proinflammatory cytokines, which results in an increase in lipolysis and a decrease in triglyceride synthesis in adipocytes.[20]

Lipotoxicity

These actions in turn result in an increase in the circulating concentration of free fatty acids. Liver increases the production of apo-B-containing particles that carry triglycerides to the adipose tissue.[26] This occurs very efficiently in visceral adipose tissue compared to subcutaneous adipose tissue. However, when the capacity of both locations is overwhelmed, the conversion of VLDL or similar particles is delayed and hypertriglyceridemia originates.[27] Furthermore, leptin-mediated protection against the lipotoxic metabolic syndrome diminishes in part because of leptin resistance, thereby increasing SREBP-1c expression and blocking the compensatory increase in fatty acid oxidation. Nonadipose tissues are used for lipid accumulation,[28] and as these organs are not able to store lipids without malfunctioning, the result is lipotoxicity culminating in insulin resistance, atherosclerotic vascular disease, macrophage foam cells, nonalcoholic fatty liver, and myopathy.[22]

Culinary plants and metabolic overload

Several grams of culinary plant material are ingested daily as part of a regular diet. The bioactive components of culinary plants differ remarkably in content, composition, and bioavailability but have limited uptake and bioavailability compared to macronutrients.[4] For example, the estimated absorption of polyphenols is between 1% and 60%, and the resulting peak plasma concentration of parent compound or metabolites does not exceed micromolar levels.[29] By contrast, intestinal luminal concentrations are believed to be up to 50-fold higher than plasma concentrations.[30]

However, low bioavailability of bioactive components is apparently not a disadvantage. As the gut is the major organ involved in nutrient absorption, unabsorbed bioactive components may inhibit macronutrient absorption. Therefore, these components may have a significant potential to reduce postprandial metabolic overload. In parallel with this finding, a growing body of *in vitro* and animal studies suggests that unabsorbed nutrients may stimulate the secretion of glucagon like peptide-1 (GLP-1) and glucose-dependent insulinotropic peptide (GIP) in enterocytes to suppress appetite, resulting in reduced energy intake.[31] In addition, bioactive components are broken down by the gut microflora to form a wide range of bioactive products, such as equol from soy isoflavones.[32]

Based on a large number of publications, it has become apparent that inflammation and oxidative stress are key features in metabolic overload.[12] The most well-known mechanism of culinary plants for the prevention of damage to cellular lipids, proteins, and DNA is through direct radical scavenging. However, the scavenging effect is considered unlikely to be the sole explanation for this effect.

Current evidence suggests that bioactive components may exert at least part of their beneficial effect by their interactions with specific proteins central to intracellular signaling cascades, ultimately leading to changes in gene expression encoding cytoprotective proteins.[4] The most prominent example is curcumin, the active component of turmeric, which inhibits a number of signaling pathways and molecular targets involved in inflammation and metabolic overload.[33] Curcumin can inhibit the IkappaB kinase (IKK) signaling complex, thereby inactivating nuclear factor kappa-light-chain-enhancer of activated B cells (NF-κB) in inflammation.[34] Curcumin also stimulates hem oxygenase-1 (HO-1) gene activity via inactivation of the nuclear factor erythroid-2-related factor 2-Kelch-like ECH-associating protein 1 (Nrf2-Keap1) complex, leading to increased Nrf2 binding to the resident HO-1 and the antioxidant-responsive element.[35] Curcumin activates Wingless-type mouse mammary tumor virus integration site family member (WNT)/β-catenin signaling, which blocks adipogenesis through repression of CCAAT/enhancer-binding protein-α (CEBPA) and peroxisome proliferator activated receptor γ (PPARγ). In adipocytes, curcumin increases the activity of AMPK, resulting in the downregulation of PPARγ and decreased cyclooxygenase-2 (COX-2) expression.[36] In addition, curcumin downregulates the inflammatory cytokines, resistin and leptin, and upregulates adiponectin and other associated proteins.[37] Taken together, it is reasonable to assume that multiple bioactive components in culinary plants can provide greater health benefits that may not be achievable by any single component in terms of the potential to affect multiple signal transduction pathways.

Challenges and opportunities of culinary plant research for metabolic overload

Despite the great diversity of compounds that plants synthesize, there are some obstacles to studying the metabolic health benefits of culinary plants. Further complicating matters, the adipose tissue and other organs, such as the liver, muscle, and hypothalamus, actively communicate with each other and participate in the regulation of energy homeostasis.[38]

Multicomponents
The lack of reproducibility of bioactivity is one of the major obstacles to the use of culinary plants.[39] In addition, the same components can often be found in multiple plants, complicating the interpretation of the results. *Standardization* refers to the production of a plant preparation that is consistent in terms of chemical composition and efficacy.[40] It begins with control over both the raw material supply and the manufacturing process. Full standardization of plants or their extracts is possible only when the major bioactive components are known and the range of their allowable fluctuations in the final product is established.[41] To identify the principal bioactive components, investigators first perform experiments on fractionating extracts of plants and then testing the activity of each fraction in a suitable cell culture model or high-throughput assay system.[42] An example of this is hydroxycitric acid, the bioactive component of *Garcinia cambogia* for *de novo* lipogenesis inhibition.[43] Although the process is based on simple principles, identifying active components is often a challenge. The process is even more complicated when culinary plants are involved in the activity related to multiple metabolic pathways. If little or no information is available about the active components, a less-specific approach can be taken. Identification of chromatographic

fingerprint or measurement of marker compounds can be used. Marker compounds are easy to quantify constituents, but may not be related to efficacy.[44] Additionally, biological activity and toxicity can be directly measured in different batches *in vitro*. However, such standardization is possible only when the mechanism of action is known and may involve *in vitro* enzymatic or transcriptional assays.[41]

The potential array of active ingredients in culinary plants might play additive or synergistic roles, providing more potent health benefits compared with a single component.[45] Typically, mechanistic studies performed *in vivo* and in cell cultures have utilized pure compounds or highly purified extracts. Results obtained from single components often differ from those of the whole food; however, nothing is known about the interactions between bioactive components.[45] The paper by Morré *et al.* suggests that (−)-epigallocatechin-3-gallate (EGCG), the most bioactive component of green tea, is unstable on its own but has greater biological activity in green tea because of the presence of other catechins.[46] Therefore, there is an urgent need to develop multiplex approaches capable of detecting beneficial interactions within mixtures, such as "-omics" and systems biology technologies. However these are only beginning to be realized and are not yet established.[41]

Multitargets

The multifactorial nature of many complex diseases is also an important consideration. Obesity cannot be ascribed to a single genetic or environmental change but arises from a combination of genetic, environmental, or behavioral factors. Furthermore, understanding obesity requires knowledge of the dynamic relationship between different organs and how these relationships change through time and space. Multiple bioactive components in culinary plants and their extracts utilize batteries of various factors to maintain homeostasis of the body, which interact with lower affinity.[47] However, low-affinity binding does not necessarily mean that the interactions of bioactive components with the targets are nonproductive. Most links in cellular protein, signaling, and transcriptional networks are weak, and multiplication of low-affinity binding might be sufficient to achieve a significant modification.[47] Besides, low-affinity multibinding might have an advantage for a lower prevalence of side effects.[48]

Measuring these factors requires an ability to acquire and integrate multiple types of data. Innovative technologies, such as rapidly emerging gene-expression real-time polymerase chain reaction (RT-PCR) arrays, provide a lower-throughput, mixture-friendly format by allowing simultaneous detection of the effects of culinary plant extracts on multiple genes in obesity-related pathways. [41]

Conclusion

Diverse arrays of bioactive components likely provide better health benefits via synergistic action. Low bioavailability produces local effects in the intestine and increased activity for additional benefits. The challenge of analyzing multiple targets provides opportunities to apply cutting-edge science, such as informatics and systems biology, in the field of plant-based functional food and supplement studies. Traditional approaches like bioprospecting, in which samples are collected from natural sources and tested or indigenous knowledge is utilized, will continue to be important.[41] Although promising data have been gleaned from *in vitro* and animal studies, very little data from human studies exist. Therefore, more information is needed to define the appropriate strategies for achieving the maximum health benefits from culinary plants and to understand their role in the context of the entire diet.

Conflict of interest

The authors declare no conflicts of interest.

References

1. Low Dog, T. 2006. A reason to season: the therapeutic benefits of spices and culinary herbs. *Explore (NY).* **2:** 446–449.
2. Lampe, J.W. 2003. Spicing up a vegetarian diet: chemopreventive effects of phytochemicals. *Am. J. Clin. Nutr.* **78:** 579S–583S.
3. Raskin, I. *et al.* 2002. Plants and human health in the twenty-first century. *Trends Biotechnol.* **20:** 522–531.
4. Holst, B. & G. Williamson. 2008. Nutrients and phytochemicals: from bioavailability to bioefficacy beyond antioxidants. *Curr. Opin. Biotechnol.* **19:** 73–82.
5. Mallavadhani, U.V. *et al.* 2003. Antifeedant activity of some pentacyclic triterpene acids and their fatty acid ester analogues. *J. Agric. Food Chem.* **51:** 1952–1955.
6. Demmig-Adams, B., A.M. Gilmore & W.W. Adams. 1996. Carotenoids 3: in vivo function of carotenoids in higher plants. *FASEB J.* **10:** 403–412.
7. Yang, R.Y., S. Lin & G. Kuo. 2008. Content and distribution of flavonoids among 91 edible plant species. *Asia Pac. J. Clin. Nutr.* **17**(Suppl 1): 275–279.

8. Kaefer, C.M. & J.A. Milner. 2008. The role of herbs and spices in cancer prevention. *J. Nutr. Biochem.* **19:** 347–361.

9. Kris-Etherton, P.M. *et al.* 2004. Bioactive compounds in nutrition and health-research methodologies for establishing biological function: the antioxidant and anti-inflammatory effects of flavonoids on atherosclerosis. *Annu. Rev. Nutr.* **24:** 511–538.

10. Most, M.M. 2004. Estimated phytochemical content of the dietary approaches to stop hypertension (DASH) diet is higher than in the Control Study Diet. *J. Am. Diet Assoc.* **104:** 1725–1727.

11. Mennen, L.I. *et al.* 2004. Consumption of foods rich in flavonoids is related to a decreased cardiovascular risk in apparently healthy French women. *J. Nutr.* **134:** 923–926.

12. Burton-Freeman, B. 2010. Postprandial metabolic events and fruit-derived phenolics: a review of the science. *Br. J. Nutr.* **104**(Suppl 3): S1–S14.

13. Nappo, F. *et al.* 2002. Postprandial endothelial activation in healthy subjects and in type 2 diabetic patients: role of fat and carbohydrate meals. *J. Am. Coll. Cardiol.* **39:** 1145–1150.

14. Sies, H., W. Stahl & A. Sevanian. 2005. Nutritional, dietary and postprandial oxidative stress. *J. Nutr.* **135:** 969–972.

15. Ursini, F., *et al.* 1998. Postprandial plasma lipid hydroperoxides: a possible link between diet and atherosclerosis. *Free Radic. Biol. Med.* **25:** 250–252.

16. Alipour, A. *et al.* 2007. Postprandial inflammation and endothelial dysfuction. *Biochem. Soc. Trans.* **35:** 466–469.

17. Quon, M.J. *et al.* 1994. Insulin receptor substrate 1 mediates the stimulatory effect of insulin on GLUT4 translocation in transfected rat adipose cells. *J. Biol. Chem.* **269:** 27920–27924.

18. Foufelle, F. & P. Ferré. 2002. New perspectives in the regulation of hepatic glycolytic and lipogenic genes by insulin and glucose: a role for the transcription factor sterol regulatory element binding protein-1c. *Biochem. J.* **366:** 377–391.

19. Unger, R.H. 2003. Lipid overload and overflow: metabolic trauma and the metabolic syndrome. *Trends Endocrinol. Metab.* **14:** 398–403.

20. Guilherme, A. *et al.* 2008. Adipocyte dysfunctions linking obesity to insulin resistance and type 2 diabetes. *Nat. Rev. Mol. Cell Biol.* **9:** 367–377.

21. Minokoshi, Y. & B.B. Kahn. 2003. Role of AMP-activated protein kinase in leptin-induced fatty acid oxidation in muscle. *Biochem. Soc. Trans.* **31:** 196–201.

22. Monteiro, R. & I. Azevedo. 2010. Chronic inflammation in obesity and the metabolic syndrome. *Mediators Inflamm.* Art. ID 289645.

23. Sartipy, P. & D.J. Loskutoff. 2003. Monocyte chemoattractant protein 1 in obesity and insulin resistance. *Proc. Natl. Acad. Sci. USA* **100:** 7265–7270.

24. Feinstein, R. *et al.* 1993. Tumor necrosis factor-alpha suppresses insulin-induced tyrosine phosphorylation of insulin receptor and its substrates. *J. Biol. Chem.* **268:** 26055–26058.

25. Hotamisligil, G.S., N.S. Shargill & B.M. Spiegelman. 1993. Adipose expression of tumor necrosis factor-alpha: di-

rect role in obesity-linked insulin resistance. *Science* **259:** 87–91.

26. Parhofer, K.G. & P.H. Barrett. 2006. Thematic review series: patient-oriented research. What we have learned about VLDL and LDL metabolism from human kinetics studies. *J. Lipid Res.* **47:** 1620–1630.

27. Laclaustra, M., D. Corella & J.M. Ordovas. 2007. Metabolic syndrome pathophysiology: the role of adipose tissue. *Nutr. Metab. Cardiovasc. Dis.* **17:** 125–139.

28. Sethi, J.K. & A.J. Vidal-Puig. 2007. Thematic review series: adipocyte biology. Adipose tissue function and plasticity orchestrate nutritional adaptation. *J. Lipid Res.* **48:** 1253–1262.

29. Manach, C. *et al.* 2005. Bioavailability and bioefficacy of polyphenols in humans. I. Review of 97 bioavailability studies. *Am. J. Clin. Nutr.* **81:** 230S–242S.

30. Kwon, O. *et al.* 2007. Inhibition of the intestinal glucose transporter GLUT2 by flavonoids. *FASEB J.* **21:** 366–377.

31. Yavropoulou, M.P. & J.G. Yovos. 2010. Central regulation of glucose-dependent insulinotropic polypeptide secretion. *Vitam. Horm.* **84:** 185–201.

32. Yuan, J.P., J.H. Wang & X. Liu. 2007. Metabolism of dietary soy isoflavones to equol by human intestinal microflora–implications for health. *Mol. Nutr. Food Res.* **51:** 765–781.

33. Graham, A. 2009. Curcumin adds spice to the debate: lipid metabolism in liver disease. *Br. J. Pharmacol.* **157:** 1352–1353.

34. Woo, H.M. *et al.* 2007. Active spice-derived components can inhibit inflammatory responses of adipose tissue in obesity by suppressing inflammatory actions of macrophages and release of monocyte chemoattractant protein-1 from adipocytes. *Life Sci.* **80:** 926–931.

35. Balogun, E. *et al.* 2003. Curcumin activates the haem oxygenase-1 gene via regulation of Nrf2 and the antioxidant-responsive element. *Biochem J.* **371:** 887–895.

36. Lee, Y.K. *et al.* 2009. Curcumin exerts antidifferentiation effect through AMPKalpha-PPAR-gamma in 3T3-L1 adipocytes and antiproliferatory effect through AMPKalpha-COX-2 in cancer cells. *J. Agric. Food Chem.* **57:** 305–310.

37. Shehzad, A. *et al.* 2011. New mechanisms and the anti-inflammatory role of curcumin in obesity and obesity-related metabolic diseases. *Eur. J. Nutr.* **50:** 151–161.

38. Karalis, K.P. *et al.* 2009. Mechanisms of obesity and related pathology: linking immune responses to metabolic stress. *FEBS J.* **276:** 5747–5754.

39. Cordell, G.A. 2000. Biodiversity and drug discovery–a symbiotic relationship. *Phytochemistry.* **55:** 463–480.

40. Ribnicky, D.M. *et al.* 2008. Evaluation of botanicals for improving human health. *Am. J. Clin. Nutr.* **87:** 472S–475S.

41. Schmidt, B.M. *et al.* 2007. Revisiting the ancient concept of botanical therapeutics. *Nat. Chem. Biol.* **3:** 360–366.

42. Barnes, S. *et al.* 2008. Technologies and experimental approaches at the National Institutes of Health Botanical Research Centers. *Am. J. Clin. Nutr.* **87:** 476S–480S.

43. Heymsfield, S.B. *et al.* 1998. Garcinia cambogia (hydroxycitric acid) as a potential antiobesity agent: a randomized controlled trial. *JAMA* **280:** 1596–1600.

44. AHPA Botanical Extracts Committee. 2003. *Standardization of Botanical Products.* Silverspring, MD: American Herbal Products Association.

45. Jeffery, E. 2005. Component interactions for efficacy of functional foods. *J. Nutr.* **135:** 1223–1225.

46. Morré, D.J. *et al.* 2003. Tea catechin synergies in inhibition of cancer cell proliferation and of a cancer specific cell surface oxidase (ECTO-NOX). *Pharmacol. Toxicol.* **92:** 234–241.

47. Csermely, P., V. Agoston & S. Pongor. 2005. The efficiency of multi-target drugs: the network approach might help drug design. *Trends Pharmacol. Sci.* **26:** 178–182.

48. Rogawski, M.A. 2000. Low affinity channel blocking (uncompetitive) NMDA receptor antagonists as therapeutic agents–toward an understanding of their favorable tolerability. *Amino Acids* **19:** 133–149.

Ann. N.Y. Acad. Sci. ISSN 0077-8923

ANNALS OF THE NEW YORK ACADEMY OF SCIENCES
Issue: *Nutrition and Physical Activity in Aging, Obesity, and Cancer*

Inflammation-mediated obesity and insulin resistance as targets for nutraceuticals

Myung-Sunny Kim,[1] Myeong Soo Lee,[2] and Dae Young Kown[1]

[1]Korea Food Research Institute, Gyongki-do, Republic of Korea. [2]Korea Institute of Oriental Medicine, Daejeon, Republic of Korea

Address for correspondence: Myung-Sunny Kim, Ph.D., Korea Food Research Institute, Baekhyon-dong 516, Bundang-ku, Songnam, Gyongki-do, 463-746, Republic of Korea. truka@kfri.re.kr

Obesity-induced inflammation plays an important role in the development of insulin resistance, type 2 diabetes (T2D), and metabolic dysfunctions. Chronic activation of proinflammatory pathways within insulin target cells can lead to obesity-related insulin resistance. The inflammatory mediators consist of immune cells, cytokines, adipokines, and inflammatory signaling molecules. Targeting obesity-associated inflammation has been shown to protect experimental animals and human subjects from obesity-induced insulin resistance. Modulation of the inflammatory responses associated with obesity may help prevent or improve obesity-induced metabolic dysfunctions. In this review, we introduce the beneficial effects of nutraceuticals for targeting inflammation in the treatment of obesity-induced insulin resistance and metabolic dysfunctions.

Keywords: inflammation; obesity; metabolic disease; nutraceuticals

Introduction

The growing prevalence of obesity and the pathologies associated with it has become a major threat to public health. The chronic inflammation observed in obesity appears to be a critical factor in the development of pathological disturbances such as insulin resistance, type 2 diabetes, cardiovascular disease, and other metabolic diseases. The obesity-induced alteration of biological conditions in target tissues results in systemic insulin resistance and inflammation.[1–3]

Modulating inflammatory responses in obese patients may be useful for preventing or ameliorating obesity-related pathologies. This review summarizes the molecular pathways that link inflammation and metabolic dysfunctions, and we also review evidence for the modulation of obesity-induced inflammation by various nutraceuticals.

Inflammation and insulin resistance

Many studies have shown that adipose tissue is an important initiator of the inflammatory response to obesity. The inflammation characterized by in-filtration of macrophages and other immune cells into obese white adipose tissue can cause systemic insulin resistance.[4,5]

Adipose tissue macrophages (ATMs) are a major source of proinflammatory cytokines, which can function in a paracrine and potentially an endocrine fashion to decrease insulin sensitivity. Activation of these tissue macrophages leads to the release of a variety of chemokines, which in turn recruit additional macrophages. Recent studies have detected various subsets of T lymphocytes in obese adipose tissue of humans and mice.[6–8] In obese subjects, adipose tissue T_H1 lymphocytes may help to recruit macrophages into adipose tissue; the macrophages then stimulate inflammation, leading to insulin resistance. Although the role of immune cells in adipose tissue has not been fully elucidated, it seems probable that the inflammatory response mediated by AT immune cells plays a key pathogenic role in the development of obesity-induced insulin resistance.

The proinflammatory cytokine tumor necrosis factor (TNF)-α was identified as the first molecular link between obesity, diabetes, and inflammation.[9,10] TNF-α was found to be overexpressed in

doi: 10.1111/j.1749-6632.2011.06098.x

the adipose and muscle tissues of obese mice and humans.[11–13] In experimental models, neutralization of TNF-α improved insulin sensitivity in obese *fa/fa* rats,[9,11] and the TNF-α–deficient obese mice were protected from obesity-induced insulin resistance.[14] Since these findings, obesity has been characterized by the presence of many inflammatory mediators in adipose tissue. These include leptin, resistin, plasminogen activator inhibitor type-1 (PAI-1), adiponectin, visfatin, monocyte chemoattractant protein-1 (MCP-1), interleukin (IL)-6, IL-1, serum amyloid A (SAA), retinol binding protein-4 (RBP-4), and macrophage inflammatory protein (MIP).[1–3] These play a central role in regulating energy and vascular system homeostasis by influencing various metabolic processes. There is also evidence of macrophage infiltration in the other metabolic organs, the liver, and skeletal muscle.[1] Kupffer cells, the resident macrophages of the liver, contribute to the production of inflammatory mediators that promote insulin resistance in hepatocytes.

Molecular mechanisms of inflammation and insulin resistance

Previous studies focusing on the intracellular pathways activated by inflammation have provided key insight into obesity-induced insulin resistance. Increased inflammatory stimuli in obese subjects, including cytokines and Toll-like receptor (TLR) stimulation, can activate the inhibitor of κB kinase-β/nuclear factor κB (IKKβ/NF-κB) axis and c-Jun N-terminal kinase (JNK).[15–17] The activation of these kinases in obesity highlights the overlap between metabolic and immune pathways, the latter of which are activated during the innate immune response by TLR signaling in response to lipopolysacharide (LPS), peptidoglycan, fatty acids, and other microbial products.[18] Genetic disruption of IKKβ and pharmacological inhibition of IKKβ with salicylates in obese mice have been shown to improve insulin resistance.[17] In addition, JNK1 knockout (KO) mice are protected against diet-induced insulin resistance, and inhibitors of JNK also appear to improve insulin sensitivity in models of insulin resistance.[16,19] Additionally, cellular stresses such as reactive oxygen species (ROS), endoplasmic reticulum (ER) stress, and ceramide can activate the NF-κB and JNK inflammatory pathways.[20]

Peroxisome proliferator-activated receptor (PPARγ) is a major molecular target for all insulin-sensitizing thiazolidinediones (TZD).[21] In normal adipose tissue, PPARγ senses fatty acids and regulates the expression of many genes involved in glucose metabolism and adipocyte differentiation. Although it is most highly expressed in adipocytes, PPARγ is also expressed in macrophages, where it can negatively regulate a large set of inflammatory genes.[22–25] Recently, it was demonstrated that macrophage-specific PPARγ KO mice on normal and high-fat diets showed inflammatory pathway activation, glucose intolerance, and insulin resistance.[26,27] In terms of glucose homeostasis, TZD treatment was much less effective in macrophage-specific PPARγ KO mice compared with controls, suggesting an essential role of macrophage PPARγ in the maintenance of systemic insulin activity.[26] IL-1 and TNF-α also suppress the ligand-induced transactivation of PPARγ, which is mediated through NF-κB and is activated by the TAK1/TAB1/NF-κB-inducing kinase (NIK) cascade downstream of IL-1 and TNF-α signaling.[28]

However, the immunological dysfunctions associated with obesity are not restricted to local metabolic tissues. It has been suggested that obesity alters the functions of circulating immune cells.[29–31] Circulating mononuclear cells from obese subjects are in a constitutive proinflammatory state and show an increase in intranuclear NF-κB binding and elevated transcript levels of proinflammatory genes such as IL-6, TNF-α, and migration inhibition factor, which are regulated by NF-κB.[29] Obesity has also been linked to elevated circulating leukocyte and lymphocyte subset counts, increased granulocyte phagocytosis, and higher levels of oxidative burst.[31]

Targeting inflammation by nutraceuticals in obesity and insulin resistance

There is a considerable need for safe therapeutic agents that can reduce the risk of obesity-induced metabolic dysfunctions, and the range of nutraceutical compounds with potential benefits for obese patients continues to expand. The reported anti-inflammatory properties of food-derived nutraceuticals may be crucial for the treatment of such diseases.

Curcumin

Curcumin, a yellow pigment of curry powder, has been shown to downregulate the expression of various NF-κB–regulated proinflammatory adipokines, including chemokines (MCP-1, MCP-4, and eotaxin)[32] and interleukins (IL-1, IL-6, and IL-8)[33] *in vitro*. Curcumin was also shown to suppress the expression of PAI-1 by inhibiting the transcription factor early growth response (Egr-1),[34] which has been closely linked with insulin resistance and obesity.

Animal studies have shown that curcumin administration ameliorated diabetes in obese and leptin-deficient *ob/ob* C57BL6/J mice, as indicated by glucose- and insulin-tolerance testing and the percentage glycosylated hemoglobin.[35] Curcumin also reduced macrophage infiltration in WAT, increased adipose tissue adiponectin production, decreased hepatic NF-κB activity, and reduced the expression of hepatic inflammation markers, including TNF-α, IL-1β, suppressor of cytokine signaling 3, MCP-1, and C-C motif receptor-2. Jain *et al.*[36] reported that curcumin supplementation lowered the high glucose-mediated monocyte production of inflammatory cytokines, including TNF-α, IL-6, IL-8, and MCP-1. This same study also showed that blood levels of TNF-α, MCP-1, glucose, and glycosylated hemoglobin were decreased in diabetic rats on a curcumin diet. Taken together, these data suggest that curcumin may be a useful phytochemical for attenuating obesity-induced inflammation and obesity-related metabolic complications.

Capsaicin

Capsaicin, a biologically active compound found in red pepper, has anti-inflammatory activities[37–39] and shows potential benefits for treating obesity and insulin resistance in animal models and clinical studies.[40–42] Capsaicin has diverse activities in metabolic tissues. In addition to its metabolic properties that induce thermogenesis and fat oxidation, capsaicin also shows anti-inflammatory properties.[41] A proteomic analysis showed that thermogenesis- and lipid metabolism-related proteins in white adipose tissue[43] and skeletal muscle[44] were altered upon capsaicin treatment, suggesting that capsaicin has a role in regulating energy metabolism. In addition to altering thermogenic proteins, capsaicin also reduced the expression of TNF-α in adipose tissue.[43] Capsaicin affected the secretion of inflammatory adipocytokines, such as IL-6 and MCP-1, in obese adipose tissue and isolated adipocytes by modulating the proinflammatory transcription factors NF-κB and PPARγ.[40] Capsaicin also directly suppressed the macrophage inflammatory response by inhibiting NF-κB activation *in vitro*.[37,45] In addition, our group has observed that capsaicin directly increases the insulin-stimulated uptake of glucose in muscle cells (unpublished data). These results indicate that capsaicin may be useful for the treatment of obesity-related inflammatory metabolic dysfunctions. In addition, the beneficial effects of spice-derived nutraceuticals on inflammation and obesity have been reviewed.[46]

Polyunsaturated fatty acids

Fatty acids (FAs) can function as endogenous ligands that modulate inflammatory responses. Saturated FAs promote inflammation by activating Toll-like receptor 4 (TLR4) on fat cells and macrophages,[47] and unsaturated FAs are weakly proinflammatory or neutral. However, ω-3 polyunsaturated fatty acids (PUFAs) from fish oils, such as docosahexanoic acid (DHA) and eicosapentaenoic acid (EPA), are known anti-inflammatory factors.[48,49] Recently, Oh *et al.*[50] showed that the ω-3 fatty acids DHA, EPA sense G protein–coupled receptor 120 (GPR120), which is highly expressed in adipose tissue macrophages and fat cells. The activation of this receptor by DHA attenuates the proinflammatory effects of TNF-α and LPS on macrophages. Activation of GPR120 by ω-3 fatty acids induces potent insulin sensitization and other antidiabetic effects *in vivo* by repressing macrophage-induced tissue inflammation. In addition, PPARγ activation by long chain ω-3 PUFA has been implicated in the prevention of high-fat diet-induced adipose tissue inflammation and remodeling.[51,52] Meijerink *et al.*[53] also showed that docohexaenoylethanolamine (DHEA), the ethnaolamide metabolite of DHA, modulates inflammation by reducing MCP-1 and nitric oxide (NO) production in macrophages. In conclusion, fish oil supplements can alleviate metabolic disease by modulating inflammatory signaling pathways.

Resveratrol and stillbenes

Resveratrol, a polyphenolic compound found in the skin of grapes and related food products, has been shown to prevent a number of diverse pathologic processes, including cardiovascular disease (CVD), cancer, oxidative stress, and inflammation.[54–56] Although the majority of research on metabolic dysfunctions has focused on its ability to enhance the effects of sirtuin SIRT1 in preventing cellular damage associated with aging and chronic illness,[57] there have been many reports detailing its anti-inflammatory and antiadipogenic effects.[58–60] A recent study reported that resveratrol has an anti-inflammatory effect on TNF-α–induced MCP-1 expression by inhibiting NF-κB transcriptional activity in adipocytes.[60] In animal models, resveratrol repressed TLR2- and TLR4-mediated proinflammatory signaling cascades in adipose tissue[58] and inhibited NF-κB signaling in the sciatic nerves of rats with streptozotocin-induced diabetes.[61] In human retinal epithelial cells, resveratrol showed an inhibitory effect on hyperglycemia-induced inflammation.[62] It has also shown the potential for preventing CVD by inhibiting inflammatory markers, the cyclooxygenase (COX)-1 enzyme, and polyphosphoinositide metabolism in platelets.[63] In rats, resveratrol administration prevented the decrease in vascular NO induced by inflammatory mediators, and it decreased the expression of TNF-α.[64] In addition, previous studies have shown that Vitisin A, a resveratrol tetramer purified from the skin of grape trees, has anti-inflammatory,[65,66] antiadipogenic,[67] and anticholestrolemic activities.[68] Vitisin A reduces the expression of LPS-stimulated proinflammatory markers in macrophages and decreases adipocyte differentiation by inhibiting PPARγ activation. Inhibition of cellular 3-hydroxy-3-methylgluctaryl coenzyme A (HMG CoA) reductase, the rate-limiting enzyme in cholesterol biosynthesis, can lower the levels of circulating cholesterol and several proinflammatory cytokines products of NF-κB target genes. These mechanisms demonstrate a potential for resveratrol and its tetramer in the control of obesity and metabolic disorders.

Ginger-derived components

The two major pungent compounds of ginger, 6-gingerol and 6-shogaol, have potent anti-inflammatory activities and can improve diabetes and insulin resistance.[69–71] Both molecules attenuate the effects on TNF-α–induced downregulation of adiponectin expression by different mechanisms in adipocytes; 6-shogaol functions as a potent agonist of PPARγ, but 6-gingerol does not, although

it is structurally similar to 6-gingerol. In addition, 6-shogaol inhibits the TNF-α–mediated downregulation of adiponectin expression via PPARγ transactivation. In contrast, 6-gingerol inhibits JNK signaling pathways in TNF-α–stimulated adipocytes without affecting PPARγ transactivation.[72] In addition, 6-gingerol is also a potent inhibitor of COX-2 expression and acts by blocking the activation of p38 MAPK and NF-κB[73] along with enhancing adipocyte differentiation.[71] Zingerone, a component of ginger, also suppresses the secretion of MCP-1 from adipose tissue of obese mice and inhibits macrophage inflammatory action such as migration and activation.[32] In animals, the ethanol extract of ginger protects against egg albumin–induced acute inflammation and hypoglycemia in models of diabetes.[70] Thus, these studies suggest that ginger has the potential to prevent inflammation and inflammation-linked metabolic dysfunction.

Flavonoids

Flavonoids are a polyphenol subclass widely distributed in plants and in the diet, and they exhibit a variety of health benefits. The anti-inflammatory properties of flavonoids have been extensively studied to establish and characterize their potential utility as therapeutic agents in the treatment of inflammatory diseases.[74] Antocyanins are found in red fruits and vegetables and have been shown to have anti-inflammatory activity in obese adipose tissues, which is mediated by PPARγ-dependent mechanisms.[75,76] Cyanidin 3-glucoside (C3G), a typical anthocyanin, downregulates the expression of RBP-4, which is known to contribute to insulin resistance in adipose tissue of diabetic mice,[77] and this improvement is associated with the inhibition of inflammatory mediators and stimulation of AMPK activity in adipocytes.[75] (−)-epigallocatechin-3-gallate (EGCG), a major green tea polyphenol, provides beneficial effects for metabolic syndrome. Long-term EGCG treatment impairs the development of obesity and decreases the expression of inflammatory markers, such as MCP-1, in obese mice, suggesting that EGCG-mediated reductions in mesenteric and retroperitoneal adipose tissue weight may have a beneficial impact on high fat–induced inflammation and the development of metabolic syndrome.[78] In humans, green tea consumption has been inversely correlated with liver damage and with the levels of inflammation markers.[79,80]

Conclusions

The evidence implicating inflammation in the pathogenesis of insulin resistance and type 2 diabetes suggests the possibility of targeting inflammation with pharmacological and dietary interventions. While pharmacological approaches that alter the inflammatory process are undoubtedly of great clinical importance dietary, nutraceuticals with anti-inflammatory activities can improve insulin sensitivity. These approaches may provide clinical benefits to the vast number of patients affected by the obesity epidemic and the metabolic disorders. However, preserving other innate immune functions should be considered in this approach.

Acknowledgments

This work was supported by research grants from Korea Food Research Institute and the Biofood Research Program from the National Research Foundation, Korea.

Conflicts of interest

The authors declare no conflicts of interest.

References

1. Schenk, S., M. Saberi & J.M. Olefsky. 2008. Insulin sensitivity: modulation by nutrients and inflammation. *J. Clin. Invest.* **118:** 2992–3002.

2. Stumvoll, M., B. J. Goldstein & T.W. van Haeften. 2005. Type 2 diabetes: principles of pathogenesis and therapy. *Lancet* **365:** 1333–1346.

3. Shoelson, S.E., J. Lee & A.B. Goldfine. 2006. Inflammation and insulin resistance. *J. Clin. Invest.* **116:** 1793–1801.

4. Weisberg, S.P. *et al.* 2003. Obesity is associated with macrophage accumulation in adipose tissue. *J. Clin. Invest.* **112:** 1796–1808.

5. Xu, H. *et al.* 2003. Chronic inflammation in fat plays a crucial role in the development of obesity-related insulin resistance. *J. Clin. Invest.* **112:** 1821–1830.

6. Feuerer, M. *et al.* 2009. Lean, but not obese, fat is enriched for a unique population of regulatory T cells that affect metabolic parameters. *Nat. Med.* **15:** 930–939.

7. Nishimura, S. *et al.* 2009. CD8 +effector T cells contribute to macrophage recruitment and adipose tissue inflammation in obesity. *Nat Med.* **15:** 914–920.

8. Winer, S. *et al.* 2009. Normalization of obesity-associated insulin resistance through immunotherapy. *Nat. Med.* **15:** 921–929.

9. Hotamisligil, G.S., N.S. Shargill & B.M. Spiegelman. 1993. Adipose expression of tumor necrosis factor-α: direct role in obesity-linked insulin resistance. *Science* **259:** 87–91.

10. Sethi, J.K. & G.S. Hotamisligil. 1999. The role of TNF α in adipocyte metabolism. *Semin. Cell. Dev. Biol.* **10:** 19–29.

11. Hotamisligil, G.S. *et al.* 1995. Increased adipose tissue expression of tumor necrosis factor-α in human obesity and insulin resistance. *J. Clin. Invest.* **95:** 2409–2415.

12. Kern, P.A. *et al.* (1995. The expression of tumor necrosis factor in human adipose tissue. Regulation by obesity, weight loss, and relationship to lipoprotein lipase. *J. Clin. Invest.* **95:** 2111–2119.

13. Saghizadeh, M., *et al.* 1996. The expression of TNF α by human muscle. Relationship to insulin resistance. *J. Clin. Invest.* **97:** 1111–1116.

14. Uysal, K.T. *et al.* 1997. Protection from obesity-induced insulin resistance in mice lacking TNF-α function. *Nature* **389:** 610–614.

15. Aguirre, V. *et al.* 2000. The c-Jun NH(2)-terminal kinase promotes insulin resistance during association with insulin receptor substrate-1 and phosphorylation of Ser (307). *J. Biol. Chem.* **275:** 9047–9054.

16. Hirosumi, J. *et al.* 2002. A central role for JNK in obesity and insulin resistance. *Nature* **420:** 333–336.

17. Yuan, M. *et al.* 2001. Reversal of obesity- and diet-induced insulin resistance with salicylates or targeted disruption of Ikkβ. *Science* **293:** 1673–1677.

18. Lee, J.Y. *et al.* 2001. Saturated fatty acids, but not unsaturated fatty acids, induce the expression of cyclooxygenase-2 mediated through Toll-like receptor 4. *J. Biol. Chem.* **276:** 16683–16689.

19. Vallerie, S. N. & G.S. Hotamisligil. 2010. The role of JNK proteins in metabolism. *Sci. Transl. Med.* **2:** 60rv65.

20. Summers, S. A. 2006. Ceramides in insulin resistance and lipotoxicity. *Prog. Lipid Res.* **45:** 42–72.

21. Forman, B.M. *et al.* 1995. 15-Deoxy-delta 12, 14-prostaglandin J2 is a ligand for the adipocyte determination factor PPAR γ. *Cell* **83:** 803–812.

22. Jiang, C., A. T. Ting & B. Seed. 1998. PPAR-γ agonists inhibit production of monocyte inflammatory cytokines. *Nature* **391:** 82–86.

23. Marx, N. *et al.* 1998. Macrophages in human atheroma contain PPARγ: differentiation-dependent peroxisomal proliferator-activated receptor γ (PPARγ) expression and reduction of MMP-9 activity through PPARγ activation in mononuclear phagocytes *in vitro*. *Am. J. Pathol.* **153:** 17–23.

24. Ricote, M. *et al.* 1998. Expression of the peroxisome proliferator-activated receptor γ (PPARγ) in human atherosclerosis and regulation in macrophages by colony stimulating factors and oxidized low density lipoprotein. *Proc. Natl. Acad. Sci. USA* **95:** 7614–7619.

25. Ricote, M. *et al.* 1998. The peroxisome proliferator-activated receptor-gamma is a negative regulator of macrophage activation. *Nature* **391:** 79–82.

26. Hevener, A.L. *et al.* 2007. Macrophage PPAR γ is required for normal skeletal muscle and hepatic insulin sensitivity and full antidiabetic effects of thiazolidinediones. *J. Clin. Invest.* **117:** 1658–1669.

27. Odegaard, J.I. *et al.* 2007. Macrophage-specific PPARγ controls alternative activation and improves insulin resistance. *Nature* **447:** 1116–1120.

28. Suzawa, M. *et al.* 2003. Cytokines suppress adipogenesis and PPAR-γ function through the TAK1/TAB1/NIK cascade. *Nat. Cell. Biol.* **5:** 224–230.

29. Ghanim, H. *et al.* 2004. Circulating mononuclear cells in the obese are in a proinflammatory state. *Circulation* **110:** 1564–1571.

30. Mendall, M. A. *et al.* 1997. Relation of serum cytokine concentrations to cardiovascular risk factors and coronary heart disease. *Heart* **78:** 273–277.

31. Nieman, D. C. *et al.* 1999. Influence of obesity on immune function. *J. Am. Diet. Assoc.* **99:** 294–299.

32. Woo, H.M. *et al.* 2007. Active spice-derived components can inhibit inflammatory responses of adipose tissue in obesity by suppressing inflammatory actions of macrophages and release of monocyte chemoattractant protein-1 from adipocytes. *Life Sci.* **80:** 926–931.

33. Wang, S.L. *et al.* 2009. Curcumin, a potential inhibitor of up-regulation of TNF-α and IL-6 induced by palmitate in 3T3-L1 adipocytes through NF-κB and JNK pathway. *Biomed. Environ. Sci.* **22:** 32–39.

34. Pendurthi, U.R. & L.V. Rao. 2000. Suppression of transcription factor Egr-1 by curcumin. *Thromb. Res.* **97:** 179–189.

35. Weisberg, S. P., R. Leibel & D.V. Tortoriello. 2008. Dietary curcumin significantly improves obesity-associated inflammation and diabetes in mouse models of diabesity. *Endocrinology* **149:** 3549–3558.

36. Jain, S.K. *et al.* 2009. Curcumin supplementation lowers TNF-α, IL-6, IL-8, and MCP-1 secretion in high glucose-treated cultured monocytes and blood levels of TNF-α, IL-6, MCP-1, glucose, and glycosylated hemoglobin in diabetic rats. *Antioxid. Redox. Signal.* **11:** 241–249.

37. Kim, C.S. *et al.* 2003. Capsaicin exhibits anti-inflammatory property by inhibiting IkB-a degradation in LPS-stimulated peritoneal macrophages. *Cell. Signal.* **15:** 299–306.

38. Manjunatha, H. & K. Srinivasan. 2006. Protective effect of dietary curcumin and capsaicin on induced oxidation of low-density lipoprotein, iron-induced hepatotoxicity and carrageenan-induced inflammation in experimental rats. *FEBS J.* **273:** 4528–4537.

39. Park, J.Y. *et al.* 2004. Capsaicin inhibits the production of tumor necrosis factor α by LPS-stimulated murine macrophages, RAW 264.7: a PPARγ ligand-like action as a novel mechanism. *FEBS Lett.* **572:** 266–270.

40. Kang, J.H. *et al.* 2007. Capsaicin, a spicy component of hot peppers, modulates adipokine gene expression and protein release from obese-mouse adipose tissues and isolated adipocytes, and suppresses the inflammatory responses of adipose tissue macrophages. *FEBS Lett.* **581:** 4389–4396.

41. Shin, K.O. & T. Moritani. 2007. Alterations of autonomic nervous activity and energy metabolism by capsaicin ingestion during aerobic exercise in healthy men. *J. Nutr. Sci. Vitaminol.* **53:** 124–132.

42. Suri, A. & A. Szallasi. 2008. The emerging role of TRPV1 in diabetes and obesity. *Trends Pharmacol. Sci.* **29:** 29–36.

43. Joo, J.I. *et al.* 2010. Proteomic analysis for antiobesity potential of capsaicin on white adipose tissue in rats fed with a high fat diet. *J. Proteome Res.* **9:** 2977–2987.

44. Kim, D.H. *et al.* 2010. Differential expression of skeletal muscle proteins in high-fat diet-fed rats in response to capsaicin feeding. *Proteomics* **10:** 2870–2881.

45. Singh, S., K. Natarajan & B.B. Aggarwal. 1996. Capsaicin (8-methyl-N-vanillyl-6-nonenamide) is a potent inhibitor of nuclear transcription factor-κ B activation by diverse agents. *J. Immunol.* **157:** 4412–4420.

46. Aggarwal, B.B. 2010. Targeting inflammation-induced obesity and metabolic diseases by curcumin and other nutraceuticals. *Annu. Rev. Nutr.* **30:** 173–199.

47. Shi, H. *et al.* 2006. TLR4 links innate immunity and fatty acid-induced insulin resistance. *J. Clin. Invest.* **116:** 3015–3025.

48. Batetta, B. *et al.* 2009. Endocannabinoids may mediate the ability of (n-3) fatty acids to reduce ectopic fat and inflammatory mediators in obese Zucker rats. *J. Nutr.* **139:** 1495–1501.

49. Lee, J.Y. *et al.* 2003. Differential modulation of Toll-like receptors by fatty acids: preferential inhibition by n-3 polyunsaturated fatty acids. *J. Lipid Res.* **44:** 479–486.

50. Oh, D.Y. *et al.* 2010. GPR120 is an ω-3 fatty acid receptor mediating potent anti-inflammatory and insulin-sensitizing effects. *Cell* **142:** 687–698.

51. Huber, J. *et al.* 2007. Prevention of high-fat diet-induced adipose tissue remodeling in obese diabetic mice by n-3 polyunsaturated fatty acids. *Int. J. Obes.* **31:** 1004–1013.

52. Todoric, J. *et al.* 2006. Adipose tissue inflammation induced by high-fat diet in obese diabetic mice is prevented by n-3 polyunsaturated fatty acids. *Diabetologia* **49:** 2109–2119.

53. Meijerink, J. *et al.* 2011. The ethanolamide metabolite of DHA, docosahexaenoylethanolamine, shows immunomodulating effects in mouse peritoneal and RAW264.7 macrophages: evidence for a new link between fish oil and inflammation. *Br. J. Nutr.* Feb. 4: 1–10 [Epub ahead of print]

54. Baur, J.A. & D.A. Sinclair. 2006. Therapeutic potential of resveratrol: the *in vivo* evidence. *Nat. Rev. Drug Discov.* **5:** 493–506.

55. Fremont, L. 2000. Biological effects of resveratrol. *Life Sci.* **66:** 663–673.

56. Jang, M. *et al.* 1997. Cancer chemopreventive activity of resveratrol, a natural product derived from grapes. *Science* **275:** 218–220.

57. Pillarisetti, S. 2008. A review of Sirt1 and Sirt1 modulators in cardiovascular and metabolic diseases. *Recent Pat. Cardiovasc. Drug Discov.* **3:** 156–164.

58. Kim, S. *et al.* 2011. Resveratrol exerts anti-obesity effects via mechanisms involving down-regulation of adipogenic and inflammatory processes in mice. *Biochemical Pharmacol.* **81:** 1343–1351.

59. Rayalam, S. *et al.* 2008. Resveratrol induces apoptosis and inhibits adipogenesis in 3T3-L1 adipocytes. *Phytother. Res.* **22:** 1367–1371.

60. Zhu, J. *et al.* 2008. Anti-inflammatory effect of resveratrol on TNF-α-induced MCP-1 expression in adipocytes. *Biochem. Biophys. Res. Commun.* **369:** 471–477.

61. Kumar, A. & S.S. Sharma. 2010. NF-κB inhibitory action of resveratrol: a probable mechanism of neuroprotection in experimental diabetic neuropathy. *Biochem. Biophys. Res. Commun.* **394:** 360–365.

62. Losso, J.N., R.E. Truax & G. Richard. 2010. Trans-resveratrol inhibits hyperglycemia-induced inflammation and connexin downregulation in retinal pigment epithelial cells. *J. Agric. Food Chem.* **58:** 8246–8252.

63. Szewczuk, L.M. *et al.* 2004. Resveratrol is a peroxidase-mediated inactivator of COX-1 but not COX-2: a mechanistic approach to the design of COX-1 selective agents. *J. Biol. Chem.* **279:** 22727–22737.

64. Zhang, H. *et al.* 2009. Resveratrol improves endothelial function: role of TNFα and vascular oxidative stress. *Arterioscler. Thromb. Vasc. Biol.* **29:** 1164–1171.

65. Mi Jeong, S. *et al.* 2009. Vitisin A suppresses LPS-induced NO production by inhibiting ERK, p38, and NF-κB activation in RAW 264.7 cells. *Int. Immunopharmacol.* **9:** 319–323.

66. Huang, K.S., M. Lin & G.F. Cheng. 2001. Anti-inflammatory tetramers of resveratrol from the roots of *Vitis amurensis* and the conformations of the seven-membered ring in some oligostilbenes. *Phytochemistry* **58:** 357–362.

67. Kim, S.H. *et al.* 2008. Vitisin A inhibits adipocyte differentiation through cell cycle arrest in 3T3-L1 cells. *Biochem. Biophys. Res. Commun.* **372:** 108–113.

68. Koo, M. *et al.* 2008. 3-Hydroxy-3-methylglutaryl-CoA (HMG-CoA) reductase inhibitory effect of *Vitis vinifera*. *Fitoterapia* **79:** 204–206.

69. Levy, A.S. *et al.* 2006. 6-Shogaol reduced chronic inflammatory response in the knees of rats treated with complete Freund's adjuvant. *BMC Pharmacol.* **6:** 12.

70. Ojewole, J.A. 2006. Analgesic, antiinflammatory and hypoglycaemic effects of ethanol extract of *Zingiber officinale (Roscoe) rhizomes* (Zingiberaceae) in mice and rats. *Phytother. Res.* **20:** 764–772.

71. Sekiya, K., A. Ohtani & S. Kusano. 2004. Enhancement of insulin sensitivity in adipocytes by ginger. *Biofactors* **22:** 153–156.

72. Isa, Y. *et al.* 2008. 6-Shogaol and 6-gingerol, the pungent of ginger, inhibit TNF-α mediated downregulation of adiponectin expression via different mechanisms in 3T3-L1 adipocytes. *Biochem. Biophys. Res. Commun.* **373:** 429–434.

73. Kim, S.O. *et al.* 2005. [6]-Gingerol inhibits COX-2 expression by blocking the activation of p38 MAP kinase and NF-κB in phorbol ester-stimulated mouse skin. *Oncogene* **24:** 2558–2567.

74. Garcia-Lafuente, A. *et al.* 2009. Flavonoids as anti-inflammatory agents: implications in cancer and cardiovascular disease. *Inflamm. Res.* **58:** 537–552.

75. Tsuda, T. 2008. Regulation of adipocyte function by anthocyanins: possibility of preventing the metabolic syndrome. *J. Agric. Food Chem.* **56:** 642–646.

76. Tsuda, T. *et al.* 2003. Dietary cyanidin 3-O-β-D-glucoside-rich purple corn color prevents obesity and ameliorates hyperglycemia in mice. *J. Nutr.* **133:** 2125–2130.

77. Sasaki, R. *et al.* 2007. Cyanidin 3-glucoside ameliorates hyperglycemia and insulin sensitivity due to downregulation of retinol binding protein 4 expression in diabetic mice. *Biochem. Pharmacol.* **74:** 1619–1627.

78. Bose, M. *et al.* 2008. The major green tea polyphenol, (-)-epigallocatechin-3-gallate, inhibits obesity, metabolic syndrome, and fatty liver disease in high-fat-fed mice. *J. Nutr.* **138:** 1677–1683.

79. Imai, K. & K. Nakachi. 1995. Cross sectional study of effects of drinking green tea on cardiovascular and liver diseases. *Br. Med. J.* **310:** 693–696.

80. Steptoe, A. *et al.* 2007. The effects of chronic tea intake on platelet activation and inflammation: a double-blind placebo controlled trial. *Atherosclerosis* **193:** 277–282.

Ann. N.Y. Acad. Sci. ISSN 0077-8923

ANNALS OF THE NEW YORK ACADEMY OF SCIENCES

Issue: *Nutrition and Physical Activity in Aging, Obesity, and Cancer*

Assessing estrogen signaling aberrations in breast cancer risk using genetically engineered mouse models

Priscilla A. Furth,[1,2,3] M. Carla Cabrera,[1] Edgar S. Díaz-Cruz,[1] Sarah Millman,[1] and Rebecca E. Nakles[1]

[1]Department of Oncology, Lombardi Comprehensive Cancer Center, Georgetown University, Washington, DC. [2]Department of Medicine, Lombardi Comprehensive Cancer Center, Georgetown University, Washington, DC. [3]Department of Nanobiomedical Science and WCU Research Center of Nanobiomedical Science, Dankook University, Chungnam, Korea

Address for correspondence: Priscilla A. Furth, Departments of Oncology and Medicine, Lombardi Comprehensive Cancer Center, 3970 Reservoir Rd NW, Research Bldg Room 520A, Georgetown University, Washington, DC 20057. paf3@georgetown.edu

Aberrations in estrogen signaling increase breast cancer risk. Molecular mechanisms that impact breast cancer initiation, promotion, and progression can be investigated using genetically engineered mouse models. Increasing estrogen receptor alpha (ERα) expression levels twofold is sufficient to initiate and promote breast cancer progression. Initiation and promotion can be increased by p53 haploinsufficiency and by coexpressing the nuclear coactivators amplified in breast cancer 1 (AIB1) or the splice variant AIB1Δ3. Progression to invasive cancer is found with coexpression of these nuclear coactivators as well as following a single dose of 7,12-dimethylbenz(a)anthracene. Loss of signal transducer and activator of transcription 5a reduces the prevalence of initiation and promotion but does not protect from invasive cancer development. Cyclin D1 loss completely interrupts mammary epithelial proliferation and survival when ERα is overexpressed. Loss of breast cancer gene 1 increases estrogen signaling and cooperates with ERα overexpression in initiation, promotion, and progression of mammary cancer.

Keywords: breast cancer; mouse models; estrogen signaling; ERα; BRCA1

Introduction to estrogen signaling

The estrogen signaling pathway starts with ligands—the estrogens—and receptors for these ligands—the estrogen receptors (ERs).[1–3] Estrogens are steroid hormones involved in normal development of the mammary gland,[4] but they also contribute to breast cancer growth.[5,6] The ovary is the main organ responsible for estrogen production in women during reproductive life.[1,7] With menopause, ovarian estrogen production falls, and other tissues become the primary sources.[8] Estrogens are synthesized from androgens by aromatization.[1] Increased aromatase expression in breast tissue is associated with breast cancer.[9]

Both ER alpha (α) and ER beta (β) are expressed in mammary tissue.[10] ERα is most closely linked to increasing mammary epithelial cell proliferation with the balance between ERα and ERβ regulating this activity.[11,12] When estrogen binds to ER, the complex translocates to the nucleus, binds to DNA target sequences called estrogen response elements (EREs),[13] and regulates expression of a number of downstream genes including progesterone receptor (PR), the receptor for the steroid hormone progesterone.[14–17] Breast cancers that express ERα are termed ERα positive.[18] Antiestrogens such as tamoxifen, fulvestrant, and aromatase inhibitors are used as endocrine therapy to minimize or even eliminate the growth of ERα-positive breast cancers. Tamoxifen is also approved as a preventative for women at high risk for breast cancer development.[19]

The estrogen pathway is subject to inhibitory and growth-promoting feedback at both RNA and protein levels through regulation of ERα gene promoter transcriptional activity, micro RNA expression, epigenetic mechanisms, ubiquitination, and acetylation.[20–24] In normal mammary gland growth,

doi: 10.1111/j.1749-6632.2011.06086.x

estrogen pathway activity is naturally inhibited; in breast cancer cells, this inhibitory regulation is lost.[11] Downstream genes including cyclin D1 mediate the proliferative effects of ERα signaling.[25] Illustrating the complexity of intracellular molecular interactions, overexpressed cyclin D1 also activates ERα transcriptional activity independent of estrogen binding and is subject to regulation by other cellular molecules.[26,27] Nuclear hormone receptor coactivators including amplified in breast cancer 1(AIB1) and steroid receptor coactivator (Src)-3 can modulate estrogen signaling.[28,29] Signal transducer and activator of transcription (STAT) 5 influences estrogen signaling.[30] Known tumor suppressor genes p53 and breast cancer gene 1 (BRCA1) also affect the estrogen signaling pathway.[31,32] The studies in the genetically engineered mouse models reviewed below were initiated to take observations from human breast tissue and cell lines into mechanistic investigations of breast cancer pathophysiology to determine where in the process of breast carcinogenesis[33] specific aberrations in estrogen signaling impact breast cancer risk and how this might happen.

Increased ERα expression as a cancer risk factor

Since increased expression levels of ERα in breast epithelial cells are associated with increased risk of breast cancer,[10] a genetically engineered conditional mouse model of increased ERα expression targeted to mammary epithelial cells was generated.[34] ERα expression is increased approximately twofold in mammary epithelial cells in the model and, unlike endogenous ERα, is not downregulated through inhibitory feedback following estrogen exposure, resulting in an overall increase in ERα and persistent ERα expression throughout the cell cycle. The model has tested at which stage(s) during cancer progression increased ERα expression acts (initiation, promotion, and/or progression)[33] by determining if gain of ERα promotes development and progression of mammary cancer initiated by expression of an oncoprotein[35] as well as testing if simply increasing ERα expression levels can initiate as well as promote progression to mammary cancer.[34] The model has determined that ERα overexpression can lead to the development of both ERα-positive and -negative mammary cancers and explored the collaborating

roles of proteins that directly and indirectly interact with ERα (AIB1, STAT5, p53, and BRCA1).[36–39]

This genetically engineered mouse model was constructed using the tetracycline responsive gene expression system to temporally and spatially regulate expression of mouse ERα cDNA. The system consists of one of the tetracyclines (usually doxycycline) and two transgenes: one directing expression of a transgene encoding either tetracycline transactivator (tTA) sequences[40] or reverse tetracycline transactivator (rtTA) sequences,[41] and the other encoding the ERα coding sequences.[42] A FLAG tag was genetically engineered at the 5′ end of the ERα coding sequences to facilitate identification of the transgenic RNA and protein.[35,42] The FLAG-tagged mouse ERα coding sequences were cloned downstream of a genetically engineered tetracycline-operator (tet-op) promoter containing tetracycline response elements (TREs) to generate the ERα transgene.[42,43] Spatial regulation is through the use of the mouse mammary tumor virus-long terminal repeat (MMTV) to direct expression of either tTA or rtTA to epithelial cells.[40,41] Expression of the ERα coding sequence is temporally regulated through the administration or withdrawal of exogenously administered tetracycline.[43] The compound bitransgenic model carrying the tet-op-ERα transgene under spatial regulation of MMTV is called the conditional ERα in mammary tissue (CERM model).

A triple transgenic model carrying the MMTV-tTA and tet-op-ERα transgenes in combination with a third tet-op-simian virus 40 T antigen (TAg) transgene was generated to test if increasing ERα expression levels could promote mammary cancer development initiated by the TAg oncoprotein.[35] This model coexpresses ERα and TAg in the same cells under the spatial control of the MMTV-tTA transgene. Mammary cancer development in the absence and presence of ERα overexpression was compared. In the absence of ERα overexpression, bigenic mice that carry only the MMTV-tTA and tet-op-TAg transgenes do not develop mammary cancer.[44,45] In contrast, 37% of the triple transgenic MMTV-tTA/tet-op-ERα/tet-op-TAg female mice develop mammary cancer by 12 months of age. Promotion of cancer progression by ERα in this model results in ERα-positive adenocarcinomas that demonstrate ER–steroid binding to estrogen and show estrogen-dependent growth.

To test if ERα overexpression by itself can initiate mammary cancer progression, double transgenic MMTV-rtTA/tet-op-ERα CERM mice were followed through 12 months of age for development of mammary hyperplasia indicative of the promotion stage of cancer development as well as progression to noninvasive and invasive mammary cancer.[34,36–38] ERα overexpression induces increased mammary epithelial cell proliferation, and by four months of age, between 20 and 30% of CERM mice demonstrate ductal hyperplasia and 17% show ductal carcinoma *in situ* (DCIS), a noninvasive cancer.[34,38] Progression to invasive cancer development by 12 months of age is less than 5% in the CERM model but does occur and may be increased by exposure to a single dose of DMBA or by coexpression of AIB1 or its splice variant AIB1 Δ3.[36,37] Significantly, both ERα-positive and ERα-negative invasive adenocarcinomas develop in CERM mice, and both show increased levels of cyclin D1 expression that is also found in the mammary hyperplasias.[34,36,37]

To test if cyclin D1 plays an essential role in the development of mammary hyperplasia and cancer initiated by ERα overexpression, ERα-overexpressing mice were crossed with germ-line cyclin D1 knockout mice.[46] These studies unexpectedly revealed an essential role for cyclin D1 in mammary epithelial cells when ERα is overexpressed. In contrast to germ-line cyclin D1 knockout mice and CERM mice, both of which show normal pubertal mammary gland development, pubertal development of the mammary gland in compound CERM/cyclin D1 knockout mice is completely abnormal. The mammary epithelial cells cannot proliferate and undergo apoptosis due to a DNA damage response associated with an abnormal upregulation of cyclin E expression. The surrounding mammary fat pad undergoes a transition to an almost purely collagenous stroma. The phenotype cannot be rescued upon transplantation of CERM/cyclin D1 knockout mammary epithelium into a cleared fat pad of wild-type mice, indicating that the defect is intrinsic to the mammary epithelial cells and demonstrating that a modest increase in ERα induces a requirement for cyclin D1 for puberty-associated mammary cell proliferation. Cyclin D1 inhibitors could act as anticancer agents in the breast by preferentially targeting cells with abnormally high ERα expression levels that might exhibit increased sensitivity to interrupting cyclin D1 pathways.[47]

Comparing CERM mouse and ACI rat models

The CERM model is unique in that activating the estrogen signaling pathway through ERα overexpression results in the generation of both ERα-positive and -negative invasive cancers and, significantly, while estrogen is required for disease development, exposure to exogenous 17β-estradiol (E2) does not provoke progression to invasive cancer, at least when given at four months of age.[34,37] In contrast, in the ACI rat model, mammary cancer development is increased following chronic administration of E2, and these cancers reproducibly express ERα and PR.[48] Normally in rats, like mice and humans, chronic administration of exogenous estrogen does not induce mammary cancer. However, the ACI rat is genetically predisposed to estrogen-induced mammary cancer with a median latency of approximately 20 weeks and close to 100% penetration. Administration of E2 results promotes lobuloalveolar hyperplasia, focal regions of atypical epithelial hyperplasia, and, ultimately, progression to numerous independently arising mammary cancers with ERα and PR overexpression. These mammary cancers are estrogen dependent, exhibit genomic instability, and are inhibited by ovariectomy and tamoxifen.[49,50] The majority of epithelial cells in the mammary carcinomas as well as the atypical hyperplasia exhibit a drastic downregulation of Cdkn2a and increased PR expression, suggesting that the atypical hyperplasias may be a precursor lesion to carcinoma. Tamoxifen not only decreases tumor prevalence but also restores normal mammary epithelial architecture.[50] Two genetic determinants of susceptibility to E2-induced mammary cancer have been mapped in this model, *Emca1* (estrogen-induced mammary cancer) and *Emca2* (mapped to rat chromosomes 5 and 18, respectively). The region of RNO5 containing *Emca1* is homologous to human chromosomes 1p and 9p, two regions of the human genome that have been implicated in breast cancer etiology.[51]

Effect of STAT5a loss on ERα-induced cancer promotion and progression

STAT5a/b is a signal transducer and activator of transcription that mediates the prolactin/JAK2 pathway contributing to differentiation and survival of normal mammary lobuloalveolar cells.[52,53] Nuclear-localized STAT5a is found in 40% of human ductal carcinoma *in situ* lesions and 76% of invasive breast cancers.[54,55] In CERM mice, the impact of germ-line STAT5a deficiency on mammary carcinogenesis is context dependent.[36] The absence of STAT5a on the background of ERα overexpression reduces the prevalence of preneoplasia; however, this effect does not extend to protection cancers developing after a single dose of 7,12-dimethylbenz(a)anthracene (DMBA) as a cancer initiator.

AIB1 or AIB1Δ3 with ERα in oncogenesis

AIB1 is a nuclear receptor coactivator expressed in human breast cancers.[56] AIB1Δ3 is a splice variant of AIB1 that also is expressed in human breast cancers and has higher transcriptional activity in tissue culture cells as compared to AIB1.[57,58] To test the effect of combining AIB1 or AIB1Δ3 overexpression with ERα overexpression, a series of tetracycline-responsive conditional transgenic mouse models were developed in which either AIB1 or AIB1Δ3 coding sequences were placed under the control of the tet-op promoter.[37] The outcome of either AIB1 or AIB1Δ3 overexpression was then tested and compared in both the absence and presence of ERα overexpression. Similar to *in vitro* results, AIB1Δ3 is more transcriptionally active than AIB1 *in vivo* and significantly increases expression levels of both ERα and PR downstream genes. This is associated with increased progression to a multilayered mammary epithelium. However, both AIB1 and AIB1Δ3 overexpression are sufficient to increase mammary hyperplasia and more modestly increase invasive cancer development in CERM mice. Unexpectedly, targeting AIB1 or AIB1Δ3 overexpression to mammary epithelial cells with ERα also significantly increased stromal collagen content. This experiment illustrates how genetic manipulations targeted to mammary epithelial cells can impact not only the mammary epithelial cells themselves but also the surrounding stroma, analogous to what was found in the compound CERM/cyclin D1 knockout mice.[46] The experiments are consistent with the notion that both AIB1 and AIB1Δ3 can work in combination with ERα to increase breast cancer risk.

p53 modulates the impact of ERα overexpression

The tumor suppressor p53 plays a role in mediating cell response to various stresses by induc-ing or repressing genes that regulate cell cycle arrest, senescence, apoptosis, and DNA repair.[59] Alterations to p53 are the most common changes so far detected in primary human breast tumors,[60] reported in up to 40% of human breast cancers.[61] p53 detection in benign lesions, indicative of possible mutation, has been associated with elevated cancer risk.[62] Human breast cancers with p53 mutations are frequently ERα-negative.[63] Serial transplant studies have shown that the absence of p53 in mammary epithelium is associated with ductal carcinoma *in situ* lesions and invasive cancer that progress from an ERα-positive to ERα-negative state.[64] In addition to the frequent somatic mutation of p53 in sporadic cancers, germline mutation of one allele of this gene in humans causes an inborn predisposition to cancer known as Li–Fraumeni syndrome. In families with Li–Fraumeni syndrome, early-onset female breast cancer is the most prevalent type of tumor.[65]

While both upregulation of ERα[34] and loss of p53 function[62,64,65] are implicated in the development of breast cancer independently, they can also collaborate to increase the prevalence of age-dependent mammary preneoplasia.[38] The combination of both genetic lesions results in an altered balance in the apoptosis/proliferation ratio of mammary epithelial cells with increased rates of cell proliferation and reduced rates of apoptosis. Changes in specific signaling pathways are associated with specific genetic lesions. Increased levels of extracellular signal-regulated kinase 1/2(ERK1/2) activation are associated with both p53 haploinsufficient and ERα-overexpressing mice. In contrast, changes in AKT activation are limited to mice with p53 haploinsufficiency either alone or in combination with ERα overexpression. The cell cycle inhibitor p27 has been shown to have tumor suppressor activity,[66] and its expression is documented in human ductal carcinoma *in situ* lesions.[67] Decreased levels of p27 protein are found in the p53 haploinsufficient mice independent of ERα overexpression. The combination of ERα deregulation and p53 haploinsufficiency results in a significant decrease in the percentage of mammary epithelial cells with nuclear-localized ERα, although ERα mRNA levels remain increased by twofold and PR expression levels are unchanged. c-Src phosphorylation has been shown to stimulate ERα ubiquitination and proteasome-dependent degradation,[68] and p53 has been reported to downregulate some Src functions.[69] The p53 haploinsufficient mice with ERα overexpression show high expression levels of activated p-Src (Tyr416) in mammary epithelial cells. It is possible that p-Src plays a role in the observed reduction in ERα protein expression in this genotype.

ERα and p53 as breast cancer risk factors in parity protection

Reproductive history is the strongest and most consistent risk factor outside of genetic background and age in breast cancer risk.[70] Early age at first pregnancy ($\leq$ 20 years of age) confers a 50% reduction in lifetime risk compared with the lifetime risk of breast cancer in nulliparous women.[71] Studies in mice have shown that treatment with estrogen and progesterone to mimic pregnancy and parity enhance p53-dependent responses and suppress mammary tumors in BALB/c-Trp53$^{+/-}$ mice.[72] Significantly, parity results in a noticeable decrease in mammary preneoplasia development in comparison to nulliparous mice in p53 haploinsufficient mice but not in mice with ERα overexpression alone or control wild-type mice, suggesting a possible protective effect of pregnancy in mice with disease due to loss of p53 function.[38] This parity protection effect may be due to an increased activation of p53 signaling through pregnancy that compensates for its reduced expression levels.

BRCA1, estrogen signaling, and breast cancer risk

Human breast cancer development secondary to BRCA1 mutation is successfully modeled in mice.[73] The BRCA1-deficient mouse model described below is one of several independently derived models, all of which demonstrate significant similarities in their propensity to develop triple negative mammary cancer and cooperativity with p53 haploinsufficiency in cancer promotion and progression.

The model originally developed by Xu *et al.* is the one that has been used most extensively to investigate how loss of BRCA1 function affects estrogen signaling in the mammary gland.[39,74,75] In this model, conditional deletion of exon 11 of the *Brca1* gene in mammary epithelial cells is affected using Cre recombinase (Cre)-LoxP (Lox) technology.[43] Exon 11 was selected for deletion due to the large number of proteins that interact with BRCA1 at domains mapping to exon 11.[76,77] LoxP sites were inserted into intron sequences flanking exon 11 of the *Brca1* gene. At these loxP sites, Cre recombinase binds to the LoxP DNA recognition sites and mediates DNA recombination between the sites deleting the intervening *Brca1* exon 11 sequences. Expression of Cre is targeted to mammary epithelial cells using a MMTV-Cre transgene.[78]

The incidence of mammary cancer development in this and other BRCA1 mutation models is significantly accelerated by simultaneously deleting one or more copies of the *p53* gene.[73,74] This genetic intervention is hypothesized to promote survival of mammary epithelial cells that do not have functional full-length BRCA1.[79] Consistent with this notion, *p53* mutations are frequently found in human breast cancers that develop secondary to BRCA1 mutation.[80] In the BRCA1 mutation model reviewed here, loss of full-length BRCA1 function results in the development of mammary hyperplasia in 19% and cancer in less than 5% of the mice by 12 months of age.[39,74] The addition of p53 haploinsufficiency increases the prevalence of hyperplasia to 45% and invasive cancer to 53% by 12 months of age.[39,74]

BRCA1 mutation carriers have an increased risk of developing basal or triple-negative breast cancers (ER, PR, and human epidermal growth factor receptor 2 [HER2] negative).[81] This predisposition for developing triple-negative breast cancer is found across the different genetically engineered mouse models of BRCA1 mutation.[73] In the model reviewed here, approximately 50% of the adenocarcinomas demonstrate a triple negative or basal phenotype by gene expression profiling.[82]

Estrogen signaling plays a role in the progression of BRCA1 mutation-related breast cancers, even though most cancers are ERα and PR negative.[83–87] *In vitro* BRCA1 can act as a repressor for ERα-mediated gene transcription, estrogen signaling, and reduces cell proliferation and modulates ERα acetylation and ubiquitination through a direct physical interaction.[24,32,88–91] This interaction of BRCA1 with ERα can be modulated by p300[92] and growth factor signaling[93] and antagonized by cyclin D1.[94] *In vivo*, decreasing estrogen signaling through ovariectomy decreases the risk of breast cancer development due to BRCA1 mutation in both human mutation carriers[95] and the mouse model reviewed here.[96]

Evidence of increased activity of an estrogen-stimulated proliferative pathway can be found *in vivo* during puberty in mice without full-length BRCA1 expression and in postpubertal mice in which activity of the estrogen signaling pathway is increased either by exogenous estrogen or introduction of increased ERα expression targeted to mammary epithelial cells. During puberty, mammary ductal extension through the fat pad is faster and estrogen-induced mammary cell differentiation is delayed as compared to wild-type mice.[39] When treated with exogenous estrogen postpuberty, these mice demonstrate accelerated promotion to mammary hyperplasia.[39] When full-length BRCA1 deficiency is combined with p53 haploinsufficiency and exogenous estrogen treatment, there is a further significant increase in the prevalence of hyperplasia[39] and cancer.[75] On a molecular level increased ERK1/2 phosphorylation and cyclin D1 expression is associated with this estrogen induced abnormal growth.[75] While introduction of ERα overexpression into BRCA1-deficient mice does not significantly increase cancer promotion or progression, the addition of p53 haploinsufficiency to this model results in a significant increase in both promotion and progression with 100% of the mice demonstrating hyperplasia and invasive cancers by 12 months of age.[39] In contrast to the impact of ERα overexpression with TAg oncoprotein where all of the cancers are ERα positive,[35] in the setting of BRCA1 deficiency only half of the cancers are ERα positive,[39] reminiscent of the increased distribution of ERα-negative (80%) as compared to ERα-positive (20%) breast cancers in women who carry BRCA1 mutations.[97]

Surprisingly, while cancer progression is impeded by ovariectomy in this model,[96] administration of tamoxifen increases breast cancer promotion and progression.[98] This is due to the fact that the relative agonist activity of the mixed ERα antagonist/agonist tamoxifen is increased by loss of BRCA1 expression.[98,99]

Significantly, BRCA1 also interacts with the ERα downstream gene PR to impede its activity, and loss of full-length BRCA1 results in an increased growth response to exogenous progesterone with the most abnormal response following combined estrogen and progesterone treatment.[100]

Summary

These studies illustrate that genetically engineered mouse models can be used to explore aberrations in estrogen signaling and investigate the impact of specific signaling pathways through genetic, endocrinological, and pharmacological methods. The investigations synergize with *in vitro* tissue culture cell-based, human tissue-based, and clinical investigations to increase our understanding of the molecular determinants of breast cancer risk.

Acknowledgments

This project was supported by NIH NCI RO1 CA112176 (P.A.F.), NIH NCI 2RO1 CA88041 (P.A.F.), WCU (World Class University) program through the National Research Foundation of Korea funded by the Ministry of Education, Science and Technology (R31-10069) (P.A.F.), NIH NCI 2RO1 CA88041-1OS1 (M.C.C.), Department of Defense Breast Cancer Program Predoctoral Traineeship Award BC100440 (R.E.N.), and The Susan B. Komen Breast Cancer Foundation KG080359 (E.S.D.-C.).

Conflicts of interest

The authors declare no conflicts of interest.

References

1. Santen, R.J., H. Brodie, E.R. Simpson, *et al.* 2009. History of aromatase: saga of an important biological mediator and therapeutic target. *Endocr. Rev.* **30:** 343–375.

2. Katzenellenbogen, B.S. 1996. Estrogen receptors: bioactivities and interactions with cell signaling pathways. *Biol. Reprod.* **54:** 287–293.

3. Zhao, C., K. Dahlman-Wright & J.-Å. Gustafsson. 2010. Estrogen signaling via estrogen receptor {beta}. *J. Biol. Chem.* **285:** 39575–39579.

4. Anderson, E. & R.B. Clarke. 2004. Steroid receptors and cell cycle in normal mammary epithelium. *J. Mammary Gland Biol. Neoplasia* **9:** 3–13.

5. Dickson, R.B. & G.M. Stancel. 2000. Estrogen receptor-mediated processes in normal and cancer cells. *J. Natl. Cancer Inst. Monographs.* **27:** 135–145.

6. Brisken, C. & B. O'Malley. 2010. Hormone action in the mammary gland. *Cold Spring Harb. Perspect. Biol.* **2:** a003178.

7. Edson, M.A., A.K. Nagaraja & M.M. Matzuk. 2009. The mammalian ovary from genesis to revelation. *Endocr. Rev.* **30:** 624–712.

8. Chahal, H.S. & W.M. Drake. 2007. The endocrine system and ageing. *J. Pathol.* **211:** 173–180.

9. Bulun, S.E., Z. Lin, H. Zhao, *et al.* 2009. Regulation of aromatase expression in breast cancer tissue. *Ann. N. Y. Acad. Sci.* **1155:** 121–131.

10. Khan, S.A., M.A. Rogers, K.K. Khurana, *et al.* 1998. Estrogen receptor expression in benign breast epithelium and breast cancer risk. *J. Natl. Cancer Inst.* **90:** 37–42.

11. Clarke, R.B. 2004. Human breast cell proliferation and its relationship to steroid receptor expression. *Climacteric* **7:** 129–137.

12. Sugiyama, N., R.P.A. Barros, M. Warner & J.-A. Gustafsson. 2010. ERbeta: recent understanding of estrogen signaling. *Trends Endocrinol. Metab.* **21:** 545–552.

13. Carlberg, C. & S. Seuter. 2010. Dynamics of nuclear receptor target gene regulation. *Chromosoma* **119:** 479–484.

14. Horwitz, K.B. & W.L. McGuire. 1975. Predicting response to endocrine therapy in human breast cancer: a hypothesis. *Science* **189:** 726–727.

15. Welboren, W.-J., F.C.G.J. Sweep, P.N. Span & H.G. Stunnenberg. 2009. Genomic actions of estrogen receptor alpha: what are the targets and how are they regulated? *Endocr. Relat. Cancer* **16:** 1073–1089.

16. Kok, M., & S.C. Linn. 2010. Gene expression profiles of the oestrogen receptor in breast cancer. *Neth. J. Med.* **68:** 291–302.

17. Kristensen, V.N., T. Sørlie, J. Geisler, *et al.* 2005. Gene expression profiling of breast cancer in relation to estrogen receptor status and estrogen-metabolizing enzymes: clinical implications. *Clin. Cancer Res.* **11** 878s–883s.

18. Hammond, M.E.H., D.F. Hayes, M. Dowsett, *et al.* 2010. American Society of Clinical Oncology/College of American Pathologists guideline recommendations for immunohistochemical testing of estrogen and progesterone receptors in breast cancer (unabridged version). *Arch. Pathol. Lab. Med.* **134:** e48–e72.

19. Brown, P.H. & S.M. Lippman. 2000. Chemoprevention of breast cancer. *Breast Cancer Res. Treat.* **62:** 1–17.

20. Tessel, M.A., N.L. Krett & S.T. Rosen. 2010. Steroid receptor and microRNA regulation in cancer. *Curr. Opin. Oncol.* **22:** 592–597.

21. Pathiraja, T.N., V. Stearns & S. Oesterreich. 2010. Epigenetic regulation in estrogen receptor positive breast cancer—role in treatment response. *J. Mammary Gland Biol. Neoplasia* **15:** 35–47.

22. Wu, F. & Y.-Y. Mo. 2007. Ubiquitin-like protein modifications in prostate and breast cancer. *Front. Biosci.* **12:** 700–711.

23. Hayashi, S.-I., H. Eguchi, K. Tanimoto, *et al.* 2003. The expression and function of estrogen receptor alpha and beta in human breast cancer and its clinical application. *Endocr. Relat. Cancer* **10:** 193–202.

24. Ma, Y., S. Fan, C. Hu, *et al.* 2010. BRCA1 regulates acetylation and ubiquitination of estrogen receptor-alpha. *Mol. Endocrinol.* **24:** 76–90.

25. Castoria, G., A. Migliaccio, P. Giovannelli & F. Auricchio. 2010. Cell proliferation regulated by estradiol receptor: therapeutic implications. *Steroids* **75:** 524–527.

26. Arnold, A. & A. Papanikolaou. 2005. Cyclin D1 in breast cancer pathogenesis. *J. Clin. Oncol.* **23:** 4215–4224.

27. Eisinger-Mathason, T.S.K., J. Andrade & D.A. Lannigan. 2010. RSK in tumorigenesis: connections to steroid signaling. *Steroids* **75:** 191–202.

28. Acconcia, F. & R. Kumar. 2006. Signaling regulation of genomic and nongenomic functions of estrogen receptors. *Cancer Lett.* **238:** 1–14.

29. Gojis, O., B. Rudraraju, M. Gudi, *et al.* 2010. The role of Src-3 in human breast cancer. *Nat. Rev. Clin. Oncol.* **7:** 83–89.

30. Fox, E.M., J. Andrade & M.A. Shupnik. 2009. Novel actions of estrogen to promote proliferation: integration of cytoplasmic and nuclear pathways. *Steroids* **74:** 622–627.

31. Jerry, D.J., K.A. Dunphy & M.J. Hagen. 2010. Estrogens, regulation of p53 and breast cancer risk: a balancing act. *Cell. Mol. Life Sci.* **67:** 1017–1023.

32. Fan, S., J. Wang, R. Yuan, *et al.* 1999. BRCA1 inhibition of estrogen receptor signaling in transfected cells. *Science* **284:** 1354–1356.

33. Farber, E. 1988. Cancer development and its natural history. A cancer prevention perspective. *Cancer* **62:** 1676–1679.

34. Frech, M.S., E.D. Halama, M.T. Tilli, *et al.* 2005. Deregulated estrogen receptor alpha expression in mammary epithelial cells of transgenic mice results in the development of ductal carcinoma in situ. *Cancer Res.* **65:** 681–685.

35. Tilli, M.T., M.S. Frech, M.E. Steed, *et al.* 2003. Introduction of estrogen receptor-alpha into the tTA/TAg conditional mouse model precipitates the development of estrogen-responsive mammary adenocarcinoma. *Am. J. Pathol.* **163:** 1713–1719.

36. Miermont, A.M., A.R. Parrish & P.A. Furth. 2010. Role of ERalpha in the differential response of STAT5A loss in susceptibility to mammary preneoplasia and DMBA-induced carcinogenesis. *Carcinogenesis* **31:** 1124–1131.

37. Nakles, R.E., M.T. Shiffert, E.S. Díaz-Cruz, *et al.* 2011. Altered AIB1 or AIB1{Delta}3 expression impacts ER{alpha} effects on mammary gland stromal and epithelial content. *Mol. Endocrinol.* **25:** 549–563.

38. Díaz-Cruz, E.S. & P.A. Furth. 2010. Deregulated estrogen receptor alpha and p53 heterozygosity collaborate in the development of mammary hyperplasia. *Cancer Res.* **70:** 3965–3974.

39. Jones, L.P., M.T. Tilli, S. Assefnia, *et al.* 2008. Activation of estrogen signaling pathways collaborates with loss of BRCA1 to promote development of ERalpha-negative and ERalpha-positive mammary preneoplasia and cancer. *Oncogene* **27:** 794–802.

40. Hennighausen, L., R.J. Wall, U. Tillmann, M. Li, *et al.* 1995. Conditional gene expression in secretory tissues and skin of transgenic mice using the MMTV-LTR and the tetracycline responsive system. *J. Cell. Biochem.* **59:** 463–472.

41. Gunther, E.J., G.K. Belka, G.B.W. Wertheim, *et al.* 2002. A novel doxycycline-inducible system for the transgenic analysis of mammary gland biology. *FASEB J.* **16:** 283–292.

42. Hruska, K.S., M.T. Tilli, S. Ren, *et al.* 2002. Conditional over-expression of estrogen receptor alpha in a transgenic mouse model. *Transgenic Res.* **11:** 361–372.

43. Furth, P.A. 1997. Conditional control of gene expression in the mammary gland. *J. Mammary Gland Biol. Neoplasia* **2:** 373–383.

44. Tilli, M.T., S.L. Hudgins, M.S. Frech, *et al.* 2003. Loss of protein phosphatase 2A expression correlates with

phosphorylation of DP-1 and reversal of dysplasia through differentiation in a conditional mouse model of cancer progression. *Cancer Res.* **63**: 7668–7673.

45. Ewald, D., M. Li, S. Efrat, *et al.* 1996. Time-sensitive reversal of hyperplasia in transgenic mice expressing SV40 T antigen. *Science* **273**: 1384–1386.

46. Frech, M.S., K.M. Torre, G.W. Robinson & P.A. Furth. 2008. Loss of cyclin D1 in concert with deregulated estrogen receptor alpha expression induces DNA damage response activation and interrupts mammary gland morphogenesis. *Oncogene* **27**: 3186–3193.

47. Kim, J.K. & J.A. Diehl. 2009. Nuclear cyclin D1: an oncogenic driver in human cancer. *J. Cell. Physiol.* **220**: 292–296.

48. Harvell, D.M., T.E. Strecker, M. Tochacek, *et al.* 2000. Rat strain-specific actions of 17beta-estradiol in the mammary gland: correlation between estrogen-induced lobuloalveolar hyperplasia and susceptibility to estrogen-induced mammary cancers. *Proc. Natl. Acad. Sci. USA* **97**: 2779–2784.

49. Shull, J.D., T.J. Spady, M.C. Snyder, *et al.* 1997. Ovary-intact, but not ovariectomized female ACI rats treated with 17beta-estradiol rapidly develop mammary carcinoma. *Carcinogenesis* **18**: 1595–1601.

50. Ruhlen, R.L., D.M. Willbrand, C.L. Besch-Williford, *et al.* 2009. Tamoxifen induces regression of estradiol-induced mammary cancer in the ACI.COP-Ept2 rat model. *Breast Cancer Res. Treat.* **117**: 517–524.

51. Gould, K.A., M. Tochacek, B.S. Schaffer, *et al.* 2004. Genetic determination of susceptibility to estrogen-induced mammary cancer in the ACI rat: mapping of Emca1 and Emca2 to chromosomes 5 and 18. *Genetics* **168**: 2113–2125.

52. Hennighausen, L., G.W. Robinson, K.U. Wagner & X. Liu. 1997. Developing a mammary gland is a stat affair. *J. Mammary Gland Biol. Neoplasia* **2**: 365–372.

53. Yamaji, D., R. Na, Y. Feuermann, *et al.* 2009. Development of mammary luminal progenitor cells is controlled by the transcription factor STAT5A. *Genes Dev.* **23**: 2382–2387.

54. Shan, L., M. Yu, B.D. Clark & E.G. Snyderwine. 2004. Possible role of STAT5A in rat mammary gland carcinogenesis. *Breast Cancer Res. Treat.* **88**: 263–272.

55. Cotarla, I., S. Ren, Y. Zhang, *et al.* 2004. STAT5A is tyrosine phosphorylated and nuclear localized in a high proportion of human breast cancers. *Int. J. Cancer* **108**: 665–671.

56. List, H.J., R. Reiter, B. Singh, *et al.* 2001. Expression of the nuclear coactivator AIB1 in normal and malignant breast tissue. *Breast Cancer Res. Treat.* **68**: 21–28.

57. Reiter, R., A. Wellstein & A.T. Riegel. 2001. An isoform of the coactivator AIB1 that increases hormone and growth factor sensitivity is overexpressed in breast cancer. *J. Biol. Chem.* **276**: 39736–39741.

58. Reiter, R., A.S. Oh, A. Wellstein & A. Riegel. 2004. Impact of the nuclear receptor coactivator AIB1 isoform AIB1-Delta3 on estrogenic ligands with different intrinsic activity. *Oncogene* **23**: 403–409.

59. Lacroix, M., R.-A. Toillon & G. Leclercq. 2006. p53 and breast cancer, an update. *Endocr. Relat. Cancer* **13**: 293–325.

60. Varley, J.M., W.J. Brammar, D.P. Lane, *et al.* 1991. Loss of chromosome 17p13 sequences and mutation of p53 in human breast carcinomas. *Oncogene* **6**: 413–421.

61. Elledge, R.M. & D.C. Allred. 1994. The p53 tumor suppressor gene in breast cancer. *Breast Cancer Res. Treat.* **32**: 39–47.

62. Rohan, T.E., W. Hartwick, A.B. Miller & R.A. Kandel. 1998. Immunohistochemical detection of c-erbB-2 and p53 in benign breast disease and breast cancer risk. *J. Natl. Cancer Inst.* **90**: 1262–1269.

63. Putti, T.C., D.M.A. El-Rehim, E.A. Rakha, *et al.* 2005. Estrogen receptor-negative breast carcinomas: a review of morphology and immunophenotypical analysis. *Mod. Pathol.* **18**: 26–35.

64. Medina, D., F.S. Kittrell, A. Shepard, *et al.* 2003. Hormone dependence in premalignant mammary progression. *Cancer Res.* **63**: 1067–1072.

65. Varley, J.M., D.G. Evans & J.M. Birch. 1997. Li-Fraumeni syndrome–a molecular and clinical review. *Br. J. Cancer* **76**: 1–14.

66. Vervoorts, J. & B. Lüscher. 2008. Post-translational regulation of the tumor suppressor p27(KIP1). *Cell. Mol. Life Sci.* **65**: 3255–3264.

67. Oh, Y.L., J.S. Choi, S.Y. Song, *et al.* 2001. Expression of p21Waf1, p27Kip1 and cyclin D1 proteins in breast ductal carcinoma in situ: relation with clinicopathologic characteristics and with p53 expression and estrogen receptor status. *Pathol. Int.* **51**: 94–99.

68. Chu, I., A. Arnaout, S. Loiseau, *et al.* 2007. Src promotes estrogen-dependent estrogen receptor alpha proteolysis in human breast cancer. *J. Clin. Invest.* **117**: 2205–2215.

69. Mukhopadhyay, U.K., R. Eves, L. Jia, *et al.* 2009. p53 suppresses Src-induced podosome and rosette formation and cellular invasiveness through the upregulation of caldesmon. *Mol. Cell. Biol.* **29**: 3088–3098.

70. Kelsey, J.L. & M.D. Gammon. 1991. The epidemiology of breast cancer. *CA Cancer J. Clin.* **41**: 146–165.

71. Bernstein, L. 2002. Epidemiology of endocrine-related risk factors for breast cancer. *J. Mammary Gland Biol. Neoplasia* **7**: 3–15.

72. Dunphy, K.A., A.C. Blackburn, H. Yan, *et al.* 2008. Estrogen and progesterone induce persistent increases in p53-dependent apoptosis and suppress mammary tumors in BALB/c-Trp53+/- mice. *Breast Cancer Res.* **10**: R43.

73. Díaz-Cruz, E.S., M.C. Cabrera, R.E. Nakles, *et al.* 2011. BRCA1 deficient mouse models to study pathogenesisa and therapy of triple negative breast cancer. *Breast Disease.* In press.

74. Xu, X., K.U. Wagner, D. Larson, *et al.* 1999. Conditional mutation of BRCA1 in mammary epithelial cells results in blunted ductal morphogenesis and tumour formation. *Nat. Genet.* **22**: 37–43.

75. Li, W., C. Xiao, B.K. Vonderhaar & C.-X. Deng. 2007. A role of estrogen/ERalpha signaling in BRCA1-associated tissue-specific tumor formation. *Oncogene* **26**: 7204–7212.

76. Deng, C.X. & S.G. Brodie. 2000. Roles of BRCA1 and its interacting proteins. *Bioessays* **22**: 728–737.

77. Gudmundsdottir, K. & A. Ashworth. 2006. The roles of BRCA1 and BRCA2 and associated proteins in the maintenance of genomic stability. *Oncogene* **25**: 5864–5874.

78. Wagner, K.U., R.J. Wall, L. St-Onge, *et al.* 1997. Cre-mediated gene deletion in the mammary gland. *Nucleic Acids Res.* **25:** 4323–4330.

79. Xu, X., W. Qiao, S.P. Linke, *et al.* 2001. Genetic interactions between tumor suppressors BRCA1 and p53 in apoptosis, cell cycle and tumorigenesis. *Nat. Genet.* **28:** 266–271.

80. Holstege, H., S.A. Joosse, C.T.M. van Oostrom, *et al.* 2009. High incidence of protein-truncating TP53 mutations in BRCA1-related breast cancer. *Cancer Res.* **69:** 3625–3633.

81. Podo, F., L.M.C. Buydens, H. Degani, *et al.* 2010. Triple-negative breast cancer: present challenges and new perspectives. *Mol. Oncol.* **4:** 209–229.

82. Herschkowitz, J.I., K. Simin, V.J. Weigman, *et al.* 2007. Identification of conserved gene expression features between murine mammary carcinoma models and human breast tumors. *Genome Biol.* **8:** R76.

83. Gorski, J.J., R.D. Kennedy, A.M. Hosey & D.P. Harkin. 2009. The complex relationship between BRCA1 and ERalpha in hereditary breast cancer. *Clin. Cancer Res.* **15:** 1514–1518.

84. Hu, Y. 2009. BRCA1, hormone, and tissue-specific tumor suppression. *Int. J. Biol. Sci.* **5:** 20–27.

85. Berstein, L.M. 2008. Endocrinology of the wild and mutant BRCA1 gene and types of hormonal carcinogenesis. *Future Oncol.* **4:** 23–39.

86. Rosen, E.M., S. Fan, R.G. Pestell & I.D. Goldberg. 2003. BRCA1 in hormone-responsive cancers. *Trends Endocrinol. Metab.* **14:** 378–385.

87. Rosen, E.M., S. Fan & C. Isaacs. 2005. BRCA1 in hormonal carcinogenesis: basic and clinical research. *Endocr. Relat. Cancer* **12:** 533–548.

88. Fan, S., Y.X. Ma, C. Wang, *et al.* 2001. Role of direct interaction in BRCA1 inhibition of estrogen receptor activity. *Oncogene* **20:** 77–87.

89. Razandi, M., A. Pedram, E.M. Rosen & E.R. Levin. 2004. BRCA1 inhibits membrane estrogen and growth factor receptor signaling to cell proliferation in breast cancer. *Mol. Cell. Biol.* **24:** 5900–5913.

90. Xu, J., S. Fan & E.M. Rosen. 2005. Regulation of the estrogen-inducible gene expression profile by the breast cancer susceptibility gene BRCA1. *Endocrinology* **146:** 2031–2047.

91. Ma, Y.X., Y. Tomita, S. Fan, *et al.* 2005. Structural determinants of the BRCA1: estrogen receptor interaction. *Oncogene* **24:** 1831–1846.

92. Fan, S., Y.X. Ma, C. Wang, *et al.* 2002. p300 Modulates the BRCA1 inhibition of estrogen receptor activity. *Cancer Res.* **62:** 141–151.

93. Ma, Y., C. Hu, A.T. Riegel, *et al.* 2007. Growth factor signaling pathways modulate BRCA1 repression of estrogen receptor-alpha activity. *Mol. Endocrinol.* **21:** 1905–1923.

94. Wang, C., S. Fan, Z. Li, *et al.* 2005. Cyclin D1 antagonizes BRCA1 repression of estrogen receptor alpha activity. *Cancer Res.* **65:** 6557–6567.

95. Domchek, S.M., T.M. Friebel, C.F. Singer, *et al.* 2010. Association of risk-reducing surgery in BRCA1 or BRCA2 mutation carriers with cancer risk and mortality. *JAMA* **304:** 967–975.

96. Bachelier, R., X. Xu, C. Li, *et al.* 2005. Effect of bilateral oophorectomy on mammary tumor formation in BRCA1 mutant mice. *Oncol. Rep.* **14:** 1117–1120.

97. Tung, N., A. Miron, S.J. Schnitt, *et al.* 2010. Prevalence and predictors of loss of wild type BRCA1 in estrogen receptor positive and negative BRCA1-associated breast cancers. *Breast Cancer Res.* **12:** R95.

98. Jones, L.P., M. Li, E.D. Halama, *et al.* 2005. Promotion of mammary cancer development by tamoxifen in a mouse model of BRCA1-mutation-related breast cancer. *Oncogene* **24:** 3554–3562.

99. Wen, J., R. Li, Y. Lu & M.A. Shupnik. 2009. Decreased BRCA1 confers tamoxifen resistance in breast cancer cells by altering estrogen receptor-coregulator interactions. *Oncogene* **28:** 575–586.

100. Ma, Y., P. Katiyar, L.P. Jones, *et al.* 2006. The breast cancer susceptibility gene BRCA1 regulates progesterone receptor signaling in mammary epithelial cells. *Mol. Endocrinol.* **20:** 14–34.

Ann. N.Y. Acad. Sci. ISSN 0077-8923

ANNALS OF THE NEW YORK ACADEMY OF SCIENCES

Issue: *Nutrition and Physical Activity in Aging, Obesity, and Cancer*

The role of carbon monoxide in metabolic disease

Yeonsoo Joe,[1] Min Zheng,[2] Seul-Ki Kim,[1] Sena Kim,[1] Jamal MD Uddin,[1] Tae Sun Min,[3] Do Gon Ryu,[4] and Hun Taeg Chung[1]

[1]School of Biological Sciences and [2]Department of Medical Science, University of Ulsan, Ulsan, South Korea. [3]Division of Natural Sciences, National Research Foundation of Korea, Daejeon, South Korea. [4]Department of Physiology, School of Oriental Medicine, Wonkwang University, Iksan, Chonbuk, South Korea

Address for correspondence: Hun Taeg Chung, School of Biological Sciences, University of Ulsan, Bldg 35 room 806, 102 Daehak-ro Nam-gu, Ulsan 680-749, South Korea. chung@ulsan.ac.kr

Metabolic disease is a complex disorder defined by various factors that increase the risk of cardiovascular disease and type 2 diabetes mellitus. In recent years, the incidence of chronic metabolic disease has dramatically increased throughout the world. These chronic metabolic diseases are associated with elevated inflammatory activities. In addition, endoplasmic reticulum (ER) stress leads to metabolic syndrome. Inflammation and ER stress are linked in the context of metabolic homeostasis and disease. Carbon monoxide (CO), a reaction product of heme oxygenase-1 (HO-1), reduces oxidative stress and inflammatory response and protects cells from ER stress. CO has anti-inflammatory effects via induction of HO-1 expression and prevents ER stress–induced apoptosis by inhibiting the C/EBP homologous protein expression. In addition to its anti-inflammatory effects and antiapoptotic effects, HO-1 plays an important role in insulin release and glucose metabolism. In our study, inhalation of CO gas or CO-releasing molecule injection ameliorates 30% fructose or methionine-deficient- and choline-deficient–diet-induced hepatic steatosis. Therefore, CO can be studied in the search for potential therapeutic targets for metabolic diseases via inhibition of inflammatory response and ER stress.

Keywords: carbon monoxide; inflammation; ER stress; metabolic disease; heme oxygenase-1

Carbon monoxide and inflammation

Carbon monoxide (CO) has recently been accepted as a cytoprotective molecule in various disease models. The endogenous production of CO is generated through inducible heme oxygenase-1 (HO-1)[1] and constitutive heme oxygenase-2 (HO-2). These enzymes are responsible for the rate-limiting step in the degradation of heme to CO, ferrous iron, and biliverdin. The antiapoptotic effects of both exogenous CO and HO-1–derived CO are demonstrated both *in vivo* and *in vitro*. CO treatment in cell cultures inhibits tumor necrosis factor-α (TNF-α)–induced apoptosis in mouse fibroblasts[2] and endothelial cells.[3] In several models of disease, low-dose CO treatment causes antiapoptotic effects. Anti-inflammatory effects of CO are also determined in cell culture models and septic models. CO inhibits the production of proinflammatory cytokines such as TNF-α, IL-1β, and macrophage

inflammatory protein-1β (MIP1β) in the presence of lipopolysaccharide (LPS) treatment.[4] Conversely, the production of the anti-inflammatory cytokine IL-10 is increased by CO treatment.[5] CO also inhibits the LPS-induced NF-κB activation by preventing the phosphorylation and degradation of the inhibitory subunit I-κBα.[6] One potential signal for anti-inflammatory effects of CO involves the p38 MAPK pathway; for example, murine macrophages treated with CO increase LPS-mediated p38 MAPK activation,[7] and the potent antioxidant curcumin induces HO-1 expression through p38 MAKP pathway.[8]

CO also regulates upstream Toll-like receptor (TLR) signaling pathways,[9,10] which are involved in the initial phase of microbial detection and have been implicated in the pathogenesis of inflammatory human diseases.[11] CO inhibits LPS-induced nicotinamide adenine dinucleotide phosphate (NADPH) oxidase activity and translocation

doi: 10.1111/j.1749-6632.2011.06121.x

of TLRs to lipid rafts, which is associated with the inhibition of ligand-induced reactive oxygen species production.[9] The anti-inflammatory effect of CO has also been demonstrated in inflammatory diseases such as sepsis and asthma.[5,12]

Taken together, CO has anti-inflammatory effects via various mechanisms. Inflammatory responses are involved in the pathogenesis of obesity, type 2 diabetes, and atherosclerosis, with the most apparent changes occurring in adipose tissue, the liver, pancreatic islets, the vasculature, and circulating leukocytes. The anti-inflammatory effects of CO may function as an important protective system for metabolic disease.

Carbon monoxide and endoplasmic reticulum stress

In addition to the anti-inflammatory effects of CO, CO/HO-1 has the protective effects of cells from endoplasmic reticulum (ER) stress. The ER is an organelle where secretory or membrane proteins are synthesized. Newly synthesized proteins are folded with ER chaperones in the ER, and only exact-folded proteins are transported to the Golgi apparatus.[13] Various infectious agents, environmental toxins, and abnormal metabolic conditions interface with protein folding and thereby lead to ER stress. Under these stresses, the unfolded proteins accumulated in the ER are collectively known as the unfolded protein response (UPR).

The ER also has an important role in Ca^{2+} storage and signaling. The concentration of Ca^{2+} is controlled by the sarcoplasmic reticulum Ca^{2+} ATPase (SERCA) proteins, which pump Ca^{2+} into the ER, and the inositol (1,4,5) triphosphate and ryanodine receptors that release Ca^{2+} from the ER. Chaperons, such as Grp78 (Bip), Grp94, and calreticulin, which stabilize protein folding intermediates, have a Ca^{2+}-dependent nature.[14,15,16] Thus, abnormal Ca^{2+} regulation in the ER triggers UPR. In mammalian cells, the signaling of UPR is mediated by three ER-associated transmembrane proteins, PERK (PKR-like eukaryotic initiation factor 2α kinase), IRE1 (inositol requiring enzyme 1), and ATF6 (activating transcription factor-6).[17] Under normal conditions, the N-termini of these ER-associated transmembrane proteins are held by ER chaperone Grp78, preventing their aggregation. Activation of IRE-1 and ATF6 by ER stress results in the upregulation of GRP78 that increases protein-folding activity and

prevents protein aggregation. The endoribonuclease activity of IRE1 cleaves a 26 base-pair segment form mRNA of the X box–binding protein-1 (XBP-1), which is then translated into the active, spliced form of the transcription factor (XBP1s).[18] Unfolded or misfolded proteins in the ER lumen are usually ubiquitinated and degraded by the proteasome system,[19] a process regulated by the UPR.

If unfolded or misfolded protein accumulation in the ER is not resolved, prolonged activation of the UPR can lead to programmed cell death. To prevent this, UPR-mediated PERK activation impedes protein translation via phosphorylation-dependent inhibition of eukaryotic translation initiation factor 2α (eIF 2α).[20] PERK is a Ser/Thr protein kinase that can mediate eIF2α phosphorylation. Activation of PERK by ER stress leads to activation of ATF4 via phosphorylation by eIF2α; in addition, promotion of ATF4 translation increases transcription of the ATF4 downstream target CHOP (C/EBP homologous protein); from this, PERK–CHOP–mediated signaling can lead to apoptosis under pathologically prolonged ER stress. However, under less-prolonged ER stress, IRE1 dimerizes and then alternatively splices XBP-1 mRNA to produce active XBP1s, as mentioned above. This is coupled with PERK-dependent signals leading the activation of the survival transcription factor NF-E2–related factor-2 (Nrf2) via site-specific phosphorylation.[21] In human endothelial cells, for example, the induction of HO-1 by exogenous CO administration protects the cells from ER stressors, and the mechanism by which this occurs is via PERK-dependent activation of Nrf2 by CO.[22] CO-releasing molecules or CO gas induces HO-1 expression via Nrf2 activation;[23] additionally, CO directly induces the expression of HO-1 in a MAPK/Nrf2-dependent manner; CO-induced PERK activation triggers nuclear trafficking of Nrf2 and increased HO-1 transcription.[24] Unlike its activation of PERK, CO suppresses ER stress–induced XBP-1 and ATF6 activation. Collectively, CO induces Nrf2-dependent HO-1 expression via the PERK pathway and thereby prevents ER stress–induced apoptosis via p38 MAPK dependent inhibition of CHOP expression.[22]

ER stress and metabolic disease

Recently, ER was shown to be responsible for cellular signaling leading to apoptosis, inflammation, and activation of immune responses.[13] In obese individuals, for example, increased cholesterol and saturated fatty acid levels decrease the fluidity of the ER membrane, leading to inhibition of SERCA Ca^{2+}-ATPases, depletion of ER luminal Ca^{2+} stores, inhibition of ER-resident molecular chaperons, and the accumulation of unfolded proteins, which triggers the UPR.[17,25]

Metabolic syndrome (MS) is characterized by several risk factors for type 2 diabetes mellitus and cardiovascular disease, including insulin resistance, hypertension, dyslipidemia, and visceral obesity.[26] Recently, low-grade inflammation initiated by danger-associated molecular patterns has been recognized as the most prominent pathogenic feature of MS because of its associated increase of plasma C-reactive protein, a marker of inflammation; high levels of C-reactive protein are linked to the development of cardiovascular disease and type 2 diabetes mellitus.[27] Early research identified the c-Jun amino terminal kinase (JNK1) as one of the serine kinases that inhibits insulin signaling.[28] More recently, work has demonstrated that JNK1 also is a central regulator of inflammatory and immune responses.[29] Like other members of this serine kinase network, JNK1 is activated by free fatty acids and the inflammatory cytokine, TNF-α.

In an attempt to better understand the obesity-associated events linked to JNK1, Ozcan *et al.* demonstrated that JNK1 can be triggered by ER stress.[29] Later work demonstrated, as mentioned previously, that the ER stress sensor IRE1 triggers inflammatory signaling via activation of MAP kinase modules, leading to the activation of the MAP kinase JNK and p38 and NF-κB.[30] Activation of these MAP kinases and of NF-κB by IRE1 requires its interaction with the adaptor protein TRAF2. The N-terminal effector domains and five Zn^{2+} fingers of TRAF2 are required for the activation of JNK and NF-κB. Under ER stress, TRAF2 activates the inhibitor κB kinase (IKK) and the apoptosis signal–regulating kinase (ASK1) through formation of an IRE1-TRAF2-ASK1 complex.[7,31] JNK induces inflammatory responses by potentiating the activity of the transcription factor c-Jun. In summary, obesity-induced ER stress induces the UPR, which, in turn, induces low-grade inflammation that leads to metabolic diseases. Therefore, we have studied whether ER stress and inflammation increased by metabolic dysfunction can be alleviated by the CO/HO-1 system.

Carbon monoxide and metabolic disease

Over the last decade, it has become clear that inflammation is a key factor for obesity and type 2 diabetes.[26] Inflammatory or oxidative insults exert a strong influence on obesity, insulin-resistant type 2 diabetes, and many metabolic syndromes. Interestingly, newly emerging data indicate the role of the HO system in insulin sensitivity and cellular metabolism. Among the byproducts of heme moiety by HO-1, CO and bilirubin suppress apoptosis, necrosis, inflammation, and oxidative stress, while the iron formed enhances the synthesis of the antioxidant, ferritin.[32] The role of the HO system is becoming clear in insulin sensitivity and glucose metabolism.[33] Indeed, upregulation of HO-1 by cobalt protoporphyrin (CoPP) increases adiponectin and reduces inflammatory cytokines. In Zucker diabetic fat (ZDF) rats, CoPP administration improves insulin sensitivity and visceral adipose tissue volume. Both improved insulin sensitivity and adipose tissue remodeling are accomplished by HO-1 induction through the increase of adiponectin and pAMPK levels. Thus, HO-1 has the potential as a therapeutic target for obesity and its associated health risks.[34] In addition, the administration of inducer of HO-1 protein and activity improves vascular function in diabetes.[35] CO seems to share many similarities with NO.[36] CO, like NO, is a smooth-muscle relaxant.[37,38] Ultimately, CO as the main HO-1–derived regulator has the role for the control of vascular tone and a beneficial effect on vascular function, thus improving vascular reactivity. In addition, CO stimulates insulin and glucagon release from isolated islets.[37] Additionally, hemin, the HO-1 inducer, increases glucose-stimulated insulin release by pancreatic β cells. Interestingly, CO is produced by glucose-stimulated islet, and consequently, triggers insulin release[37] as well as protects pancreatic β cells.[38]

Taken together, CO/HO-1 may play an important role in insulin resistance, type 2 diabetes, and cardiometbolic complications. In addition, the features of various metabolic syndromes are clearly associated with non-alcoholic fatty liver disease (NAFLD), one of the most common chronic liver diseases. Hepatic steatosis is the earliest and most common type of liver disease, which progresses to more severe complications, such as steatohepatitis, cirrhosis, and hepatocellular carcinoma. A number of emerging

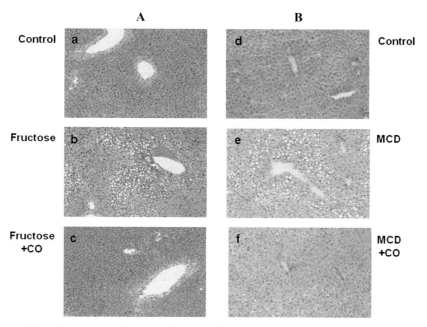

Figure 1. Effect of CO on lipid accumulation in the liver. Steatohepatitis was induced by feeding on C57bl/c with 30% fructose for eight weeks or the methionine choline–deficient (MCD) diet for three weeks. Liver sections were stained with hematoxylin and eosin. Mice were exposed to CO gas at a concentration of 250 ppm. Mice were maintained in the CO cage for the duration of CO exposure for 6 h/day. (A) In fructose-induced NAFLD models, animals ($n = 4$–7 per group) had either free excess to tap water or tap water containing 30% fructose; (a) tap water, (b); 30% fructose, (c); 30% fructose with CO gas. (B) In MCD-induced NAFLD models, mice were fed control (MCS) or MCD diets for 21 days; (a) normal diet, (b) MCD diet, (c) MCD diet with CO gas. The fructose- or MCD-treated group increases lipid accumulation in liver (b, d). Inhalation of CO ameliorates fructose or MCD-induced steatohepatitis (c, e).

reports have emphasized the link between the ER stress response and hepatic lipid metabolism.[39,40] In mouse models, the UPR is increased in obesity. Enhanced ER stress leads to suppression of insulin receptor signaling via JNK activation, presumably IRE1 α dependent, and insulin resistance, in turn, is induced by JNK-mediated inhibitory phosphorylation of serine residue 307 of insulin receptor substrate 1(IRS-1). The interconnectedness of ER stress and hepatic steatosis has been proven through genetic modulation of the eEF2α phosphorylation pathway, the IRE1α-XBP1 pathway.[39,40]

On the other hand, TLR4 signaling plays an important role in the pathogenesis of steatohepatitis. That is, methionine-deficient and choline-deficient (MCD) diet–induced steatohepatitis induces TLR-4 expression as well as the TLR accessory molecules MD-2 and CD14. In TLR-4 mutant mice, injury and inflammation are markedly attenuated, and MCD diet–induced fibrogenesis was also protected. Therefore, TLR-4 modulates lipid accumulation and fibrosis.[41] In our previous report, CO protects en-

dothelial cells from ER stress–induced apoptosis.[22] Additionally, CO inhibits TLR signaling pathways by inhibiting translocation of TLR to lipid rafts. As shown in Figure 1, hepatic steatosis was detected in two NAFLD models, 30% fructose-induced hepatic lipid accumulation and MCD-induced NAFLD. Inhalation of CO gas or CO-releasing molecule (CORM) injection ameliorates hepatic lipid accumulation. Therefore, our data indicate the novel role of CO in metabolic disease.

Summary

CO, a by-product of heme catabolism by HO, confers potent anti-inflammatory effects. Its effect on anti-inflammatory response is dependent on the p38 MAPK pathway. Additionally, CO inhibits the TLR signaling pathway by inhibiting translocation of TLR to lipid rafts and protects cells from ER stress–induced apoptosis. In addition, CO induces Nrf2-dependent HO-1 expression via the PERK pathway and prevents ER stress–induced apoptosis via the p38 MAPK–dependent inhibition of CHOP expression. CO/HO-1 improves vascular function on diabetes and stimulates insulin release from islets. Inhalation of CO gas or CORM injection alleviates hepatic steatosis induced by 30% fructose for eight weeks or MCD diet for three weeks. Therefore, we suggest that CO may play an important role in the regulation of cellular metabolism.

Acknowledgment

This work was supported by grants from the Korea Research Foundation Grant funded by the Korean Government (MOEHRD) (BRL-2009-0087350).

Conflicts of interest

The authors declare no conflicts of interest.

References

1. Tenhunen, R., H.S. Marver & R. Schmid. 1968. The enzymatic conversion of heme to bilirubin by microsomal heme oxygenase. *Proc Natl. Acad. Sci. USA* **61:** 748–755.

2. Petrache, I. *et al.* 2000. Heme oxygenase-1 inhibits TNF-alpha-induced apoptosis in cultured fibroblasts. *Am. J. Physiol. Lung Cell Mol. Physiol.* **278:** L312–319.

3. Brouard, S. *et al.* 2000. Carbon monoxide generated by heme oxygenase 1 suppresses endothelial cell apoptosis. *J. Exp. Med.* **192:** 1015–1026.

4. Morse, D. & J. Sethi. 2002. Carbon monoxide and human disease. *Antioxid. Redox Signal* **4:** 331–338.

5. Otterbein, L.E. *et al.* 2000. Carbon monoxide has anti-inflammatory effects involving the mitogen-activated protein kinase pathway. *Nat. Med.* **6:** 422–428.

6. Sarady, J.K. *et al.* 2002. Carbon monoxide modulates endotoxin-induced production of granulocyte macrophage colony-stimulating factor in macrophages. *Am. J. Respir. Cell Mol. Biol.* **27:** 739–745.

7. Wang, X.M. *et al.* 2006. Caveolin-1 confers antiinflammatory effects in murine macrophages via the MKK3/p38 MAPK pathway. *Am. J. Respir. Cell Mol. Biol.* **34:** 434–442.

8. Jeong, G.S. *et al.* 2006. Comparative effects of curcuminoids on endothelial heme oxygenase-1 expression: orthomethoxy groups are essential to enhance heme oxygenase activity and protection. *Exp. Mol. Med.* **38:** 393–400.

9. Nakahira, K. *et al.* 2006. Carbon monoxide differentially inhibits TLR signaling pathways by regulating ROS-induced trafficking of TLRs to lipid rafts. *J. Exp. Med.* **203:** 2377–2389.

10. Wang, X.M. *et al.* 2009. The heme oxygenase-1/carbon monoxide pathway suppresses TLR4 signaling by regulating the interaction of TLR4 with caveolin-1. *J. Immunol.* **182:** 3809–3818.

11. Akira, S. & K. Takeda. 2004. Toll-like receptor signaling. *Nat. Rev. Immunol.* **4:** 499–511.

12. Chapman, J.T. *et al.* 2001. Carbon monoxide attenuates aeroallergen-induced inflammation in mice. *Am. J. Physiol. Lung Cell Mol. Physiol.* **281:** L209–216.

13. Kaufman, R.J. 2002. Orchestrating the unfolded protein response in health and disease. *J. Clin. Invest.* **110:** 1389–1398.

14. Bertolotti, A. *et al.* 2000. Dynamic interaction of BiP and ER stress transducers in the unfolded-protein response. *Nat. Cell Biol.* **2:** 326–332.

15. Chen, X., J. Shen & R. Prywes. 2002. The luminal domain of ATF6 senses endoplasmic reticulum (ER) stress and causes translocation of ATF6 from the ER to the Golgi. *J. Biol. Chem.* **277:** 13045–13052.

16. Hidalgo, C. 2005. Cross talk between Ca2+ and redox signalling cascades in muscle and neurons through the combined activation of ryanodine receptors/Ca2+ release channels. *Philos. Trans. R. Soc. Lond. B Biol. Sci.* **360:** 2237–2246.

17. Zhang, K. & R.J. Kaufman. 2004. Signaling the unfolded protein response from the endoplasmic reticulum. *J. Biol. Chem.* **279:** 25935–25938.

18. Sidrauski, C. & P. Walter. 1997. The transmembrane kinase Ire1p is a site-specific endonuclease that initiates mRNA splicing in the unfolded protein response. *Cell* **90:** 1031–1039.

19. Werner, E.D., J.L. Brodsky & A.A. McCracken. 1996. Proteasome-dependent endoplasmic reticulum-associated protein degradation: an unconventional route to a familiar fate. *Proc. Natl. Acad. Sci. USA* **93:** 13797–13801.

20. Harding, H.P. *et al.* 2000. Perk is essential for translational regulation and cell survival during the unfolded protein response. *Mol. Cell* **5:** 897–904.

21. Cullinan, S.B. *et al.* 2003. Nrf2 is a direct PERK substrate and effector of PERK-dependent cell survival. *Mol. Cell Biol.* **23:** 7198–7209.

22. Kim, K.M. *et al.* 2007. Carbon monoxide induces heme oxygenase-1 via activation of protein kinase R-like endoplasmic reticulum kinase and inhibits endothelial cell apoptosis triggered by endoplasmic reticulum stress. *Circ. Res.* **101:** 919–927.

23. Lee, B.S. *et al.* 2006. Carbon monoxide mediates heme oxygenase 1 induction via Nrf2 activation in hepatoma cells. *Biochem. Biophys. Res. Commun.* **343:** 965–972.

24. Cullinan, S.B. & J.A. Diehl. 2004. PERK-dependent activation of Nrf2 contributes to redox homeostasis and cell survival following endoplasmic reticulum stress. *J. Biol. Chem.* **279:** 20108–20117.

25. Zheng, X. & S.J. Hu. 2005. Effects of simvastatin on cardiac performance and expression of sarcoplasmic reticular calcium regulatory proteins in rat heart. *Acta. Pharmacol. Sin.* **26:** 696–704.

26. Wellen, K.E. & G.S. Hotamisligil. 2005. Inflammation, stress, and diabetes. *J. Clin. Invest.* **115:** 1111–1119.

27. Hotamisligil, G.S. 2006. Inflammation and metabolic disorders. *Nature* **444:** 860–867.

28. Hirosumi, J. *et al.* 2002. A central role for JNK in obesity and insulin resistance. *Nature* **420:** 333–336.

29. Ozcan, U. *et al.* 2004. Endoplasmic reticulum stress links obesity, insulin action, and type 2 diabetes. *Science* **306:** 457–461.

30. Urano, F. *et al.* 2000. Coupling of stress in the ER to activation of JNK protein kinases by transmembrane protein kinase IRE1. *Science* **287:** 664–666.

31. Matsukawa, J. *et al.* 2004. The ASK1-MAP kinase cascades in mammalian stress response. *J. Biochem.* **136:** 261–265.

32. Hintze, K.J. & E.C. Theil. 2006. Cellular regulation and molecular interactions of the ferritins. *Cell Mol. Life Sci.* **63:** 591–600.

33. Li, M. *et al.* 2008. Treatment of obese diabetic mice with a heme oxygenase inducer reduces visceral and subcutaneous adiposity, increases adiponectin levels, and improves insulin sensitivity and glucose tolerance. *Diabetes* **57:** 1526–1535.

34. Nicolai, A. *et al.* 2009. Heme oxygenase-1 induction remodels adipose tissue and improves insulin sensitivity in obesity-induced diabetic rats. *Hypertension* **53:** 508–515.

35. Di Pascoli, M. *et al.* 2006. Chronic CO levels have a beneficial effect on vascular relaxation in diabetes. *Biochem. Biophys. Res Commun.* **340:** 935–943.

36. Moncada, S., R.M. Palmer & E.A. Higgs. 1991. Nitric oxide: physiology, pathophysiology, and pharmacology. *Pharmacol. Rev.* **43:** 109–142.

37. Henningsson, R. *et al.* 1999. Heme oxygenase and carbon monoxide: regulatory roles in islet hormone release: a biochemical, immunohistochemical, and confocal microscopic study. *Diabetes* **48:** 66–76.

38. Ye, J. & S.G. Laychock. 1998. A protective role for heme oxygenase expression in pancreatic islets exposed to interleukin-1beta. *Endocrinology* **139:** 4155–4163.

39. Lee, A.H. *et al.* 2008. Regulation of hepatic lipogenesis by the transcription factor XBP1. *Science* **320:** 1492–1496.

40. Ye, J. *et al.* 2000. ER stress induces cleavage of membrane-bound ATF6 by the same proteases that process SREBPs. *Mol. Cell* **6:** 1355–1364.

41. Rivera, C.A. *et al.* 2007. Toll-like receptor-4 signaling and Kupffer cells play pivotal roles in the pathogenesis of non-alcoholic steatohepatitis. *J. Hepatol.* **47:** 571–579.

Ann. N.Y. Acad. Sci. ISSN 0077-8923

ANNALS OF THE NEW YORK ACADEMY OF SCIENCES

Issue: *Nutrition and Physical Activity in Aging, Obesity, and Cancer*

Combinatorial strategies employing nutraceuticals for cancer development

Yogeshwer Shukla and Jasmine George

Proteomics Laboratory, Indian Institute of Toxicology Research (CSIR), Lucknow, Uttar Pradesh, India

Address for correspondence: Yogeshwer Shukla, Proteomics Laboratory, Indian Institute of Toxicology Research (CSIR), Mahatma Gandhi Marg, Lucknow 226001, Uttar Pradesh, India. yogeshwer_shukla@hotmail.com; yshukla@iitr.res.in

Cancer is the second leading cause of death worldwide. Therefore, the fight against cancer is one of the most important areas of research in medicine, and one that possibly contributes to the increased interest in chemoprevention as an alternative approach to the control of cancer. Cancer prevention by nutraceuticals present in fruits and vegetables has received considerable attention because of their low cost and wide safety margin. A substantial amount of evidence from human, animal, and cell culture studies has shown cancer chemopreventive effects from these natural products. However, single-agent intervention has failed to produce the expected outcome in clinical trials; therefore, combinations of nutraceuticals are gaining increasing popularity. Thus, combinations of nutraceuticals that mimic real-life situations and are competent in targeting multiple targets with very little or virtually no toxicity are needed. In this review, we summarize the results of those studies that report combinatorial cancer chemopreventive action of various nutraceuticals and their combinations with anticancer drugs.

Keywords: nutraceuticals; cancer; chemoprevention; anticancer drugs; clinical trials

Introduction

Worldwide, about 12.7 million cases of and 7.6 million deaths from cancer are estimated to have occurred in 2008, with 56% of the cases and 64% of the deaths in economically developing countries. It is estimated that there will be 16 million new cases every year by 2020.[1] Epidemiological and laboratory data clearly indicate that cancer is linked to not only genetics, but also lifestyle, including dietary and environmental exposure.[2]

It has been estimated that more than two thirds of human cancer cases could be prevented by lifestyle modifications, including dietary habits.[3] Substantial epidemiologic and experimental data exist to suggest that a healthy diet, that is, one high in fruits and vegetables, decreases the risk of a variety of chronic diseases, including cancer. To date, hundreds of natural and synthetic compounds have been shown to possess promising cancer-preventive properties. Despite this, both the incidence and cure rate of cancer have not improved much and thus have necessitated that some modifications be made to improve efficacy with minimized toxicity. Nowadays, an emphasis has been placed on the development of novel combination therapies/chemoprevention using nutraceuticals that are competent in targeting multiple targets against cancer. Many plant-derived products, in combination with one another, have been shown to increase the efficacy of cancer control and have a broader spectrum of activity.[4] They may act together to give either a synergistic action to combat tumors through regulation of different signaling pathways or compensation for the opposite properties in cancer cell proliferation or apoptosis. In this paper, the data for using nutraceuticals in combination to combat a variety of cancers are reviewed.

Nutraceuticals

The term *nutraceutical* was coined from "nutrition" and "pharmaceutical" by Stephen DeFelice in 1989. A nutraceutical can be defined as "a food (or part of a food) that provides medical or health benefits, including the prevention and/or treatment of a

doi: 10.1111/j.1749-6632.2011.06104.x

Ann. N.Y. Acad. Sci. 1229 (2011) 162–175 © 2011 New York Academy of Sciences.

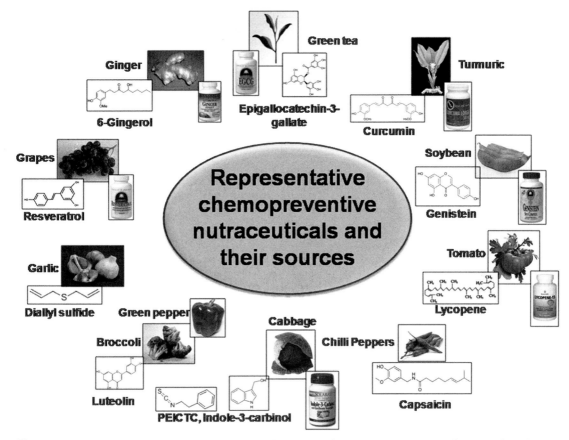

Figure 1. Common sources of nutraceuticals known to exhibit cancer-chemopreventive properties along with their chemical structures.

disease."[5,6] Such products may range from isolated nutrients, dietary supplements, and specific diets to genetically engineered designer foods, herbal products, and processed foods such as cereals, soups, and beverages. In addition, these products are less expensive, safer, and more readily available than are synthetic agents.[7] Some nutraceuticals are currently under clinical trials, but many have already been approved for clinical use.[5,8,9] In the past decade, a number of nutraceuticals have been identified with diverse chemical structures to fight against cancer (Fig. 1).

Role of nutraceuticals against neoplastic development

In the last two decades, much evidence has emerged indicating that, at the molecular level, most chronic diseases, including cancer, are caused by a dysregulated inflammatory response.[10] Inflammation is often linked to neoplastic development and acts as a driving force in premalignant and malignant transformation of cells.[11] There is now growing evidence supporting the notion that chronic inflammation may lead to malignancies of different organs including the skin, stomach, colon, breast, prostate, and pancreas.[12–14] One of the most important links between inflammation and cancer is proinflammatory transcription factor nuclear factor-kappa B (NF-κB).[15] NF-κB is a ubiquitous and evolutionarily conserved transcription factor that regulates the expression of genes involved in the transformation, survival, proliferation, invasion, angiogenesis, and metastasis of cancer cells. Many nutraceuticals are shown to exert chemopreventive/anticancer activity by suppressing the NF-κB signaling pathway.[16–19]

Humans are unknowingly exposed to environmental insults such as pesticides, fumes, automobile exhaust, ionizing, ultraviolet radiation, etc., which cause the formation of oxidants by metabolic activity within cells. When in excess, these oxidants can cause an imbalance, leading to production of reactive oxygen species (ROS) or oxidative stress.[20] Normally, there is equilibrium between ROS generation and antioxidant defense systems, and any imbalance between them can lead to oxidative stress. Oxidative stress can alter the structure of cellular components such as DNA, proteins, and lipids, which, when left unrepaired, can induce cell death or cancer development through various mechanisms.[21] Imbalance of oxidative stress has been shown to be able to trigger the activation of multiple signaling pathways, including the activation of various transcription factors (e.g., NF-κB) and phosphorylation cascades of mitogen-activated protein kinases (MAPKs).[22] Thus, cancer control can be achieved by decreasing the rate of oxidative stress and enhancing antioxidant defense mechanisms. The potential role of dietary antioxidants present in nutraceuticals in reducing the risk of cancer by suppressing the state of oxidative stress has been well documented in the literature.[23–25]

Another major cause of neoplastic development is the dysregulation of body homeostasis, a fundamental characteristic of living beings. The balance between cell proliferation and apoptosis is a critical step in the maintenance of homeostasis.[26,27] The dysregulation of apoptosis is a hallmark of cancer and is critical for cancer development and tumor cell survival.[28] Cancer cells can invade apoptosis mainly through two signaling pathways: extrinsic (receptor mediated) and intrinsic (mitochondria mediated). The extrinsic pathway is triggered by a complex set of antiapoptotic and proapototic proteins, including caspase family proteins, Bax, B cell lymphoma (Bcl)-2 family proteins, cytochrome c, apoptotic protease activating factor (Apaf)-1, and death receptors (APO-1/TRAIL). The intrinsic pathway is initiated by cellular developmental signals or as a result of severe cellular stress, including DNA damage. Some antiapoptotic proteins, such as Bcl-2 and Bcl-2 extra large (Bcl-xL),[29] are overexpressed in many cancer types. Therefore, selective downregulation of antiapoptotic proteins and upregulation of proapoptotic proteins in cancer cells offer promising therapeutic interventions for cancer treatment. A number of nutraceuticals, mostly phytochemicals derived from dietary or medicinal plants, have shown potential to reduce cancer incidence by inducing apoptosis with the use of various mechanisms in multiple types of cancer cells.[30]

Nutraceuticals in combination

Nutraceuticals have proven very promising in detoxifying and inhibiting anti-inflammatory and anti-cell growth signaling pathways that can culminate in apoptosis and/or cell cycle arrest as mentioned above. A synergistic therapeutic effect is defined as a stronger effect by the combination of two or more compounds compared to individual compounds. It is believed that chemotherapeutic/chemopreventive combinational approaches have been used to reduce drug toxicity, to delay the development of cancer cells, and to reach a greater effect than with one active agent alone.

Nutraceuticals may act independently or in combination as anticancer agents. The additive and synergistic effects of nutraceuticals may be responsible for their potent antioxidant and anticancer activities, and the benefit of a diet rich in fruits and vegetables is attributed to the complex mixture of nutraceuticals present in whole foods.[31] This hypothesis partially explains why a single antioxidant cannot replace the combination of natural nutraceuticals in achieving health benefits. Limited knowledge is available regarding any interaction between/among nutraceuticals in suppressing neoplastic development. Some of the combinatorial effects of nutraceuticals against neoplastic development are described in the following sections.

Prostate cancer (PCa)

PCa is the most prevalent malignancy in men, with an expected 217,730 new cases and 32,059 deaths due to this cancer in 2010 in the United States alone.[32] Prostate carcinogenesis has been viewed as a multistage and complex process consisting of initiation, promotion, and progression. Despite surgical and diagnostic advances, the incidence of PCa is expected to rise in the near future. Both the high rate of occurrence and the long latency period to clinically significant disease make PCa an ideal disease for pharmacologic or nutritional chemoprevention.[33,34]

Cruciferous vegetables are a group of vegetables named by their cross-shaped flowers and include broccoli, Brussel sprouts, watercress, cabbage, kale, cauliflower, kohlrabi, and turnips. Compared with

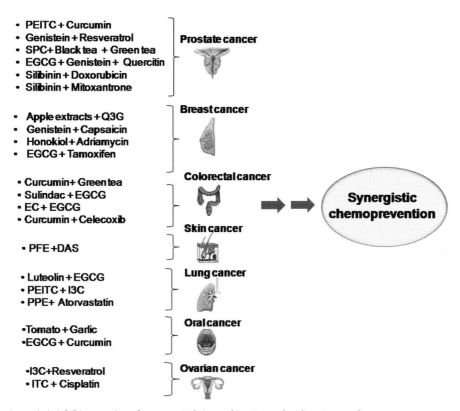

- PEITC + Curcumin
- Genistein + Resveratrol
- SPC+ Black tea + Green tea
- EGCG + Genistein + Quercitin
- Silibinin + Doxorubicin
- Silibinin + Mitoxantrone

Prostate cancer

- Apple extracts + Q3G
- Genistein + Capsaicin
- Honokiol + Adriamycin
- EGCG + Tamoxifen

Breast cancer

- Curcumin+ Green tea
- Sulindac + EGCG
- EC + EGCG
- Curcumin + Celecoxib

Colorectal cancer

Skin cancer

- PFE +DAS

- Luteolin + EGCG
- PEITC + I3C
- PPE+ Atorvastatin

Lung cancer

- Tomato + Garlic
- EGCG + Curcumin

Oral cancer

- I3C+Resveratrol
- ITC + Cisplatin

Ovarian cancer

Synergistic chemoprevention

Figure 2. Synergistic inhibitory action of nutraceuticals in combination and with anticancer drugs against various cancers.

other families of vegetables, they contain a significant amount of isothiocyanates, and strong anticarcinogenic activities of cruciferous vegetables have thus been attributed to the high abundance of isothiocyanates.[35] Phenylethylisoathiocyanate (PEITC) is one such naturally occurring isothiocyanate compound that has attracted a great deal of attention due to its remarkable cancer-chemopreventive properties. The mechanisms by which PEITC protects against cancer have been shown to involve the deletion of preneoplastic cells through induction of cell cycle arrest and apoptosis[36,37] and inhibition of carcinogen activation via modulation of cytochrome P450-dependent monooxygenases and enhancement of the antioxidant response element-dependent carcinogen detoxification enzyme.[38] Curcumin (diferuloyl-methane), the yellow phenolic pigment found in the spice turmeric, extracted from the rhizome of the plant *Curcuma longa*, has been shown to possess strong antioxidant and anti-inflammatory effects.[39] Due to these properties, curcumin has been very widely investigated for its potential chemopreventive activity. Treat-

ment with curcumin caused apoptosis and cell cycle arrest but inhibited cell growth, activation of signal transduction, and transforming activities in both androgen-dependent and androgen-independent PCa cells in culture.[40] Curcumin has been shown to inhibit the induction of cancers of the skin, forestomach, duodenum, and colon in models of chemical carcinogenesis in mice and rats.[41–43] The combined treatment of low doses of PEITC and curcumin has been shown to suppress human PCa cell growth *in vitro* as well as in immunodeficient (Nu/Nu) mice bearing xenografts of androgen-independent human PCa cells (PC-3) and in the TRAMP mouse model of PCa by inhibition of Akt and NF-κB signaling pathways (Fig. 2).[44,45]

Another nutraceutical from soy, genistein, has gained popularity in the fight against cancer within the last decade.[46] Epidemiological evidence indicates that there are positive associations between chemoprevention and the main source of genistein, soy consumption.[47,48] Soy has been found to inhibit the growth of transplantable human prostate carcinomas and tumor angiogenesis in mice.[49]

Resveratrol, a polyphenolic phytoalexin found in red wine and grape-derived products, has also recently received much attention in regards to cancer prevention. Reports have shown that resveratrol suppressed chemically induced mammary cancer in rats.[50–52] Genistein and resveratrol, alone and in combination, suppress PCa development in the SV-40 Tag rats by reducing cell proliferation and insulin-like growth factor-1 protein expression and by increasing apoptosis in the prostate (Fig. 2).[53]

Tea from the *Camellia sinensis* species of the *Theaceae* family is one of the most ancient and, after water, is the most widely consumed beverage in the world. Tea is rich in polyphenolic constituents, which have strong anti-inflammatory, antioxidant, anticarcinogenic, as well as antimutagenic properties in a variety of biological systems. Tea polyphenols are also reported to inhibit proliferation and increase apoptosis in PCa cells in *in vitro*.[54] Soy phytochemical concentrate, black tea, and green tea combinations at low doses are reported to have significantly reduced tumorigenicity rate, primary tumor growth, tumor proliferation index and microvessel density, serum androgen level, and metastases to lymph nodes in androgen-sensitive human prostate tumors in mice than either or their alone doses.[55] Combination of epigallocatechin gallate (EGCG) and genistein, derived from green tea and soy products, with quercetin, present in abundance in fruits and vegetables, exert synergy in controlling the proliferation and expression of androgen receptor and tumor suppressor p53 gene expression in CWR22Rv1 PCa cells.[56] These studies thus show that the intake of whole foods could significantly affect PCa tumorigenesis and that the combination of whole foods may be superior in slowing cancer growth.

Breast cancer

Breast cancer (BC) is the most frequently diagnosed cancer in women. Approximately one million women are estimated to be newly diagnosed with BC each year worldwide. Although a great deal of work has been done on the prevention and treatment of BC, the results are not satisfactory and need to be greatly improved. For example, one drug, tamoxifen, has been demonstrated to be effective in only one third of BC patients.[57] Therefore, exploring new approaches in the prevention and treatment of BC is of great interest.

Apples are widely and commonly consumed and are one of the main contributors of phytochemicals in the human diet. They are rich in hydroxycinnamic acids, dihydrochalcones, flavan-3-ols/procyanidins, anthocyanins, and flavonols. Quercetin 3-glycosides (Q3G), chlorogenic acid, catechin, epicatechin and their dimers, phloridzin, and cyanidin 3-glycosides are the main individual phenolics in apples. Apple consumption has been linked to a lowered risk of cancer, coronary heart disease, asthma and pulmonary function problems, and type II diabetes.[58] The synergistic effects of apple extracts and Q3G were assessed by measurement of the inhibition of MCF-7 human BC cells proliferation (Fig. 2).[59]

The chemopreventive potential of genistein, as mentioned above, has attracted considerable interest because of its inhibitory activity on cellular events associated with carcinogenesis. On the basis of its potential anticancer activity, genistein has been extensively studied for exerting its efficacy through regulation of various cell signaling pathways.[60] Genistein, in combination with capsaicin, exerts anti-inflammatory and anticarcinogenic properties through the modulation of MAPK family proteins and COX-2 synergistically or nonsynergistically (Fig. 2).[61]

Colon cancer

Colon cancer (CC) is a malignant tumor with high morbidity and mortality. With 639,000 deaths worldwide per year, it is the fourth most common form of cancer and the third leading cause of cancer-related death worldwide.[62] Epidemiological studies have demonstrated that CC development is closely associated with dietary habits and lifestyle, that is, the consumption of food high in fat and carbohydrates, which could promote the growth of tumors.[63]

Curcumin, which is widely used as a food additive, inhibits proliferation and metastasis and induces apoptosis in various malignant tumors, including CC, by modulating several different signal pathways.[64–66] Epidemiologic studies suggest that the consumption of tea, especially green tea, is linked to a decreased incidence of various cancers including CC.[67–69] Over 40 experimental studies in rodents have shown that green tea or its constituents can either inhibit carcinogenesis or the growth of established cancers at various organ sites, including the colon.[70] Green tea contains several polyphenolic compounds including the following catechins: EGCG, (–)-epigallocatechin (EGC), epicatechin-3-gallate (ECG), and epicatechin (EC). EGCG is one of the major constituents of green tea, and it seems to be the most potent compound in tea with respect to inhibiting cell proliferation and inducing apoptosis in cancer cells.[71,72] Recently, the chemopreventive effects of curcumin and green tea catechins individually and in combination on 1,2-dimethylhydrazine (DMH)-induced colon carcinogenesis were studied in male Wistar rats by inhibiting the total number of aberrant crypt foci (ACF) per rat suggest that the combination of curcumin and catechins may produce a synergistic CC-preventative effect that would be more potent than each of the compounds alone (Fig. 2).[73] Ohishi et al. demonstrated that sulindac, a promising cancer-preventive agent for CC, synergistically suppressed ACF formation without notable side effects when used in combination with EGCG (Fig. 2).[74] The combination of only 1 mg/mL of EC and 10 mg/mL of EGCG showed synergistic effects on growth inhibition and induction of apoptosis in human CC cells (Fig. 2). Mechanistic studies showed that this is due to the inhibition of transcriptional activity of the activator protein 1 (AP-1), c-fos, NF-κB, and cyclinD1 promoters.[75]

Skin cancer

Our laboratory is also actively investigating the hypothesis that combinations of food-based cancer prevention strategies will be a highly effective strategy for the reduction/prevention of carcinogenesis. We have chosen to focus our experimental efforts on pomegranate fruit extract (PFE) and garlic constituent (diallyl sulfide [DAS]), two foods widely consumed and frequently cited to have potential human health benefits.[76–79]

Pomegranate (Punica granatum Linn.; Punicaceae) fruit is widely consumed fresh and in beverage forms as juice and wines.[80] The juice and peel of pomegranates possess marked antioxidant capacity[80,81] with high content of polyphenols, in particular, ellagitannins, condensed tannins, and anthocyanins,[80,82] and both have been shown to have chemopreventive, chemotherapeutic, and anti-inflammatory efficacy.[83,84] DAS, a organosulfur component of garlic (Allium sativum; Alliaceae) has been demonstrated to exert a potential chemopreventive activity against human cancers, such as that of the colon and lung.[85] Recently, we reported

that the combination of PFE and DAS synergistically inhibited mouse skin tumor growth, which was accompanied by a reduction in nick formation, regression of tumor volume, decrease in proliferation markers, inhibition of MAPKs and NF-κB signaling, and induction of apoptotic cell death (Fig. 2).[86] Therefore, we assert that the use of combination therapy in the management of skin cancer proves to be more beneficial over individual agents.

Lung cancer

Among various cancers, lung cancer is the leading cause of cancer-related mortality in the United States, and it is also one of the most common cancers worldwide.[1] Although new advancements have been made in lung cancer diagnosis and treatment, the overall 5-year survival rate is still less than 5%. The poor lung cancer survival statistics suggest that, in addition to smoking cessation, there is an urgent need for additional approaches for the prevention of this deadly disease.

Luteolin, 3′,4′,5,7-tetrahydroxyflavone, is a natural antioxidant that usually occurs in its glycosylated form in several green vegetables such as artichoke, celery, broccoli, cauliflower, green pepper, cabbage, and spinach.[87] It exhibits a wide range of pharmacological properties ranging from anti-inflammation to anticancer effects.[88] Studies have shown that the combination of luteolin and EGCG more effectively induced apoptosis of both lung cancer and squamous cell carcinoma of the head and neck cancer cell lines and inhibited tumor growth in nude mice xenograft models (Fig. 2). Their combination activated both mitochondria-dependent and -independent pathways of apoptosis to varying degrees in the cell lines tested. Moreover, lung cancer cell lines expressing wild-type p53 showed higher sensitivity to the combination than those with mutant or no p53. Moreover, knockdown of p53 using shRNA strongly inhibited apoptosis, suggesting activation of p53-dependent apoptotic pathways by the combination of luteolin and EGCG.[89]

Inhibitory effects of N-acetyl-S-(PEITC)-L-cysteine (PEITC-NAC), myo-inositol (MI), and indole-3-carbinol (I3C) or 3,3′-diindolylmethane (DIM), alone and in combination, have been studied by Kassie et al.[90] on 4-(methylnitrosamino)-1-(3-pyridyl)-1-butanone (NNK) plus benzo[a]pyrene-induced A/J mouse lung tumorigenesis and proliferation of A549 cells and human bronchial epithelial cells (HBECs) (Fig. 2). Combinatorial treatment with these agents caused marked reductions in mice lung tumor multiplicity. Combinatorial treatment also caused reduction in activation of Akt, ERK, and NF-κB in lung tumor tissues; CSC-pretreated HBEC; and A549 cells. This study demonstrated the promise of combinations of PEITC-NAC, I3C/DIM, and MI for the chemoprevention of lung carcinogenesis.

Oral cancer

Oral cancer is a major health problem in developing countries such as India. The high incidence of oral cancer and oral precancerous lesions in India have long been linked with the habit of betel quid chewing incorporating tobacco.[91] Oral leukoplakia is the most common premalignant lesion of oral cancer, and up to 20% of the patients with leukoplakia develop invasive carcinoma.[92] There is increasing evidence for an association between a high consumption of fruits and vegetables and reduced risk of oral cancer.[93,94]

Epidemiologic studies have provided evidence that increased intake of tomato and garlic are associated with decreased cancer risk.[95,96] Tomatoes and tomato products contain rich sources of an antioxidant carotenoid called lycopene, reported to be the most powerful of all the dietary carotenoids. Recently, researchers have found that dietary intake of lycopene was linked to a lower risk of cell proliferation in prostate and oral cancer.[97,98] Bhuvneswari et al.[99] showed that a combination treatment of tomato and garlic inhibits 7,12-dimethylbenz[a]anthracene (DMBA)-induced bone marrow nuclei, genotoxicity, and oxidative stress in Swiss albino mice. The same group also showed that this combined treatment synergistically suppressed the incidence and mean tumor burden of DMBA-induced hamster buccal pouch carcinomas at lower doses by modulating xenobiotic-metabolizing enzymes in the pouch and liver with a decreased incidence of bone marrow micronuclei (Fig. 2).[100]

As stated above, curcumin is traditionally well known to have therapeutic effects on various types of diseases.[64–66] The combination of EGCG and curcumin showed synergistic interactions in growth inhibition and increased sigmoidicity of the dose-effect curves in human oral epithelial cells (Fig. 2).[101] Synergism between a combination of EGCG

and curcumin was also seen in the inhibition of chemically induced oral carcinogenesis in hamsters through suppression of cell proliferation, induction of apoptosis, and inhibition of angiogenesis.[102] The combinations of these nutraceuticals may be explored as chemopreventive agents for humans at high risk of oral cancer, such as those with erythroplakia and leukoplakia.

Ovarian cancer

Ovarian cancer accounts for nearly 3% of all cancers among women. It is the ninth most common cancer and the fifth most common cause of cancer-related deaths in women. In 2010, an estimated 21,880 new cases and 13,850 deaths in women in the United States were due to ovarian cancer.[32]

I3C is a compound present in cruciferous vegetables such as broccoli, cabbage, and cauliflower. Its ability to cause G1 arrest of cell cycle, induce apoptosis, and interfere with signal transduction pathways has been demonstrated in a variety of cancers, including that of prostate, melanoma, and BC cell lines.[103–105] Due to its broad spectrum of activities combined with its low toxicity, I3C has been acclaimed as a potent chemopreventive and anticancer agent.[106] Another nutraceutical, resveratrol, is a powerful antioxidant present in the skin and seeds of grapes. These two compounds belong to a group of potential chemopreventive agents of dietary origin. For the first time, Raj et al.[107] demonstrated the effects of I3C on ovarian cancer cells (SK-OV-3 cells) and its synergism with resveratrol (Fig. 2). SK-OV-3 cells underwent profound morphological changes upon combination treatment with I3C or resveratrol, inhibited cell proliferation, and caused cell contraction and apoptosis. Analysis of apoptosis-associated genes revealed an inhibition of retinoblastoma protein and survivin gene expression. This was accompanied by elevation of p21, a tumor suppressor. The cell cycle was inhibited at both G1 and G2/M by individual treatments and was accentuated by a combination. This will provide a foundation for the use of these compounds in combination for chemoprevention of ovarian cancers.

Other combinatorial effects: nutraceuticals and anticancer drugs

It has been suggested that chemotherapy could favorably be combined with dietary agents in anticancer strategies, since combination treatment enhances the therapeutic ratio of chemotherapy by targeting both tumor cells and tumor vessels. Moreover, these combined treatment modalities are achieved without increased toxicity compared with chemotherapy alone.[108,109]

Honokiol, an active compound purified from magnolia, has drawn much attention for its antiangiogenesis and apoptosis properties. Previous reports have demonstrated that honokiol inhibited mouse skin tumor promotion in an *in vivo* two-stage carcinogenesis[110] and induced apoptosis of human CC cell RKO via p53-independent pathways.[111] Adriamycin (ADR), a DNA-intercalating agent, is a significant active chemotherapy medicine for the treatment of a variety of human and murine tumors.[112,113] ADR could induce the apoptosis of tumor cells by inhibiting DNA polymerases, topoisomerases, and RNA synthesis.[114–117] When combined with ADR, Honokiol encapsulated with liposome inhibited the proliferation of mouse 4T1 BC cells via apoptosis and significantly decreased tumor growth through increased apoptosis in mouse breast tumor model also as compared with either treatment alone (Fig. 2).[118]

Atorvastatin, an inhibitor of 3-hydroxy- 3-methylglutaryl CoA (HMG-CoA) reductase, is a commonly used drug for the treatment of hypercholesterolemia. In addition to inhibiting cholesterol biosynthesis, atorvastatin also inhibits the biosyntheses of farnesyl pyrophosphate and geranyl pyrophosphate, which are required in higher amounts by malignant cells than normal cells for their growth.[119,120] A synergistic inhibitory effect of a novel combination of polyphenon E (PPE, a standardized green tea polyphenol preparation) and atorvastatin was studied in a mouse 4-(methylnitrosaminao)-1-(3-pyridyl)-1-butanone–induced lung tumorigenesis and in human lung cancer H1299 and H460 cell lines (Fig. 2). PPE and atorvastatin at low doses synergistically inhibited lung tumorigenesis in mice as well as the growth of lung cancer cells, possibly through enhanced apoptosis.[121] Additional studies are needed to determine whether lower levels of PPE and atorvastatin can prevent lung cancer in animal models and humans.

In 2001, Weinstein's group reported that EGCG at 0.1 μg/mL markedly enhanced the growth inhibitory effects of 5-fluorouracil on human head and neck squamous cell carcinoma lines, YCU-N861 and YCU-H891, by inhibiting the epidermal growth factor receptor signaling pathway.[122] Interestingly, YCU-H891 cells that are resistant to 5-fluorouracil became sensitive to the drug when combined with EGCG.[122] They also reported that treatment with EGCG inhibited the growth of both YCU-H891 cells and BC cell line BT-474 more strongly than that with taxol alone.[123] Liang *et al.*[124] reported that treatment with EGCG significantly reduced the IC50 value for doxorubicin (DOX) from 36 to 1.9 μg/mL, and that for ECG to 2.3 μg/mL in human hepatocellular carcinoma cells BEL-7404/DOX. Additionally, the combination of EGCG and DOX clearly enhanced the reduction of tumor volumes in an *in vivo* xenograft model inoculated with BEL-7404/DOX cells. Furthermore, combination treatment with EGCG and tamoxifen was synergistically cytotoxic and enhanced apoptosis in MDA-MB-231 human BC cells and decreased tumor growth in a MCF-7 cell xenograft model (Fig. 2).[125,126]

Milk thistle (*Silybum marianum*) has a long history of use in humans and is commonly used in the treatment of liver disease.[127] Silymarin, the name of the crude milk thistle extract, is composed of several stereoisomers including silibinin (or silybin), silychristin, and silydianin.[128] Silibinin and silymarin have been shown to have anticancer effects in several *in vitro* and *in vivo* cancer models.[129–134] Silibinin's antineoplastic actions appear to work through several different pathways.[135] One of the most prominent effects seen in preclinical studies of silibinin is G1 arrest and apoptosis[136] with an increase of the cyclin-dependent kinase inhibitors kip1/p27 and cip1/p21.[134] Further study has shown that silibinin causes decreased phosphorylation of retinoblastoma protein leading to stability of the complex formed with E2F.[137] Silibinin increases the efficacy of several chemotherapy agents both *in vitro* and *in vivo*. It acts synergistically with DOX to inhibit growth via apoptosis in the human PCa cells (DU145)[138] and sensitizes these same cells to the antineoplastic effects of cisplatin and carboplatin.[139] The combination of silibinin and mitoxantrone (anthracenedione and topoisomerase II inhibitor) exhibits a pattern of synergy in reducing cell viability with increased apoptosis in human PCa cells PC-3.[140]

Shpitz *et al.*[141] examined the chemopreventive effects of celecoxib, a specific COX-2 inhibitor, and curcumin alone and in combination using the DMH-induced CC in rats (Fig. 2). Curcumin and celecoxib decreased the average number of ACF per rat colon, and the most efficient effect was observed when rats received both agents. Curcumin potentiates the antitumor effects of gemcitabine in pancreatic cancer by suppressing proliferation, angiogenesis, NF-κB, and NF-κB–regulated gene products.[142] Curcumin synergistically augments the growth inhibition inserted by celecoxib in pancreatic cancer cells (P-34, MIAPaCa, and Panc-1) expressing COX-2. This synergistic effect was mediated through inhibition of COX-2.[143] This may enable the use of gemcitabine and celecoxib at lower and safer concentrations and may pave the way for a more effective treatment in this devastating disease.

The synthetic isothiocyanate derivative indole-3-ethyl isothiocyanate (ITC), a popular chemopreventive agent present in cruciferous vegetables, exerts synergy to stimulate apoptosis in combination with the chemotherapeutic drug cisplatin in human ovarian carcinoma cells.[144] Thus, there may be worth in future studies in assessing the value of ITC in the treatment of ovarian cancer and in elucidating the mechanisms of its action.

Clinical trials

To date, very few nutraceuticals in combination or with anticancer drugs have been successful in clinical trials for the treatment of cancer. In the recent past, vitamin E and selenium (Se) have received attention for the management of PCa.[145–147] Present in a variety of food products and available as dietary supplements, Se is an essential micronutrient that occurs predominantly as selenomethionine (SeMet), whereas vitamin E (or α-tocopherol) is a fat-soluble physiological antioxidant, and both are required for normal health.[148–150] The ongoing Se and vitamin E chemoprevention trial (SELECT), sponsored by the National Cancer Institute, is an intergroup phase III, randomized, double-blind, placebo-controlled, population-based clinical trial designed to test the efficacy of Se and vitamin E alone and in combination in the prevention of PCa.[151] However, a recent study by McCormick et al.[152] demonstrated that the combination of selenium and vitamin E did not significantly reduce the incidence of PCa in a rat model of androgen-dependent PCa and thus do not

support the hypothesis that Se and vitamin E are effective agents for PCa chemoprevention.

Recently, a study by Vidlar et al.[153] demonstrated that the combination of 570 mg of silymarin and 250 μg of Se daily for 6 months significantly reduced two markers of lipid metabolism known to be associated with PCa progression, low-density lipoproteins and total cholesterol in the blood of men after radical prostatectomy, with no adverse effects. These findings suggest that a dietary intervention with a SM–Se combination could benefit both patients after radical prostatectomy and those who are at risk of PCa progression.

Conclusions and future directions

Clearly, research on the combined action of nutraceuticals and with anticancer drugs is influencing the processes involved in the progression and metastasis of common cancers. Many of these nutraceuticals are reported to act synergistically, which may explain why some food items or diets may show cancer-preventive effects that cannot be explained based on individual bioactive ingredients. It is interesting to note that many of these nutraceuticals are already commercially available as dietary herbal supplements or in the form of pills. Still many of these nutraceuticals have not been approved by the Food and Drug Administration (FDA) and are not indicated for specific diseases, but are being sold simply as nutritional supplements for general health and immune function maintenance. This underscores an immediate need to further establish the efficacy and toxicity profiles of combinations of active compounds and use them based on logically derived synergistic combinations. The development of new supplement regimens, cancer therapies, and nutraceuticals may especially benefit from improved insight into the mechanisms behind synergistic effects of both natural and synthetic chemopreventive compounds.

Conflicts of interest

The authors declare no conflicts of interest.

References

1. Jemal, A. et al. 2011. Global cancer statistics. CA. Cancer J. Clin. **61:** 69–90.
2. Wogan, G.N. et al. 2004. Environmental and chemical carcinogenesis. Semin. Cancer Biol. **14:** 473–486.
3. Surh, Y.J. 2003. Cancer chemoprevention with dietary phytochemicals. Nat. Rev. Cancer **3:** 768–780.

4. de Kok, T.M., S.G. van Breda & M.M. Manson. 2008. Mechanisms of combined action of different chemopreventive dietary compounds: a review. *Eur. J. Nutr.* **2:** 51–59.

5. Brower, V. 1998. Nutraceuticals: poised for a healthy slice of the healthcare market? *Nat. Biotechnol.* **16:** 728–731.

6. Zeisel, S.H. 1999. Regulation of "nutraceuticals." *Science* **285:** 185–186.

7. Camire, M.E. 2003. Nutraceuticals for health promotion and disease prevention. *Council for Agricultural and Technology*, Issue paper no. 24.

8. Amin, A.R. *et al.* 2009. Perspectives for cancer prevention with natural compounds. *J. Clin Oncol.* **27:** 2712–2725.

9. Martinez, M.E., J.R. Marshall & E. Giovannucci. 2008. Diet and cancer prevention: the roles of observation and experimentation. *Nature Rev. Cancer* **8:** 694–703.

10. Aggarwal, B.B. & P. Gehlot. 2009. Inflammation and cancer: how friendly is the relationship for cancer patients? *Curr. Opin. Pharmacol.* **9:** 351–369.

11. Philip, M. *et al.* 2004. Inflammation as a tumor promoter in cancer induction. *Semin. Cancer Biol.* **14:** 433–439.

12. Li, Q., S. Withoff & I.M. Verma. 2005. Inflammation-associated cancer: NF-kB is the lynchpin. *Trends Immunol.* **26:** 318–325.

13. Marx, J. 2004. Cancer research. Inflammation and cancer: the link grows stronger. *Science* **306:** 966–968.

14. Karin, M. & F.R. Greten. 2005. NF-κB: linking inflammation and immunity to cancer development and progression. *Nature Rev. Immunol* **5:** 749–759.

15. Karin M. 2009. NF-kappaB as a critical link between inflammation and cancer. *Cold Spring Harb. Perspect. Biol.* **1:** a000141.

16. Shishodia, S. & B.B. Aggarwal. 2004. Guggulsterone inhibits NF-kappaB and IkappaBalpha kinase activation, suppresses expression of anti-apoptotic gene products, and enhances apoptosis. *J. Biol. Chem.* **279:** 47148–47158.

17. Siddiqui, I.A. *et al.* 2008. Suppression of NFkappaB and its regulated gene products by oral administration of green tea polyphenols in an autochthonous mouse prostate cancer model. *Pharm. Res.* **25:** 2135–2142.

18. Bhui, K. *et al.* 2009. Bromelain inhibits COX-2 expression by blocking the activation of MAPK regulated NF-kappa B against skin tumor-initiation triggering mitochondrial death pathway. *Cancer Lett.* **282:** 167–176.

19. Roy, P. *et al.* 2009. Resveratrol enhances ultraviolet B-induced cell death through nuclear factor-kappaB pathway in human epidermoid carcinoma A431 cells. *Biochem. Biophys. Res. Comm.* **384:** 215–220.

20. Galli, F. *et al.* 2005. Oxidative stress and reactive oxygen species. *Contrib. Nephrol.* **149:** 240–260.

21. Ames, B.N., M.K. Shigenaga & L.S. Gold. 1993. DNA lesions, inducible DNA repair, and cell division: the three key factors in mutagenesis and carcinogenesis. *Environ. Health Perspect.* **101**(Suppl 5): 35–44.

22. Thannickal, V.J. & B.L. Fanburg. 2000. Reactive oxygen species in cell signaling. *Am. J. Physiol. Lung Cell Mol. Physiol.* **279:** L1005-L1028.

23. Chu, Y-F. *et al.* 2002. Antioxidant and antiproliferative activities of vegetables. *J. Agric. Food Chem.* **50:** 6910–6916.

24. Dragsted, L.O., M. Strube & J.C. Larsen. 1993. Cancer-protective factors in fruits and vegetables: biochemical and biological background. *Pharmacol. Toxicol.* **72:** 116–135.

25. Liu, R.H. & D.L. Felice. 2007. Antioxidants and whole food phytochemicals for cancer prevention. Antioxidant measurement and mechanism. *ACS Symposium Series* Vol. 956, Chapter 3, pp 15–34.

26. Green, D.R. 2000. Apoptotic pathways: paper wraps stone blunts scissors. *Cell* **102:** 1–4.

27. Meier, P., A. Finch & G. Evan. 2000. Apoptosis in development. *Nature* **407:** 796–801.

28. Hanahan, D., & R.A. Weinberg. 2000. The hallmarks of cancer. *Cell* **100:** 57–70.

29. Wang, S., D. Yang & M.E. Lippman. 2003. Targeting Bcl-2 and Bcl-XL with nonpeptidic small-molecule antagonists. *Semin. Oncol.* **30:** 133–142.

30. Gosslau, A., & K.Y. Chen. 2004. Nutraceuticals, apoptosis, and disease prevention. *Nutrition* **1:** 95–102.

31. Liu, R.H. 2004. Potential synergy of phytochemicals in cancer prevention: mechanism of action. *J. Nutr.* **134**(12 Suppl): 3479S–3485S.

32. Jemal, A. *et al.* 2010. Cancer statistics. *CA Cancer J. Clin.* **60:** 277–300.

33. Schmid, H.P., J.E. McNeal & T.A. Stamey. 1993. Observations on the doubling time of prostate cancer. The use of serial prostate-specific antigen in patients with untreated disease as a measure of increasing cancer volume. *Cancer* **71:** 2031–2040.

34. Ries, L. *et al.* 2004. *SEER Cancer Statistics Review*, 1975–2004. National Cancer Institute. Bethesda, MD.

35. Zhang, Y. 2004. Cancer-preventive isothiocyanates: measurement of human exposure and mechanism of action. *Mutat. Res.* **555:** 173–190.

36. Singh, A.V. *et al.* 2004. Sulforaphane induces caspase-mediated apoptosis in cultured PC-3 human prostate cancer cells and retards growth of PC-3 xenografts in vivo. *Carcinogenesis* **25:** 83–90.

37. Xiao, D. *et al.* 2005. Caspase-dependent apoptosis induction by phenethyl isothiocyanate, a cruciferous vegetable-derived cancer chemopreventive agent, is mediated by Bak and Bax. *Clin. Cancer Res.* **11:** 2670–2679.

38. Rushmore, T.H. & A.N. Kong. 2002. Pharmacogenomics, regulation and signaling pathways of phase I and II drug metabolizing enzymes. *Curr. Drug Metab.* **3:** 481–490.

39. Sharma, O.P. 1976. Antioxidant activity of curcumin and related compounds. *Biochem. Pharmacol.* **25:** 1811–1812.

40. Chaudhary, L.R. & K.A. Hruska. 2003. Inhibition of cell survival signal protein kinase B/Akt by curcumin in human prostate cancer cells. *J. Cell. Biochem.* **89:** 1–5.

41. Huang, M.T. *et al.* 1988. Inhibitory effect of curcumin, chlorogenic acid, caffeic acid, and ferulic acid on tumor promotion in mouse skin by 12-O-tetradecanoylphorbol-13-acetate. *Cancer Res.* **48:** 5941–596.

42. Huang, M.T. *et al.* 1992. Inhibitory effects of curcumin on tumor initiation by benzo[a]pyrene and 7,12-dimethylbenz4 [a]anthracene. *Carcinogenesis.* **13:** 2183–2186.

43. Huang, M.T. *et al.* 1994. Inhibitory effects of dietary curcumin on forestomach, duodenal, and colon carcinogenesis in mice. *Cancer Res.* **54:** 5841–5847.

44. Kim, J.H. *et al.* 2006. Inhibition of EGFR signaling in human prostate cancer PC-3 cells by combination treatment with beta-phenylethyl isothiocyanate and curcumin. *Carcinogenesis* **27:** 475–482.

45. Khor, T.O. *et al.* 2006. Combined inhibitory effects of curcumin and phenethyl isothiocyanate on the growth of human PC-3 prostate xenografts in immunodeficient mice. *Cancer Res.* **66:** 613–621.

46. Ravindranath, M.H. *et al.* 2004. Anticancer therapeutic potential of soy isoflavone, genistein. *Adv. Exp. Med. Biol.* **546:** 121–165.

47. De Lemos, M.L. 2001. Effects of soy phytoestrogens genistein and daidzein on breast cancer growth. *Ann. Pharmacother.* **35:** 1118–1121.

48. Mccue, P. & K. Shetty. 2004. Health benefits of soy isoflavonoids and strategies for enhancement: a review. *Crit. Rev. Food Sci. Nutr.* **44:** 361– 367.

49. Zhou, J.R. *et al.* 1999. Soybean phytochemicals inhibit the growth of transplantable human prostate carcinoma and tumor angiogenesis in mice. *J. Nutr.* **19:** 1628–1635.

50. Banerjee, S., C. Bueso-Ramos & B.B. Aggarwal. 2002. Suppression of 7,12- dimethylbenz(a)anthracene-induced mammary carcinogenesis in rats by resveratrol: role of nuclear factor-kappaB, cyclooxygenase 2, and matrix metalloprotease 9. *Cancer Res.* **17:** 4945–4954.

51. Bhat, K.P. *et al.* 2001. Estrogenic and antiestrogenic properties of resveratrol in mammary tumor models. *Cancer Res.* **20:** 7456–7463.

52. Whitsett, T.M., Carpenter & C.A. Lamartiniere. 2006. Resveratrol, but not EGCG, in the diet suppresses DMBA-induced mammary cancer in rats. *J. Carcinog.* **5:** 15–25.

53. Harper, C.E. *et al.* 2009. Genistein and resveratrol, alone and in combination, suppress prostate cancer in SV-40 tag rats. *Prostate* **15:** 1668–1682.

54. Klein, R.D. & S.M. Fischer. 2002. Black tea polyphenols inhibit IGF-I-induced signaling through Akt in normal prostate epithelial cells and Du145 prostate carcinoma cells. *Carcinogenesis* **23:** 217–221.

55. Zhou, J.R. *et al.* 2003. Soy phytochemicals and tea bioactive components synergistically inhibit androgen-sensitive human prostate tumors in mice. *J. Nutr.* **133:** 516–521.

56. Hsieh, T. & M.J. Wu. 2009. Targeting cwr22rv1 prostate cancer cell proliferation and gene expression by combinations of the phytochemicals egcg, genistein and quercetin. *Anticancer Res.* **29:** 4025–4032.

57. Forbes, J.F. 1997. The control of breast cancer: the role of tamoxifen. *Semin. Oncol.* **24:** 15–19.

58. Boyer, J. & R.H. Liu. 2004. Apple phytochemicals and their health benefits. *Nutr. J.* **3:** 1–45.

59. Yang, J. & R.H. Liu. 2009. Synergistic effect of apple extracts and quercetin 3-β-d-glucoside combination on antiproliferative activity in MCF-7 human breast cancer cells in vitro. *J. Agric. Food Chem.* **57:** 8581–8586.

60. Kousidou, O., G.N. Tzanakakis & N.K. Karamanos. 2006. Effects of the natural isoflavonoid genistein on growth,

signaling pathways and gene expression of matrix macromolecules by breast cancer cells. *Mini Rev. Med. Chem.* **6:** 331–337.

61. Hwang, J.T. *et al.* 2009. Anti-inflammatory and anticarcinogenic effect of genistein alone or in combination with capsaicin in TPA-treated rat mammary glands or mammary cancer cell line. *Ann. N. Y. Acad. Sci.* **1171:** 415–420.

62. World Health Organization (WHO), 2009. Cancer Fact sheet n 297.

63. Pisani, P., F. Bray & D.M. Parkin. 2002. Estimates of the world-wide prevalence of cancer for 25 sites in the adult population. *Int. J. Cancer* **97:** 72–81.

64. Aggarwal, B.B., A. Kumar & Bharti A.C. 2003. Anticancer potential of curcumin: preclinical and clinical studies. *Anticancer Res.* **23:** 363–398.

65. Johnson, J.J. & H. Mukhtar. 2007. Curcumin for chemoprevention of colon cancer. *Cancer Lett.* **255:** 170–181.

66. Anand, P. *et al.* 2008. Curcumin and cancer: an "old-age" disease with an "age-old" solution. *Cancer Lett.* **267:** 133–164.

67. Yang, C.S. & Z.Y. Wang. 1993. Tea and cancer. *J. Natl. Cancer Inst.* **85:** 1038–1049.

68. Stoner, G.D. & H. Mukhtar. 1995. Polyphenols as cancer chemopreventive agents. *J. Cell Biochem.* **22**(Suppl.): 169–180.

69. Ji, B.T. *et al.* 1997. Green tea consumption and the risk of pancreatic and colorectal cancers. *Int. J. Cancer* **70:** 255–258.

70. Yang, C.S., P. Maliakal & X. Meng. 2002. Inhibition of carcinogenesis by tea. *Annu. Rev. Pharmacol. Toxicol.* **42:** 25–54.

71. Ahmad, N. *et al.* 1997. Green tea constituent epigallocatechin-3- gallate and induction of apoptosis and cell cycle arrest in human carcinoma cells. *J. Natl. Cancer Inst.* **89:** 1881–1886.

72. Yang, G.Y. *et al.* 1998. Inhibition of growth and induction of apoptosis in human cancer cell lines by tea polyphenols. *Carcinogenesis* **19:** 611–616.

73. Xu, G. *et al.* 2010. Combination of curcumin and green tea catechins prevents dimethylhydrazine-induced colon carcinogenesis. *Food Chem. Toxicol.* **1:** 390–395.

74. Ohishi, T. *et al.* 2002. Synergistic effects of (_)-epigallocatechin gallate with sulindac against colon carcinogenesis of rats treated with azoxymethane. *Cancer Lett.* **177:** 49–56.

75. Shimizu, M. *et al.* 2005. (-)-Epigallocatechin gallate and polyphenon E inhibit growth and activation of the epidermal growth factor receptor and human epidermal growth factor receptor-2 signaling pathways in human colon cancer cells. *Clin. Cancer Res.* **7:** 2735–2746.

76. Kim, N.D. *et al.* 2002. Chemopretevive and adjuvant therapeutic potential of pomegranate (Punica granatum) for human breast cancer. *Breast Cancer Res. Treat.* **71:** 203–217.

77. Pantuck, A.J. *et al.* 2006. Phase-II study of pomegranate juice for men with rising prostate-specific antigen following surgery or radiation for prostate cance. *Clin. Cancer Res.* **12:** 4018–4026.

78. Afaq, F. *et al*. 2005. Anthocyanin- and hydrolysable tannin-rich pomegranate fruit extract modulates MAPK and NF-KB pathways and inhibits skin tumorigenesis in CD-1 mice. *Int. J. Cancer* **113:** 423–433.

79. Fleischauer, A.T., C. Poole & L. Arab. 2000. Garlic consumption and cancer prevention: meta-analyses of colorectal and stomach cancers. *Am. J. Clin. Nutr.* **72:** 1047–1052.

80. Gil, M.I. *et al*. 2000. Antioxidant activity of pomegranate juice and its relationship with phenolic composition and processing. *J. Agric. Food Chem.* **48:** 4581–4589.

81. Kaur, G. *et al*. 2006. Punica granatum (pomegranate) flower extract possesses potent antioxidant activity and abrogates Fe- NTA induced hepatotoxicity in mice. *Food Chem. Toxicol.* **44:** 984–993.

82. Seeram, N.P. *et al*. 2005. In vitro antiproliferative, apoptotic and antioxidant activities of punicalagin, ellagic acid and a total pomegranate tannin extract are enhanced in combination with other polyphenols as found in pomegranate juice. *J. Nutr. Biochem.* **16:** 360–367.

83. Adams, L.S. *et al*. 2006. Pomegranate juice, total pomegranate ellagitannins, and punicalagin suppress inflammatory cell signaling in colon cancer cells. *J. Agric. Food Chem.* **54:** 980–985.

84. Malik, A. *et al*. 2005. Pomegranate fruit juice for chemoprevention and chemotherapy of prostate cancer. *Proc. Natl. Acad. Sci. USA* **102:** 14813–14818.

85. Dausch, J.G. & D.W. Nixon. 1990. Garlic: a review of its relationship to malignant disease. *Prev. Med.* **19:** 346–361.

86. George, J. *et al*. 2011. Synergistic growth inhibition of mouse skin tumors by pomegranate fruit extract and diallyl sulfide: evidence for inhibition of activated MAPKs/NF-κB and reduced cell proliferation. *Food Chem. Toxicol.* **49:** 1511–1520.

87. Miean, K.H. & S. Mohamed. 2001. Flavonoid (myricetin, quercetin, kaempferol, luteolin, and apigenin) content of edible tropical plants. *J. Agric. Food. Chem.* **49:** 3106–3112.

88. Shimoi, K. *et al*. 2000. Metabolic fate of luteolin and its functional activity at focal site. *Biofactors* **12:** 181–186.

89. Amin, A.R. *et al*. 2010. Enhanced anti-tumor activity by the combination of the natural compounds (-)-epigallocatechin-3-gallate and luteolin: potential role of p53. *J. Biol. Chem.* **45:** 34557–34565.

90. Kassie, F. *et al*. (2010. Inhibition of lung carcinogenesis and critical cancer-related signaling pathways by N-acetyl-S-(N-2-phenethylthiocarbamoyl)-l-cysteine, indole-3-carbinol and myo-inositol, alone and in combination. *Carcinogenesis* **9:** 1634–1641.

91. Sankaranarayanan, R. 1990. Oral caner in India: an epidemiologic and clinical review. *Oral Sirg. Oral Med. Oral Path.* **69:** 325–330.

92. Silverman, S. Jr., M. Gorsky & F. Lozada. 1984. Oral leukoplakia and malignant transformation. A follow-up study of 257 patients. *Cancer* **3:** 563–568.

93. Morse, D.E. *et al*. 2000. Food group intake and the risk of oral epithelial dysplasia in a United States population. *Cancer Causes Control* **8:** 713–720.

94. La Vecchia, C. *et al*. 1997. Epidemiology and prevention of oral cancer. *Oral Oncol.* **5:** 302–312.

95. Giovannucci, E. 1999. Tomatoes, tomato-based products, lycopene, and cancer: review of the epidemiologic literature. *J. Natl. Cancer Inst.* **91:** 317–331.

96. Thomson, M. & M. Ali. 2003. Garlic (*Allium sativum*): a review of its potential use as an anti-cancer agent. *Curr. Cancer Drug Targets* **3:** 67– 81.

97. Yang, C.M. *et al*. 2011. Lycopene inhibits the proliferation of androgen-dependent human prostate tumor cells through activation of PPARγ-LXRα-ABCA1 pathway. *J. Nutr. Biochem.* **3:** 67–81.

98. Lu, R. *et al*. 2011. Lycopene: features and potential significance in the oral cancer and precancerous lesions. *J. Oral Pathol. Med.* **5:** 361–368.

99. Bhuvaneswari, V. *et al*. 2004. Tomato and garlic by gavage modulate 7,12-dimethylbenz[a]anthracene-induced genotoxicity and oxidative stress in mice. *Braz. J. Med. Biol. Res.* **7:** 1029–1034.

100. Bhuvaneswari, V., S.K. Abraham & S. Nagini. 2005. Combinatorial antigenotoxic and anticarcinogenic effects of tomato and garlic through modulation of xenobiotic-metabolizing enzymes during hamster buccal pouch carcinogenesis. *Nutrition* **6:** 726–731.

101. Khafif, A. *et al*. 1998. Quantitation of chemopreventive synergism between (-)-epigallocatechin-3-gallate and curcumin in normal, premalignant and malignant human oral epithelial cells. *Carcinogenesis* **3:** 419–424.

102. Li, N. *et al*. 2002. Inhibition of 7,12-dimethylbenz[a]anthracene (DMBA)– induced oral carcinogenesis in hamsters by tea and curcumin. *Carcinogenesis* **23:** 1307–1313.

103. Chinni, S.R. *et al*. 2001. Indole-3-Carbinol induced cell growth inhibition, G1 cell cycle arrest and apoptosis in prostate cancer cells. *Oncogene* **20:** 2927–2936.

104. Kim, D.S. *et al*. 2006. Indole-3-carbinol enhances ultraviolet B-induced apoptosis by sensitizing melanoma cells. *Cell. Mol. Life. Sci.* **63:** 2661–2668.

105. Kim, Y.S. & J.A. Milner. 2005. Targets for indole-3-carbinol in cancer prevention. *J. Nutr. Biochem.* **16:** 65– 73.

106. Weng, J.R. *et al*. 2008. Indole-3-carbinol as a chemopreventive and anti-cancer agent. *Cancer Lett.* **262:** 153–163.

107. Raj, M.H. *et al*. 2008. Synergistic action of dietary phytoantioxidants on survival and proliferation of ovarian cancer cells. *Gynecol. Oncol.* **3:** 432–438.

108. Suganuma, M., A. Saha & H. Fujiki. 2011. New cancer treatment strategy using combination of green tea catechins and anticancer drugs. *Cancer Sci.* **2:** 317–323.

109. Qiu M, C. Yi & M. Hou. 2006. Combined low-dose chemotherapy inhibiting angiogenesis and growth of Lewis lung carcinoma xenografts in mice. *J. Sichuan. Univ.* **37:** 534–537.

110. Konoshima, T. *et al*. 1991. Studies on inhibitors of skin tumor promotion, IX: neolignans from *Magnolia officinalis*. *J. Nat. Prod.* **54:** 816–822.

111. Wang, T. *et al*. 2004. Honokiol induces apoptosis through p53-independent pathway in human colorectal cell line RKO. *World J. Gastroenterol.* **10:** 2205–2208.

112. Feleszko, W. *et al*. 2002. Lovastatin potentiates antitumor activity of doxorubicin in murine melanoma via an apoptosis-dependent mechanism. *Int. J. Cancer* **100:** 111–118.

113. Safrit, J.T. & B. Bonavida. 1992. Sensitivity of resistant human tumor cell lines to tumor necrosis factor and adriamycin used in combination: correlation between downregulation of tumor necrosis factor-messenger RNA induction and overcoming resistance. *Cancer Res.* **52:** 6630–6637.

114. Cutts, S.M. *et al.* 1996. Adriamycininduced DNA adducts inhibit the DNA interactions of transcription factors and RNA polymerase. *J. Biol. Chem.* **271:** 5422–5429.

115. Tanaka, M. & S. Yoshisa. 1980. Mechanism of the inhibition of calf thymus DNA polymerase α and β by daunomycin and adriamycin. *J. Biochem.* **87:** 911–918.

116. Tewey, K.M. *et al.* 1984. Adriamycin-induced DNA damage mediated by mammalian DNA topoisomerase II. *Science* **226:** 466–468.

117. Zhu, K. *et al.* 1999. Adriamycin inhibits human RH II/Gu RNA helicase activity by binding to its substrate. *Biochem. Biophys. Res. Commun.* **266:** 361–365.

118. Hou W, *et al.* 2008. Synergistic antitumor effects of liposomal Honokiol combined with Adriamycin in breast cancer models. *Phytother. Res.* **22:** 1125–1132.

119. Buchwald, H. 1992. Cholesterol inhibition, cancer, and chemotherapy. *Lancet* **339:** 1154–1156.

120. Larsson, O. 1996. HMG-CoA reductase inhibitors: role in normal and malignant cells. *Crit. Rev. Oncol. Hematol.* **22:** 197–212.

121. Lu, G. *et al.* 2008. Synergistic inhibition of lung tumorigenesis by a combination of green tea polyphenols and atorvastatin. *Clin. Cancer Res.* **15:** 4981–4988.

122. Masuda, M.M. Suzui & I.B. Weinstein. 2001. Effects of epigallocatechin-3-gallate of growth, epidermal growth factor receptor signaling pathways, gene expression, and chemosensitivity in human head and neck squamous cell carcinoma cell lines. *Clin. Cancer Res.* **7:** 4220–4229.

123. Masuda, M. *et al.* 2003. Epigallocatechin-3-gallate inhibits activation of HER-2/ neu and downstream signaling pathways in human head and neck and breast carcinoma cells. *Clin. Cancer Res.* **9:** 3486–3491.

124. Liang, G. *et al.* 2010. Green tea catechins augment the antitumor activity of doxorubicin in an in vivo mouse model for chemoresistant liver cancer. *Int. J. Oncol.* **37:** 111–123.

125. Stuart, E.C., L. Larsen & R.J. Rosengren. 2007. Potential mechanisms for the synergistic cytotoxicity elicited by 4-hydroxytamoxifen and epigallocatechin gallate in MDA-MB-231cells. *Int. J. Oncol.* **30:** 1407–1412.

126. Sartippour, M.R. *et al.* 2006. The combination of green tea and tamoxifen is effective against breast cancer. *Carcinogenesis* **27:** 2424–2433.

127. Flora, K. *et al.* 1998. Milk thistle (Silybum marianum) for the therapy of liver disease. *Am. J. Gastroenterol.* **93:** 139–143.

128. Wagner, H., L. Horhammer & M. Seitz 1968. [Chemical evaluation of a silymarin-containing flavonoid concentrates from Silybum marianum (L.) Gaertn]. *Arzneimittelforschung* **18:** 696–698.

129. Zhu, W., J.S. Zhang & C.Y. Young. 2001. Young Silymarin inhibits function of the androgen receptor by reducing nuclear localization of the receptor in the human prostate cancer cell line LNCaP. *Carcinogenesis* **22:** 1399–1403.

130. Tyagi, A. *et al.* 2004. Silibinin causes cell cycle arrest and apoptosis in human bladder transitional cell carcinoma cells by regulating CDKI-CDK-cyclin cascade, and caspase 3 and PARP cleavages. *Carcinogenesis* **25:** 1711–1720.

131. Yang, S.H. *et al.* 2003. Anti-angiogenic effect of silymarin on colon cancer LoVo cell line. *J. Surg. Res.* **113:** 133–138.

132. Singh, R.P. *et al.* 2002. Dietary feeding of silibinin inhibits advance human prostate carcinoma growth in athymic nude mice and increases plasma insulin-like growth factor-binding protein-3 levels. *Cancer Res.* **62:** 3063–3069.

133. Lahiri-Chatterjee, M. *et al.* 1999. A flavonoid antioxidant, silymarin, affords exceptionally high protection against tumor promotion in the SENCAR mouse skin tumorigenesis model. *Cancer Res.* **59:** 622–632.

134. Zi, X., D.K. Feyes & R. Agarwal. 1998. Anticarcinogenic effect of a flavonoid antioxidant, silymarin, in human breast cancer cells MDA-MB 468: induction of G1 arrest through an increase in Cip1/p21 concomitant with a decrease in kinase activity of cyclin-dependent kinases and associated cyclins. *Clin. Cancer Res.* **4:** 1055–1064.

135. Singh R.P. & R. Agarwal. 2004. Prostate cancer prevention by silibinin. *Curr. Cancer Drug Targets* **4:** 1–11.

136. Zi, X. & R. Agarwal. 1999. Silibinin decreases prostate-specific antigen with cell growth inhibition via G1 arrest, leading to differentiation of prostate carcinoma cells: implications for prostate cancer intervention. *Proc. Natl. Acad. Sci. USA* **96:** 7490–7495.

137. Tyagi, A., C. Agarwal & R. Agarwal. 2002. Inhibition of retinoblastoma protein (Rb) phosphorylation at serine sites and an increase in Rb-E2F complex formation by silibinin in androgen-dependent human prostate carcinoma LNCaP cells: role in prostate cancer prevention. *Mol. Cancer Ther.* **1:** 525–532.

138. Tyagi, A.K. *et al.* 2002. Silibinin strongly synergizes human prostate carcinoma DU145 cells to doxorubicin- induced growth inhibition, G2-M arrest, and apoptosis. *Clin. Cancer Res.* **8:** 3512–3519.

139. Dhanalakshmi, S. *et al.* 2003. Silibinin sensitizes human prostate carcinoma DU145 cells to cisplatin- and carboplatin- induced growth inhibition and apoptotic death. *Int. J. Cancer* **106:** 699–705.

140. Flaig, T.W. *et al.* 2007. Silibinin synergizes with mitoxantrone to inhibit cell growth and induce apoptosis in human prostate cancer cells. *Int. J. Cancer* **19:** 2028–2033.

141. Shpitz, B. *et al.* 2006. Celecoxib and curcumin additively inhibit the growth of colorectal cancer in a rat model. *Digestion* **74:** 140–144.

142. Kunnumakkara, A.B. *et al.* 2007. Curcumin potentiates antitumor activity of gemcitabine in an orthotopic model of pancreatic cancer through suppression of proliferation, angiogenesis, and inhibition of nuclear factor kappa B-regulated gene products. *Cancer Res.* **67:** 3853–3861.

143. Lev-Ari, S. *et al.* 2005. Curcumin synergistically potentiates the growth inhibitory and pro-apoptotic effects of celecoxib in pancreatic adenocarcinoma cells. *Biomed. Pharmacother.* **59**(Suppl. 2): S276–S280.

144. Stehlik, P., H. Paulikova & L. Hunakova. 2010. Synthetic isothiocyanate indole-3-ethyl isothiocyanate (homoITC) enhances sensitivity of human ovarian carcinoma cell lines

A2780 and A2780/CP to cisplatin. *Neoplasma* **5:** 473–481.

145. Crispen, P.L. *et al.* 2007. Vitamin E succinate inhibits NF-kappaB and prevents the development of a metastatic phenotype in prostate cancer cells: implications for chemoprevention. *Prostate* **67:** 582–590.

146. Ip, C. *et al.* 2000. In vitro and in vivo studies of methylseleninic acid: evidence that a monomethylated selenium metabolite is critical for cancer chemoprevention. *Cancer Res.* **60:** 2882–2886.

147. Venkateswaran, V., N.E. Fleshner & L.H. Klotz. 2004. Synergistic effect of vitamin E and selenium in human prostate cancer cell lines. *Prostate Cancer Prostatic Dis.* **7:** 54–56.

148. Morris, V.C. & O.A. Levander. 1970. Selenium content of foods. *J. Nutr.* **100:** 1383–1388.

149. Schrauzer, G.N. 2001. Nutritional selenium supplements: product types, quality, and safety. *J. Am. Coll. Nutr.* **20:** 1–4.

150. Harris, P.L., M.L. Quaife & W.J. Swanson. 1950. Vitamin E content of foods. *J. Nutr.* **40:** 367–381.

151. Lippman, S.M. *et al.* 2009. Effect of selenium and vitamin E on risk of prostate cancer and other cancers: the Selenium and Vitamin E Cancer Prevention Trial (SELECT). *JAMA* **301:** 39–51.

152. McCormick, D.L. *et al.* 2010. Null activity of selenium and vitamin e as cancer chemopreventive agents in the rat prostate. *Cancer Prev. Res (Phila).* **3:** 381–392.

153. Vidlar, A. *et al.* 2010. The safety and efficacy of a silymarin and selenium combination in men after radical prostatectomy: a six month placebo-controlled double-blind clinical trial. *Biomed. Pap. Med. Fac. Univ. Palacky. Olomouc. Czech. Repub.* **3:** 239–244.

Ann. N.Y. Acad. Sci. ISSN 0077-8923

ANNALS OF THE NEW YORK ACADEMY OF SCIENCES

Issue: *Nutrition and Physical Activity in Aging, Obesity, and Cancer*

Effects of physical activity on cancer prevention

Hye-Kyung Na and Sergiy Oliynyk

[1]Department of Food and Nutrition, College of Human Ecology, Sungshin Women's University, Seoul, South Korea

Address for correspondence: Hye-Kyung Na, Department of Food and Nutrition, College of Human Ecology, Sungshin Women's University, 147, Mia-dong, Kangbuk-gu, Seoul 149-100, South Korea. nhk1228@sungshin.ac.kr

Results of most epidemiological and laboratory studies suggest an inverse relationship between regular exercise and the risk of certain malignancies, such as intestinal, colon, pancreatic, breast, lung, skin, mammary, endometrial, and prostate cancer. However, physical activity can have different influence on carcinogenesis, depending on energy supply and the age of the subject as well as strength, frequency, and length of exercise. The biochemical and molecular basis of the interaction between aerobic physical activity and tumorigenic processes remains poorly understood. Physical activity may generate reactive oxygen species (ROS) to a different extent. Mild oxidative stress caused by moderate physical activity can activate cellular stress response signaling and potentiate cellular antioxidant defense capacity. However, accumulation of relatively large amounts of ROS as a consequence of exhaustive exercise can either directly damage DNA, causing mutation, or promote tumorigenesis by activating proinflammatory signaling. This review highlights the effects of physical activity on various malignancies in the context of redox status modulated during exercise.

Keywords: physical activity; cancer prevention; carcinogenesis; reactive oxygen species

Introduction

Multiple lines of compelling evidence suggest that physical activity reduces the risk of different types of malignances, especially those of the colon, breast, prostate, endometrial, and lung.[1–5] Friedenreich and colleagues analyzed more than 250 epidemiological studies on the association between physical activity and cancer prevention. Based on this analysis, it has been concluded that physical activity is convincingly associated with the reduced risk of developing colon and breast cancers, probably contributes to the reduced risk of endometrial cancer, and possibly lowers the risk of prostate and lung cancers.[6,7]

Table 1 summarizes the results of some representative animal studies evaluating the effects of physical activity on experimentally induced carcinogenesis. Despite the large number of investigations conducted on physical activity and cancer, the results have been discordant and even conflicting. This is largely due to incomplete assessments of exercise duration and frequency as well as intensity and the type of diet consumed during exercise. The molec-

ular basis for such differential effects of physical activity remains largely unresolved.

The purpose of this paper is to summarize the key findings on the cancer-preventive or opposite effects of physical activity and to suggest possible underlying mechanisms.

Colon and intestinal cancer

Several epidemiological studies have shown that regular exercise can delay the onset of colon and intestinal cancer.[7] Physical activity (long-term aerobic training) has been shown to significantly protect against chemically induced colon carcinogenesis (Table 1).[8–13] Rats subjected to free-wheel running developed markedly reduced incidence (percentage of animals with tumors) and multiplicity (tumors/animal) of colon adenocarcinomas, and the formation of small intestinal adenocarcinomas and liver foci was also lowered in the exercise group.[10] However, there was no difference in body mass between exercise and sedentary groups.

The protective effect of physical activity on colon carcinogenesis may depend on the type of exercise

doi: 10.1111/j.1749-6632.2011.06105.x

Table 1. Effects of exercise on experimentally induced intestinal, colon, and pancreatic carcinogenesis

Exercise type	Protocol	Effects on carcinogenesis	Ref.
Wheel	33 cm diameter, 20 wk	Decreased the DMH-induced colon tumor incidence in Sprague–Dawley male rats	8
Treadmill	120 min/d, 10 m/min, 5 d/wk	Decreased the DMH-induced colon tumor incidence and multiplicity in F344 male rats	9
Wheel	13.5 inch diameter, 38 wk	Decreased the AOM-induced colon tumor incidence and multiplicity in F344 male rats	10
Treadmill	5 h/d, 7 m/min, 5 d/wk, 38 wk	Decreased the AOM-induced colon tumor multiplicity in Fischer male rats	11 12
Swimming	Single exhaustive swimming bout in untrained rats	Increased the number of aberrant crypt foci	18
Swimming	8 wk, 5 d/wk	Inhibited the cell proliferation during DMH-induced colon carcinogenesis	13
Swimming	20 min/d, 5 d/wk, 35 wk	No significant effect on DMH-induced colon carcinogenesis in Wistar male rats	17
Treadmill	60 min/d, 18–21 m/min, 5% gradient, 5 d/wk, 7 wk	No significant effect in $Apc^{Min/+}$ male and female mice	22
Wheel and Treadmill	45 min/d, 20 m/min, 5% gradient, 5 d/wk; 3 wk wheel running, 5 wk on treadmill	No significant effect in $Apc^{Min/+}$ male and female mice	23
Treadmill and Wheel	60 min/d, 18 m/min, 5% gradient, 6 d/wk; 9 wk; 9.5 inch diameter, 9 wk	Treadmill training—decreased the total number of intestinal polyps only in male $Apc^{Min/+}$ mice; wheel training—no significant effect in $Apc^{Min/+}$ male & female mice	14
Wheel	16 wk	Inhibited the intestinal tumorigenesis in $Apc^{Min/+}$ male and female mice	15
Treadmill	60 min/d, 18 m/min, 6 d/wk; 10 wk	Inhibited intestinal tumorigenesis in Apc$^{Min+/-}$ male and emale mice	19
Treadmill	30–60 min/d, < or = 21 m/min, 5 d/wk, < or = 12 wk	Inhibited intestinal tumorigenesis in Apc$^{Min+/-}$ male and female mice	24
Aerobic exercise	6 wk	Inhibited intestinal tumorigenesis in Balb/c male mice	16
Wheel	0.95 km/day (M), 2.73 km/day (F)	Prevented against azaserine-induced pancreatic carcinogenesis in Lewis male and F344 female rats	21
Treadmill	15–20 min/d, 3–5 d/wk	Protected against azaserine-induced pancreatic carcenogenesis in Lewis male rats	20

and the gender. The number of large polyps (≥ 1 mm diameter) in male $Apc^{Min/+}$ mice was reduced by 38% after treadmill running (49 +/− 6; $P = 0.005$) compared with male controls (79 +/− 6), but these effects were not observed in female $Apc^{Min/+}$ mice.[14] Moreover, the crypt depth-to-villus height ratio in the intestine, an indirect marker of intestinal inflammation, decreased by 21% and 24%, respectively, in male and female treadmill runners but not in wheel runners.[14] In another study, voluntary exercise inhibited intestinal tumorigenesis in $Apc^{Min/+}$ mice and azoxymethane (AOM) plus dextran sulfate sodium (DSS)–treated mice, and this effect was associated with the decreased IGF-1/IGFBP-3 ratio, aberrant β-catenin signaling, and altered arachidonic acid metabolism.[15] Demarzo et al. reported a significant increase in the proliferating cell nuclear antigen-labeling index in 1,2-dimethyl-hydrazine (DMH)–treated rats, which was significantly lowered in the physical activity group.[13] Regular aerobic exercise suppressed the formation of aberrant crypt foci induced by AOM in the colon of rats.[16] Although the level of cyclooxygenase-2 (COX-2) was not changed, expression of inducible nitric oxide synthase (iNOS) was decreased in the exercise group compared with that in sedentary mice with concomitant reduction of the nitrotyrosine level. In addition, the level of tumor necrosis factor-alpha (TNF-α) was decreased following exercise in the colonic mucosa and plasma. However, exercise did not affect body mass and colon cancer development as well as expression of antioxidant enzyme and chaperon proteins in the colon.[16] It has been shown that the load of exercise is critical to confer the cancer-preventive effects in DMH-induced colon carcinogenesis.[17] In this work, aerobic swimming training (5 days/week, 35 weeks) with 2% body weight of load protected against the formation of DMH-induced aberrant crypt foci, while 4% body weight of load was less effective. However, a single bout of exhaustive swimming in untrained rats significantly increased the number of aberrant crypt foci compared to the nonexercise group.[18]

The preventive effect of physical activity on colon carcinognesis is influenced to some extent by diet. Chemopreventive effects of physical activity were observed in high-fat diet-induced colon carcinogenesis. Of the rats fed a high-fat corn oil diet, moderate exercise (running 2 km/day on weekdays for 38 weeks) reduced the number of animals developing carcinomas in the colon (sedentary, 10; exercise, 0) and in the small intestine (sedentary, 5; exercise, 0).[12] In another study, exercise reduced the total intestinal polyp number by 50% and the number of large polyps (>1 mm diameter) by 67% in standard diet-fed $Apc^{Min/+}$ mice. The western-style diet increased the polyp number by 75% in the $Apc^{Min/+}$ mice, but exercise neither decreased the polyp number nor altered the polyp size in mice fed the western-style diet.[19] Moreover, mice fed the western-style diet suffered from more severe inflammation and immunosuppression, which were not completely ameliorated by exercise. These data suggest that the cancer-preventive effect of physical activity is dependent on the type of diet.

Thus, it is likely that exercise can be protective, or does not affect, or aggravate colon carcinogenesis, depending on the type, the intensity, and duration of exercise, as well as the type of diet.

Pancreatic cancer

The diagnosis of pancreatic cancer usually occurs late in the course of disease development; thus, the prognosis is poor, with <1% of patients surviving five years. It has been demonstrated that the age of animals can influence the final effect of regular aerobic exercise on pancreatic carcinogenesis.[20] In this study, when treadmill exercise began at the 6th week of age, food intake was reduced by 15% compared to that in the sedentary group fed ad libitum. Under the same experimental conditions, the burden of azaserine-induced foci was decreased by approximately 37%. However, when the higher intensity of treadmill exercise began at the 13th week of age, this exercise group had an increased focal burden, compared to their sedentary pair-fed controls.[20] Notably, such enhancement occurred despite a reduction in food intake and body fat stores in the treadmill exercise group. These findings indicate that exercise may suppress or promote carcinogenesis, depending upon the age (stage in the life cycle) of the animal. Effects of calorie restriction also rely on age: the decrease in the azaserine-induced foci in the rat trained at the 6th week of age for 20 weeks (but not 13 weeks of age) is attributed to reduced caloric intake in young rats.

The length of the training course is also important for determining the cancer-preventive effect of exercise. Voluntary exercise (running wheels) reduced the growth rate of azaserine-induced pancreatic foci in F344 rats at 4 months postinitiation, but such a protective effect was not observed at 2 months postinitiation.[21] Generally, regular aerobic exercise may have a protective effect against pancreatic carcinogenesis, but this effect depends on the age and the duration of the training course. Perhaps calorie restriction may enhance this effect in young age.

Mammary cancer

Breast cancer is the most common malignancy diagnosed among women in the world. The 2008 NIH Report on Physical Activity and Health concludes that the evidence is strong that a reduction in the risk for breast cancer is associated with moderate-to-vigorous physical activity.[25] In addition, population-based studies have generated a large body of data supporting that physical activity (total physical activity, occupational and recreational) is protective against breast cancer in both pre- and postmenopausal women, although the evidence is stronger in postmenopausal women.[26] Moreover, it has been reported that moderate and vigorous physical activity can improve the quality of life in breast cancer survivors and ameliorate the treatment-related symptoms and mood in women with breast cancer receiving chemotherapy.[27,28] Thus, it appears that physical activity may play an important role in preventing breast cancer in both pre- and postmenopausal women, as well as delaying the onset of breast cancer in women with genetic susceptibility and improving survival in women after a breast cancer diagnosis.

Physical activity can enhance or inhibit the development of chemically induced mammary cancer in rodents depending on the intensity of exercise.[29,30] Although the molecular mechanisms underlying the cancer-preventive effects of physical activity on breast carcinogenesis are not clearly elucidated, three hypotheses are considered: (1) the mTOR network hypothesis, where physical activity inhibits carcinogenesis by suppressing the activation of the mTOR signaling network in mammary carcinomas; (2) the hormesis hypothesis, where the carcinogenic response to physical activity is nonlinear, which is attributable to the physiological cellular stress response; and (3) the metabolic reprogramming hypothesis, where physical activity limits the amount of glucose and glutamine required for the growth of mammary cancer cells, thereby inducing apoptosis.[31] In addition, exposure to estrogen is an important determinant of breast cancer risk, and exercise reduces estrogen levels. This may lead to decreased accumulation of DNA adducts formed by estrogen metabolites in the breast tissues and reduced promoter hypermethylation of breast tumor suppressor genes.[32,33]

In addition, physical activity has been known to change the metabolic profile of estrogen. Some estrogen metabolites have been found to reduce hormonal activity compared with their parent molecule, estradiol. It has been known that 2-methoxyestradiol and 2-hydroxy-3-methoxyestradiol inhibit the proliferation of estrogen receptor (ER)-positive and ER-negative breast cancer cells.[34] 2-methoxyestradiol/2-hydroxy-estradiol and 4-methoxyestradiol/4-hydroxyestra-diol ratios were higher after training over two consecutive menstrual cycles, suggesting that physical activity may suppress the proliferation of breast epithelial cells.[35] Moreover, physical activity is considered to reduce the breast cancer risk not only by decreasing the endogenous estrogen level due to the decreased body fat, but also by increasing the amount of circulating sex estrogen-binding globulin.[36,37]

Calorie restriction, the most commonly recommended dietary strategy in humans to prevent or reverse obesity, dramatically inhibits spontaneous, chemically, or virally induced mammary tumorigenesis in diverse animal models. Cohen et al. observed a decrease in the fat stores of exercised rats compared with sedentary rats.[38] This effect was not directly dependent on food consumption; in this study, the exercised rats actually increased their food consumption and calorie intake, but tumorigenesis was still suppressed. In addition, comparison of gene expression profiles between ad libitum and 30% calorie restriction groups revealed 425 statistically significant changes, whereas analysis of ad libitum versus ad libitum plus exercise group showed 45 changes, with only three changes included among the same genes, indicating that calorie restriction and exercise differentially influence expression patterns in noncancerous mammary tissue.[39] Differential expression was observed in genes related to breast cancer stem cells, the epithelial–mesenchymal transition, and the growth and survival of breast cancer cells.[39] Thus, calorie restriction and exercise seem to exert their effects on mammary carcinogenesis through distinct pathways.[39] However, a decrease in body weight may also contribute to the cancer-preventive effect of regular physical activity.

Skin cancer

Voluntary running wheel exercise delayed the onset and reduced the number and the volume of tumors in ultraviolet B (UVB)-induced mouse skin carcinogenesis model.[40] Running wheel exercise decreased the number of nonmalignant tumors (primarily keratoacanthomas) by 34% and the number of tumors per mouse by 32%, respectively, in UVB-initiated short-term and long-term carcinogenesis models.[40]

Moreover, running wheel exercise decreased the formation of squamous cell carcinomas in the UVB-induced long-term carcinogenesis model by 27%. In addition, the size of keratoacanthoma and squamous cell carcinoma was reduced substantially in short-term and long-term UVB-induced skin carcinogenesis models. Animals with running wheel exercise exhibited decreases in parametrial fat pad weight and thickness of the dermal fat layer.[40] Physical activity with controlled calorie intake also exhibited significantly reduced body weight and body fat as well as the modified phospholipid profile.[41] Alterations in the membrane lipid fatty acid composition may also be involved in cancer progression. Phosphatidylinositols (PIs) and their derivatives have been found to play an important role in carcinogenic processes.[41] Physical activity with calorie intake reduced the levels of PIs as well as expression of phosphatidylinositol 3-kinase (PI3-K) in phorbol ester-treated mouse epidermis. In addition, the level of long-chain polyunsaturated fatty acids and omega-3 fatty acids in the phospholipids were enhanced in phorbol ester-treated mouse epidermis.[41]

Double-edged sword of physical activity: role of ROS

Physical activity can have different influences on carcinogenesis, depending on energy supply as well as strength and frequency of exercise loads. Moderate regular exercise exhibits cancer-preventive potential as well as other health-beneficial effects, whereas single exhaustive exercise may increase the risk of some cancer development. The molecular mechanisms underlying the cancer-preventive or cancer-promoting effects of physical activity have not yet been resolved. One of the reasons for such controversy may be attributed to the degree of exercise-mediated oxidative stress, which differentially affects health.

ROS are formed continuously as a consequence of metabolic reactions or other biochemical processes as well as by environmental stressors. During metabolic stress, ROS production increases, and the subsequent removal of ROS depends on the capacities of endogenous ROS scavengers and antioxidant defense. Such antioxidant defense mechanism is essential for cellular protection against oxidative and inflammatory insults. Antioxidants include enzymes such as superoxide dismutase

(SOD), glutathione peroxidase (GPX), catalase (CAT), and heme oxygenase-1.

During exercise, a 10- to 40-fold increase in oxygen uptake occurs relative to the resting state, which can cause increased formation of ROS. Numerous studies have demonstrated that both sustained and intensive acute physical loads cause oxidative stress, which can result in cellular damage.[42–48] It has been known that exhaustive exercise diminishes antioxidants levels and consequently augments generation of oxygen free radicals, leading to oxidative stress and inflammation.[49] ROS may play a key role in carcinogenesis by causing DNA base modifications. For instance, hydroxyl radical can attack DNA to form 8-hydroxyguanine (8-OH-dG).[50] While exhausting exercise is reported to increase DNA damage,[51–53] moderate aerobic exercise does not increase, but may rather alleviate oxidative DNA damage.[54] The basal levels of 8-OH-dG were significantly lower in physically active subjects than those of sedentary ones.[54] After mild exercise for 30 min, the 8-OH-dG levels of the sedentary subjects were significantly decreased. Physical activity of submaximum power induced acidosis, which was caused by an excess level of lactate in the anaerobic zone of energy supply.[55]

It has been reported that mild exercise (50% VO_2 max) increases the expression of SOD, a representative antioxidant enzyme, and human MutT homolog (hMTH), an 8-oxo-dGTPase.[54] Habitual exercise (swimming with weight, 60 min/day, 7 weeks) decreased the formation of 8-OH-dG in the kidney of rats compared to that of the control animals following treatment with Fe-nitrilotriacetic acid (Fe-NTA), an ROS-generating carcinogen that induces oxidative stress and cancer in the kidney. The formation of 8-OH-dG was inversely related to loads of activity.[54] The rat treated with Fe-nitrilotriacetic acid (Fe-NTA) showed the low level of SOD expression. However, the rat that performed habitual exercise exhibited increased expression of SOD, but not CAT and GPx activity.

Besides directly damaging DNA, ROS can stimulate inflammatory signal transduction pathways via activation of redox-sensitive transcription factors such as NF-κB, which functions as a tumor promoter and has been known to be involved in inflammation-associated carcinogenesis. NF-κB is a major transcription factor regulating cyclooxygenase-2 (COX-2), a rate-limiting enzyme in prostaglandin biosynthesis. Abnormal upregulation of COX-2 has been implicated in many inflammation-associated chronic disorders, including cancer. A single bout of exercise accelerates NF-κB activation and COX-2 expression in an intensity-dependent manner in human peripheral blood mononuclear cells.[56] As exercise intensity increased, both COX-2 expression and NF-κB DNA binding activity were enhanced. Vigorous exercise (100% of heart rate reserve, treadmill) also induces the phosphorylation of both IKKα and IκBα.

The induction of antioxidant and phase-2 enzymes represents an important cellular defense in response to oxidative and electrophilic insults. Nuclear transcription factor erythroid 2p45 (NF-E2)–related factor 2 (Nrf2) plays a crucial role in regulating phase-2 detoxifying/antioxidant gene induction. Exercise in old rats decreased the malondialdehyde levels and increased the total SOD activity and Cu/ZnSOD protein in renal proximal tubules.[57] In addition, exercise (treadmill, 15 m/min, 15-degree grade, 5 d/wk, for 6 wks) increased the nuclear localization of Nrf2 and subsequent binding to antioxidant response elements in renal proximal tubules.[57] Moreover, people who carry the ATG haplotype in Nrf2 gene had 57.5% higher training response in VO_2 at running economy than noncarriers.[58] Polymorphisms in *Nrf2* may explain some of the individual differences in endurance capacity.[58]

Taking the above findings together, it is speculated that levels of ROS dependent on the load of physical activity differentially regulate the redox-sensitive transcription factors such as Nrf2 or NF-κB. Moderate physical activity induces antioxidant gene expression through activation of Nrf2, which confers tolerance to the oxidative stress induced by carcinogenic insult. In contrast, exhaustive physical activity may induce oxidative damage beyond the antioxidant capacity of cells, thereby activating NF-κB. This, in turn, stimulates the expression of genes involved in carcinogenesis.

Conclusion

Many epidemiological, clinical, and experimental studies have revealed an inverse relationship between physical activity and the frequency of various cancers. Several plausible biological mechanisms have been proposed to explain the cancer-preventive effects of exercise. These include changes in endogenous metabolic or sex hormone levels and growth factors, decreased obesity and central adiposity, and alterations in immune functions. Weight control may play a particularly important role because links between excess weight and an increased cancer risk have been established in various malignancies, including colon and breast cancer. Moreover, central adiposity has also been implicated in promoting metabolic conditions amenable to carcinogenesis.

Although the molecular mechanism underlying cancer-preventive effects of physical activity is not clear, induction of antioxidant enzymes and suppression of inflammation-related gene expression through activation of Nrf2 and suppression of NF-κB signaling, respectively, are relatively well defined. Paradoxically, exercise can cause oxidative stress and inflammation. During exercise, substantial production of ROS occurs as a consequence of the increase in oxygen uptake. Therefore, physical activity regulates a greater flux of oxygen-free radicals that could alter cellular redox status, depending on the type, intensity, duration, and frequency of physical activity together with the type of diet consumed. Considering the fact that physical activity is one of the few potentially modifiable factors in preventing various malignancies, the determination of the optimal load of physical activity that can elicit cancer-preventive effects merits further investigation.

Acknowledgments

The authors thank Dr. Young-Joon Surh (College of Pharmacy, Seoul National University, South Korea) for the editorial support in the preparation of the manuscript. This work was supported by the Sungshin Women's University Research Grant (2009-1-21-004).

Conflicts of interest

The authors declare no conflicts of interest.

References

1. Shephard, R.J. 1990. Physical activity and cancer. *Int. J. Sports Med.* **11:** 413–420.
2. Shephard, R.J. 1993. Exercise in the prevention and treatment of cancer. An update. *Sports Med.* **15:** 258–280.
3. Tamakoshi, K. *et al.* 2001. Epidemiology and primary prevention of colorectal cancer. *Gan To Kagaku Ryoho.* **28:** 146–150.
4. Thune, I. & A.S. Furberg. 2001. Physical activity and cancer risk: dose-response and cancer, all sites and site-specific.

Med. Sci. Sports Exerc. **33**: S530–S550; discussion S609–510.

5. Moore, S.C. *et al.* 2010. Physical activity, sedentary behaviours, and the prevention of endometrial cancer. *Br. J. Cancer* **103**: 933–938.

6. Friedenreich, C.M. 2001. Physical activity and cancer prevention: from observational to intervention research. *Cancer Epidemiol. Biomarkers Prev.* **10**: 287–301.

7. Friedenreich, C.M. & M.R. Orenstein. 2002. Physical activity and cancer prevention: etiologic evidence and biological mechanisms. *J. Nutr.* **132**: 3456S–3464S.

8. Andrianopoulos, G. *et al.* 1987. The influence of physical activity in 1,2 dimethylhydrazine induced colon carcinogenesis in the rat. *Anticancer Res.* **7**: 849–852.

9. Fuku, N. *et al.* 2007. Effect of running training on DMH-induced aberrant crypt foci in rat colon. *Med. Sci. Sports Exerc.* **39**: 70–74.

10. Reddy, B.S., S. Sugie & A. Lowenfels. 1988. Effect of voluntary exercise on azoxymethane-induced colon carcinogenesis in male F344 rats. *Cancer Res.* **48**: 7079–7081.

11. Thorling, E.B., N.O. Jacobsen & K. Overvad. 1993. Effect of exercise on intestinal tumour development in the male Fischer rat after exposure to azoxymethane. *Eur. J. Cancer Prev.* **2**: 77–82.

12. Thorling, E.B., N.O. Jacobsen & K. Overvad. 1994. The effect of treadmill exercise on azoxymethane-induced intestinal neoplasia in the male Fischer rat on two different high-fat diets. *Nutr. Cancer* **22**: 31–41.

13. Demarzo, M.M. *et al.* 2008. Exercise reduces inflammation and cell proliferation in rat colon carcinogenesis. *Med. Sci. Sports Exerc.* **40**: 618–621.

14. Mehl, K.A. *et al.* 2005. Decreased intestinal polyp multiplicity is related to exercise mode and gender in $Apc^{Min/+}$ mice. *J. Appl. Physiol.* **98**: 2219–2225.

15. Ju, J. *et al.* 2008. Voluntary exercise inhibits intestinal tumorigenesis in $Apc^{Min/+}$ mice and azoxymethane/dextran sulfate sodium-treated mice. *BMC Cancer* **8**: 316–323.

16. Aoi, W. *et al.* 2010. Regular exercise reduces colon tumorigenesis associated with suppression of iNOS. *Biochem. Biophys. Res. Commun.* **399**: 14–19.

17. Lunz, W. *et al.* 2008. Long-term aerobic swimming training by rats reduces the number of aberrant crypt foci in 1,2-dimethylhydrazine-induced colon cancer. *Braz. J. Med. Biol. Res.* **41**: 1000–1004.

18. Demarzo, M.M. & S.B. Garcia. 2004. Exhaustive physical exercise increases the number of colonic preneoplastic lesions in untrained rats treated with a chemical carcinogen. *Cancer Lett.* **216**: 31–34.

19. Baltgalvis, K.A. *et al.* 2009. The interaction of a high-fat diet and regular moderate intensity exercise on intestinal polyp development in *Apc* $^{Min/+}$ mice. *Cancer Prev. Res. (Phila).* **2**: 641–649.

20. Craven-Giles, T. *et al.* 1994. Dietary modulation of pancreatic carcinogenesis: calories and energy expenditure. *Cancer Res.* **54**: 1964s–1968s.

21. Roebuck, B.D., J. McCaffrey & K.J. Baumgartner. 1990. Protective effects of voluntary exercise during the postinitiation phase of pancreatic carcinogenesis in the rat. *Cancer Res.* **50**: 6811–6816.

22. Colbert, L.H. *et al.* 2000. Exercise and tumor development in a mouse predisposed to multiple intestinal adenomas. *Med. Sci. Sports Exerc.* **32**: 1704–1708.

23. Colbert, L.H. *et al.* 2003. Exercise and intestinal polyp development in APCMin mice. *Med. Sci. Sports Exerc.* **35**: 1662–1669.

24. Basterfield, L. & J.C. Mathers. 2010. Intestinal tumours, colonic butyrate and sleep in exercised Min mice. *Br. J. Nutr.* **104**: 355–363.

25. Physical Activity Guidelines Advisory Committee. 2008. *Physical Activity Guidelines Advisory Committee Report*. US Department of Health and Human Services. Washington, DC.

26. World Cancer Research Fund/American Institute for Cancer Research. 2007. In *Food, Nutrition, Physical Acitivity, and the Prevention of Cancer: A Global Perspective*. American Institute for Cancer Research, Washington, DC.

27. Mandelblatt, J.S. *et al.* 2011. Associations of physical activity with quality of life and functional ability in breast cancer patients during active adjuvant treatment: the Pathways Study. *Breast Cancer Res. Treat* [Epub ahead of print].

28. Yang, C.Y. *et al.* 2011. Effects of a home-based walking program on perceived symptom and mood status in postoperative breast cancer women receiving adjuvant chemotherapy. *J. Adv. Nurs.* **67**: 158–168.

29. Thompson, H.J. 1992. Effect of amount and type of exercise on experimentally induced breast cancer. *Adv. Exp. Med. Biol.* **322**: 61–71.

30. Thompson, H.J. *et al.* 1995. Exercise intensity dependent inhibition of 1-methyl-1-nitrosourea induced mammary carcinogenesis in female F-344 rats. *Carcinogenesis* **16**: 1783–1786.

31. Thompson, H.J. *et al.* 2009. Candidate mechanisms accounting for effects of physical activity on breast carcinogenesis. *IUBMB Life* **61**: 895–901.

32. Coyle, Y.M. 2008. Physical activity as a negative modulator of estrogen-induced breast cancer. *Cancer Causes Control* **19**: 1021–1029.

33. Coyle, Y.M. *et al.* 2007. Role of physical activity in modulating breast cancer risk as defined by *APC* and *RASSF1A* promoter hypermethylation in nonmalignant breast tissue. *Cancer Epidemiol. Biomarkers Prev.* **16**: 192–196.

34. Zhu, B.T. & A.H. Conney. 1998. Functional role of estrogen metabolism in target cells: review and perspectives. *Carcinogenesis* **19**: 1–27.

35. De Cree, C. *et al.* 1997. Responses of catecholestrogen metabolism to acute graded exercise in normal menstruating women before and after training. *J. Clin. Endocrinol. Metab.* **82**: 3342–3348.

36. McTiernan, A. *et al.* 2004. Effect of exercise on serum estrogens in postmenopausal women: a 12-month randomized clinical trial. *Cancer Res.* **64**: 2923–2928.

37. Shephard, R.J. 1995. Exercise and cancer: linkages with obesity? *Int. J. Obes. Relat. Metab. Disord.* **19**(Suppl 4): S62–S68.

38. Cohen, L.A. *et al.* 1992. Voluntary exercise and experimental mammary cancer. *Adv. Exp. Med. Biol.* **322**: 41–59.

39. Padovani, M. *et al.* 2009. Distinct effects of calorie restriction and exercise on mammary gland gene expression in C57BL/6 mice. *Cancer Prev. Res. (Phila)* **2**: 1076–1087.

40. Michna, L. *et al.* 2006. Inhibitory effects of voluntary running wheel exercise on UVB-induced skin carcinogenesis in SKH-1 mice. *Carcinogenesis* **27:** 2108–2115.

41. Ouyang, P. *et al.* 2010. Weight Loss via exercise with controlled dietary intake may affect phospholipid profile for cancer prevention in murine skin tissues. *Cancer Prev. Res. (Phila)* **3:** 466–477.

42. Marzatico, F. *et al.* 1997. Blood free radical antioxidant enzymes and lipid peroxides following long-distance and lactacidemic performances in highly trained aerobic and sprint athletes. *J. Sports Med. Phys. Fitness.* **37:** 235–239.

43. Kostka, T. 1999. Aging, physical activity and free radicals. *Pol Merkur Lekarski.* **7:** 202–204.

44. Selamoglu, S. *et al.* 2000. Aerobic and anaerobic training effects on the antioxidant enzymes of the blood. *Acta Physiol. Hung.* **87:** 267–273.

45. Bloomer, R.J. & A.H. Goldfarb. 2004. Anaerobic exercise and oxidative stress: a review. *Can. J. Appl. Physiol.* **29:** 245–263.

46. Bloomer, R.J. *et al.* 2005. Effects of acute aerobic and anaerobic exercise on blood markers of oxidative stress. *J. Strength. Cond. Res.* **19:** 276–285.

47. Bloomer, R.J. & W.A. Smith. 2009. Oxidative stress in response to aerobic and anaerobic power testing: influence of exercise training and carnitine supplementation. *Res. Sports Med.* **17:** 1–16.

48. Fisher-Wellman, K. & R.J. Bloomer. 2009. Acute exercise and oxidative stress: a 30 year history. *Dyn. Med.* **8:** 1–25.

49. Cooper, C.E. *et al.* 2002. Exercise, free radicals and oxidative stress. *Biochem. Soc. Trans.* **30:** 280–285.

50. Floyd, R.A. 1990. Role of oxygen free radicals in carcinogenesis and brain ischemia. *FASEB J.* **4:** 2587–2597.

51. Inoue, T. *et al.* 1993. Effect of physical exercise on the content of 8-hydroxydeoxyguanosine in nuclear DNA prepared from human lymphocytes. *Jpn. J. Cancer Res.* **84:** 720–725.

52. Poulsen, H.E., S. Loft & K. Vistisen. 1996. Extreme exercise and oxidative DNA modification. *J. Sports Sci.* **14:** 343–346.

53. Poulsen, H.E., A. Weimann & S. Loft. 1999. Methods to detect DNA damage by free radicals: relation to exercise. *Proc. Nutr. Soc.* **58:** 1007–1014.

54. Sato, Y. *et al.* 2003. Increase of human MTH1 and decrease of 8-hydroxydeoxyguanosine in leukocyte DNA by acute and chronic exercise in healthy male subjects. *Biochem. Biophys. Res. Commun.* **305:** 333–338.

55. Bentley, D.J. *et al.* 2007. Incremental exercise test design and analysis: implications for performance diagnostics in endurance athletes. *Sports Med.* **37:** 575–586.

56. Kim, S.Y. *et al.* 2009. Effects of exercise on cyclooxygenase-2 expression and nuclear factor-κB DNA binding in human peripheral blood mononuclear cells. *Ann. N. Y. Acad. Sci.* **1171:** 464–471.

57. Asghar, M. *et al.* 2007. Exercise decreases oxidative stress and inflammation and restores renal dopamine D1 receptor function in old rats. *Am. J. Physiol. Renal Physiol.* **293:** F914–F919.

58. He, Z. *et al.* 2007. NRF2 genotype improves endurance capacity in response to training. *Int. J. Sports Med.* **28:** 717–721.

Ann. N.Y. Acad. Sci. ISSN 0077-8923

Regulation of the Keap1/Nrf2 system by chemopreventive sulforaphane: implications of posttranslational modifications

Young-Sam Keum

Department of Biochemistry, College of Pharmacy, Dongguk University, 813 Siksa-dong, Goyang, Kyunggi-do, 410-773, Republic of Korea

Address for correspondence: Young-Sam Keum, Ph.D., Department of Biochemistry, College of Pharmacy, Dongguk University, 813 Siksa-dong, Goyang, Kyunggi-do, Republic of Korea, 410-773. keum03@dongguk.edu

The chemopreventive agent sulforaphane is an isothiocyanate derived from cruciferous vegetables. Transcriptional activation of antioxidant response element (ARE)-regulated phase II detoxification and antioxidant genes through the induction of transcription factor NF-E2-related factor-2 (Nrf2) is considered as the prime mechanism of its chemopreventive action. Cellular level of Nrf2 is tightly regulated by proteolysis through Cullin3 (Cul3)/Kelch-like ECH-associated protein 1 (Keap1)-dependent polyubiquitination. Sulforaphane is an electrophile that can react with protein thiols to form thionoacyl adducts and is believed to affect the Cys residues in Keap1 protein. In addition, sulforaphane might affect the activity of a variety of intracellular kinases to phosphorylate Nrf2 proteins, which dictates the nucleocytoplasmic trafficking of Nrf2 or modulates the Nrf2 protein stability. This review is designed to briefly account for the regulatory mechanism of Nrf2 protein expression by Cul3/Keap1 E3 ligase and for the possible roles of posttranslational modifications of cellular Keap1 or Nrf2 proteins by sulforphane in the regulation of ARE-dependent gene activation.

Keywords: sulforaphane; antioxidant response element (ARE); posttranslational modifications

Sulforaphane as a putative chemopreventive agent

The consumption of naturally occurring dietary compounds prevents the development of various types of cancer. *Chemoprevention* is defined as the use of natural or synthetic compounds to delay or prevent carcinogenesis in humans.[1] Tumor formation comprises three stages of biological processes: initiation, promotion, and progression. It is well accepted that an appropriate interruption of tumor initiation and promotion steps by chemopreventive agents can reduce the incidence of tumor development in many experimental models. This has led to a conceptual classification of chemopreventive agents into two types: suppressing agents and blocking agents.[2] Unlike many dietary chemopreventive compounds (e.g., curcumin, resveratrol, and epigallocatechin gallate [EGCG]) that

possess polyphenolic moiety, natural chemopreventive isothiocyanates are characterized by the N=C=S functional group. Dietary chemopreventive isothiocyanates, including sulforaphane, phenethyl isothiocyanate (PEITC), and indole-3 carbinol (I3C), are abundantly found in cruciferous vegetables such as broccoli, brussels sprouts, cauliflower, and cabbage. Sulforaphane was identified in broccoli by monitoring the induction of quinone reductase activity in murine hepatoma cells and was later found to be a monofunctional inducer: it selectively increases phase II enzyme activities without apparently affecting the arylhydrocarbon receptor-dependent cytochrome P-450s (phase I enzymes).[3] Sulforaphane exists as a precursor form of thioglucoside, e.g., glucoraphanin, in broccoli. Upon consumption, glucoraphanin is hydrolyzed into sulforaphane in our

doi: 10.1111/j.1749-6632.2011.06092.x

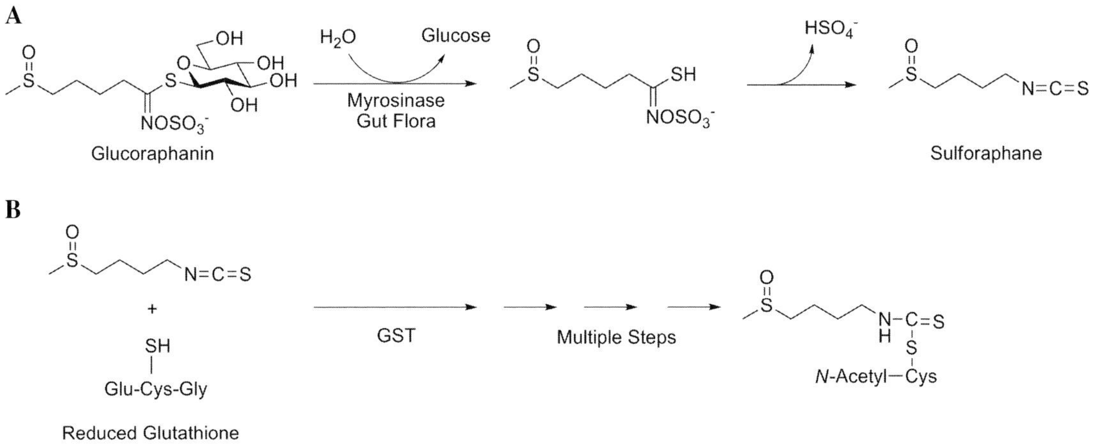

Figure 1. (A) Sulforaphane is produced from its precursor, glucoraphanin, by an enzymatic action of plant-specific myrosinase or gut microflora after consumption of cruciferous vegetables, including broccoli. (B) Sulforaphane is conjugated with reduced glutathione (GSH) in cells by glutathione S-transferase (GST), which undergoes several enzymatic transformations to produce *N*-acetyl-sulforaphane (sulforaphane-NAC). This pathway is referred to as the mercapturic acid pathway.

body by the enzymatic action of plant-specific myrosinase or unidentified microflora in the gut (Fig. 1). Sulforaphane is then directly conjugated to reduced glutathione (GSH) and metabolized via the mercapturic acid pathway.[4]

Sulforaphane is protective against the formation of various types of tumor in rodent models. Administration of sulforaphane significantly suppressed gastrointestinal adenoma formation in ApcMin/+ mice.[5] Topical application of sulforaphane suppressed 7,12-dimethylbenz(a)anthracene (DMBA) and 12-O-tetradecanoylphorbol-13-acetate (TPA)-induced papilloma formation in mouse skin.[6] Likewise, administration of sulforaphane-containing broccoli sprouts was found to be effective in suppressing the growth of prostate tumors in TRAMP mice.[7] Epidemiological studies have demonstrated an inverse relationship between consumption of cruciferous vegetables and incidence of tumors in humans.[8] In agreement with this fact, Kensler *et al.* have demonstrated that consumption of broccoli sprouts in hot water reduced the urinary formation of aflatoxin-DNA adduct in residents of Qidong, the Republic of China, where hepatocellular carcinoma is prevalent due to aflatoxin contamination.[9] Because sulforaphane is metabolized by the mercapturic acid pathway, it was conceived that individuals with a lower level of glutathione S-transferase (GST) enzymes would have a slower rate of metabolic excretion of sul-

foraphane and, therefore, receive greater chemopreventive benefits from a dietary intake of cruciferous vegetables. Indeed, the subjects with GSTT1-null genotype, given cruciferous vegetables, had a significant increase in the area under the time–concentration curve (AUC) of isothiocyanates in blood, with a reduced risk of colorectal cancer.[10,11] Presently, several small-scale clinical trials of sulforaphane are currently ongoing (the reader is directed to the NIH website [http://clinicaltrials.gov/ct2/search] for more information).

Regulation of phase II detoxification gene expression by Cullin3/Keap1 E3 ligase

Sulforaphane suppresses carcinogenesis through multiple biological mechanisms of actions, such as suppression of cell cycle, apoptotic induction, suppression of reactive oxygen species (ROS) generation, and inhibition of histone deacetylases.[12] In particular, sulforaphane is a strong inducer of phase II detoxification enzymes. Incubation of cells with sulforaphane results in the induction of Nrf2 protein in a short time period (less than 30 min) with a concomitant transcriptional activation of its target genes, such as heme oxygenase-1 (HO-1), NAD[P]H: quinone oxidoreductases (NQOs), glutathione S-transferases (GSTs), and UDP-glucuronosyltransferases (UGTs).[13] It is noteworthy that Nrf2 mRNA level is unaffected by treatment with sulforaphane, suggesting that cellular expression of Nrf2 protein is posttranscriptionally regulated.[14] It is known that Nrf2 is constantly degraded in the cytoplasm under basal conditions. Upon exposure to oxidative stress or electrophiles, degradation of the Nrf2 protein is halted, which makes it stabilized and free to translocate into the nucleus, thereby activating target genes by binding to the *cis*-acting element, termed antioxidant response element (ARE). Nrf2 is a 597 amino acid residue protein that possesses six conserved Nrf2-ECH homology (Neh) domains. It serves as a critical transcription factor for ARE-mediated gene expression, as Nrf2 knockout mice do exhibit an impairment of the induction of phase II detoxification enzymes in the liver and intestine.[15] Analysis of domain functions of Nrf2 illustrates that the Neh1 domain is a basic leucine-zipper (bZIP) structure, required for DNA binding in association with small Maf proteins and that the Neh4 and Neh5 constitute transactivation domains that contribute to ARE activation by binding to coactivators, such as CBP and p300.[16]

Keap1 (Kelch-like ECH-associated protein 1) is a cytosolic repressor protein of Nrf2 that was initially identified by a yeast two-hybrid assay, using the Neh2 domain as a bait.[17] Keap1, a 626 amino acid residue protein, possesses the BTB (bric-à-brac, tramtrack, and broad) domain in the N-terminal region and six Kelch domains in the C-terminal region. Examination of domain–domain interactions between Nrf2 and Keap1 has identified that C-terminal Kelch region of Keap1 is responsible for binding to the Neh2 domain in Nrf2. As mentioned above, the Nrf2 protein is intrinsically unstable. After the identification of the BTB domain as a component of Cullin3 (Cul3)-based E3 ligase,[18] it was soon realized that the BTB domain is a required module for an efficient binding of Keap1 to Cul3 and that Keap1 acts as an adaptor protein to target multiple lysine residues within the Neh2 domain of Nrf2 for ubiquitin-mediated protein degradation.[19] Yamamoto *et al.* have provided a model, the so-called hinge and latch model, in order to explain the molecular interactions between the Nrf2 and Keap1 proteins. According to this model, the ratio between Keap1 and Nrf2 binding is 2:1, and two Keap1 proteins seem to simultaneously associate with a single Nrf2 protein through the ETGE and DLG motifs, located in the Neh2 domain.[20] Be-

cause the affinity of ETGE motif to Keap1 is stronger than that of DLG motif, the ETGE motif and DLG motifs were coined as a hinge and latch, respectively. While the hinge and latch model is currently accepted as a prevailing model of Nrf2/Keap1 interaction, Hannink *et al.* have provided another interesting observation, in which two Keap1 proteins simultaneously bind to Nrf2 and phosphoglycerate mutase family member 5 (PGAM5) through a conserved E(S/T)GE motif, resulting in the formation of a ternary complex.[21] As such, knocking down not only Keap1 but also PGAM5 substantially increased Nrf2-dependent gene expression, suggesting a possibility that PGAM5 might constitute an important component of inducible cytoprotective gene expression by Nrf2.

Posttranslational mofidication of Keap1/Nrf2 proteins by sulforaphane

According to the hinge and latch model, reactive cysteine (Cys) residues in Keap1 are proposed as sensors in response to an exposure to electrophiles. There are 27 Cys residues in the human Keap1 protein and individual Cys residues seem to differentially respond to electrophiles, depending on the types. This led to a recent classification of ARE inducers into six classes, so-called cysteine code.[22] Less than a decade ago, Zhang *et al.* demonstrated that mutation of Cys (C) into Ser (S) in Keap1 led to a perturbation of Keap1-mediated repression of Nrf2 under basal conditions (C273S or C288S) or a disruption of the activity of Nrf2 to escape from Keap1-mediated repression (C151S). In addition, they showed that sulforaphane-mediated ARE-luciferase activation was abrogated when HA-Keap1-C151S plasmid, but not HA-Keap1-C273S or HA-Keap1-C288S plasmids, was overexpressed.[23] In an attempt to find out whether sulforaphane can form a direct adduct with the Keap1 protein, Hong *et al.* have exposed sulforaphane to a recombinant Keap1 protein and observed that Keap1-sulforaphane adduct was labile and that the Cys residues of the recombinant Keap1 protein that form an adduct with sulforaphane varied, depending on the workup conditions or the concentration of sulforaphane used in the experiment.[24] Recently, Hu *et al.* have conducted a similar *in vitro* study and found that sulforaphane indeed formed a covalent adduct with a recombinant Keap1 protein at Cys-151, when iodoacetamide was omitted from the protocol and sample preparation time was reduced.[25] To the best of our knowledge, it is still unknown, however, whether sulforaphane can form a stable adduct with endogenous Keap1 protein in cells and, if so, which residue(s) it is conjugated to is yet to be elucidated.

Contrary to Keap1, a number of investigators have focused on studying the functional outcomes of Nrf2 phosphorylation. There exist a number of putative kinases that are reported to directly phosphorylate the Nrf2 protein and affect its cellular location or stability. Pickett *et al.* have demonstrated that protein kinase C (PKC) can directly phosphorylate the Nrf2 protein at Ser-40, although its functional significance is yet unclear. Likewise, p38δ mitogen-activated protein kinase (MAPK) was shown to directly phosphorylate the recombinant GST-tagged Nrf2 protein, and this phosphorylation promoted the interaction of recombinant protein with endogenous Keap1 *in vitro*.[26] On the contrary, there is another report demonstrating that all MAPKs, including p38α isoform, can directly phosphorylate the Nrf2 protein, but Nrf2 phosphorylation by MAPKs seemed to have a minimal effect on Nrf2 stability or its subcellular localization.[27] The reason for this discrepancy might stem from the difference of p38 MAPK isoforms, used in each of the studies as well as a failure to pinpoint the exact residue in the Nrf2 protein to be phosphorylated by p38 MAPK. Although it is still uncertain whether ERK and JNK can directly phosphorylate the Nrf2 protein, there are a significant number of papers showing that sulforaphane is a strong inducer of ERK and JNK phosphorylation and that these two signaling kinases are critically involved in the activation of ARE-dependent gene expression.[28] The question of how the activation of ERK and JNK by sulforaphane contributes to the activation of genes, thereby encoding phase II detoxification enzymes, merits further investigation. On the other hand, Jain and Jaiswal have shown that Fyn kinase can directly phosphorylate Nrf2 protein at Tyr-568 and promotes its nuclear export and degradation, thereby contributing to the suppression of ARE-mediated gene expression.[29] Later, they showed that GSK3β acts as a direct upstream regulatory kinase of Fyn that contributes to Nrf2 phosphorylation at Tyr-568.[30] Very recently, Cuadrado *et al.* have provided an intriguing result showing that GSK3β acts as a direct kinase that phosphorylates Serine cluster, located within the Neh6 domain of the Nrf2 protein, thereby facilitating Nrf2 protein degradation by Cullin1/F-box (βTrCP) E3 ligase complex, but not by Cul3/Keap1 E3 ligase.[31] This study signifies the existence of dual Nrf2-targeting E3 ligase machinery. While the effect of sulforaphane on Fyn kinase activity and/or expression is unavailable at present, Rojo *et al.* have demonstrated that sulforaphane-mediated ARE activation is abrogated by overexpression of active GSK3β,[32] suggesting a possibility that regulation of Fyn and/or GSK3β activity might constitute another route to activate ARE-dependent gene expression by sulforaphane.

Future perspectives

Posttranslational modifications of Keap1 and Nrf2 proteins seem to play an important role in the regulation of ARE-dependent gene expression. While the Cys modifications of Keap1 are believed to function as a sensor in response to various electrophiles, the functional significance of Nrf2 phosphorylation is not yet well understood, except for the fact that GSK3β can phosphorylate Nrf2 to promote its nuclear exclusion or proteolysis. In addition, it is imperative to know whether sulforaphane can indeed affect the Cys (or possibly other amino acid) residue(s) of cellular Keap1 protein and, if it is so, then whether it would bring out the conformation changes of Keap1 protein, thereby resulting in the release of Nrf2 protein. However, unlike an *in vitro* condition, it has been difficult to detect endogenous sulforaphane-Keap1 adduct formation in cells until now. In the same tenet, the experimental attempts to elucidate the exact phosphorylation-prone residues in Nrf2 protein and the upstream regulatory kinase(s), both of which are directly or indirectly altered by sulforaphane, are currently required. Together, these studies will enable us to understand, at least in part, how somatic mutations of Keap1 and Nrf2, found in several human cancers, contribute to variable individual chemopreventive susceptibility after consumption of cruciferous vegetables.

Acknowledgement

This research was supported by Basic Research Program through the National Research Foundation of Korea (NRF) funded by the Ministry of Education, Science and Technology (2011-0013733). The author thanks Dr. Joydeb Kumar Kundu (School of

Pharmacy, Seoul National University, Republic of Korea) for his kind help editing this manuscript.

Conflicts of interest

The author declares no conflicts of interest.

References

1. Surh, Y.J. 2003. Cancer chemoprevention with dietary phytochemicals. *Nat. Rev. Cancer* **3:** 768–780.
2. Surh, Y. 1999. Molecular mechanisms of chemopreventive effects of selected dietary and medicinal phenolic substances. *Mutat. Res.* **428:** 305–327.
3. Zhang, Y. *et al.* 1992. A major inducer of anticarcinogenic protective enzymes from broccoli: isolation and elucidation of structure. *Proc. Natl. Acad. Sci. USA* **89:** 2399–2403.
4. Shapiro, T.A. *et al.* 2001. Chemoprotective glucosinolates and isothiocyanates of broccoli sprouts: metabolism and excretion in humans. *Cancer Epidemiol. Biomarkers Prev.* **10:** 501–508.
5. Hu, R. *et al.* 2006. Cancer chemoprevention of intestinal polyposis in ApcMin/+ mice by sulforaphane, a natural product derived from cruciferous vegetable. *Carcinogenesis* **27:** 2038–2046.
6. Xu, C. *et al.* 2006. Inhibition of 7,12-dimethylbenz(a)anthracene-induced skin tumorigenesis in C57BL/6 mice by sulforaphane is mediated by nuclear factor E2-related factor 2. *Cancer Res.* **66:** 8293–8296.
7. Keum, Y.S. *et al.* 2009. Pharmacokinetics and pharmacodynamics of broccoli sprouts on the suppression of prostate cancer in transgenic adenocarcinoma of mouse prostate (TRAMP) mice: implication of induction of Nrf2, HO-1 and apoptosis and the suppression of Akt-dependent kinase pathway. *Pharm Res.* **26:** 2324–2331.
8. Zhang, Y. 2004. Cancer-preventive isothiocyanates: measurement of human exposure and mechanism of action. *Mutat. Res.* **555:** 173–190.
9. Kensler, T.W. *et al.* 2005. Effects of glucosinolate-rich broccoli sprouts on urinary levels of aflatoxin-DNA adducts and phenanthrene tetraols in a randomized clinical trial in He Zuo township, Qidong, People's Republic of China. *Cancer Epidemiol. Biomarkers Prev.* **14:** 2605–2613.
10. Seow, A. *et al.* 1998. Urinary total isothiocyanate (ITC) in a population-based sample of middle-aged and older Chinese in Singapore: relationship with dietary total ITC and glutathione S-transferase M1/T1/P1 genotypes. *Cancer Epidemiol. Biomarkers Prev.* **7:** 775–781.
11. Seow, A. *et al.* 2002. Dietary isothiocyanates, glutathione S-transferase polymorphisms and colorectal cancer risk in the Singapore Chinese Health Study. *Carcinogenesis* **23:** 2055–2061.
12. Clarke, J.D., R.H. Dashwood & E. Ho. 2008. Multi-targeted prevention of cancer by sulforaphane. *Cancer Lett.* **269:** 291–304.
13. Thimmulappa, R.K. *et al.* 2002. Identification of Nrf2-regulated genes induced by the chemopreventive agent sulforaphane by oligonucleotide microarray. *Cancer Res.* **62:** 5196–5203.
14. McMahon, M. *et al.* 2003. Keap1-dependent proteasomal degradation of transcription factor Nrf2 contributes to the negative regulation of antioxidant response element-driven gene expression. *J. Biol. Chem.* **278:** 21592–21600.
15. Itoh, K. *et al.* 1997. An Nrf2/small Maf heterodimer mediates the induction of phase II detoxifying enzyme genes through antioxidant response elements. *Biochem. Biophys. Res. Commun.* **236:** 313–322.
16. Taguchi, K., H. Motohashi & M. Yamamoto. 2011. Molecular mechanisms of the Keap1-Nrf2 pathway in stress response and cancer evolution. *Genes. Cells* **16:** 123–140.
17. Itoh, K. *et al.* 1999. Keap1 represses nuclear activation of antioxidant responsive elements by Nrf2 through binding to the amino-terminal Neh2 domain. *Genes Dev.* **13:** 76–86.
18. Xu, L. *et al.* 2003. BTB proteins are substrate-specific adaptors in an SCF-like modular ubiquitin ligase containing CUL-3. *Nature* **425:** 316–321.
19. Zhang, D.D. *et al.* 2004. Keap1 is a redox-regulated substrate adaptor protein for a Cul3-dependent ubiquitin ligase complex. *Mol. Cell Biol.* **24:** 10941–10953.
20. Tong, K.I. *et al.* 2006. Two-site substrate recognition model for the Keap1-Nrf2 system: a hinge and latch mechanism. *Biol. Chem.* **387:** 1311–1320.
21. Lo, S.C. & M. Hannink. 2008. PGAM5 tethers a ternary complex containing Keap1 and Nrf2 to mitochondria. *Exp. Cell Res.* **314:** 1789–1803.
22. Kobayashi, M. *et al.* 2009. The antioxidant defense system Keap1-Nrf2 comprises a multiple sensing mechanism for responding to a wide range of chemical compounds. *Mol. Cell Biol.* **29:** 493–502.
23. Zhang, D.D. & M. Hannink. 2003. Distinct cysteine residues in Keap1 are required for Keap1-dependent ubiquitination of Nrf2 and for stabilization of Nrf2 by chemopreventive agents and oxidative stress. *Mol. Cell Biol.* **23:** 8137–8151.
24. Hong, F., M.L. Freeman & D.C. Liebler. 2005. Identification of sensor cysteines in human Keap1 modified by the cancer chemopreventive agent sulforaphane. *Chem. Res. Toxicol.* **18:** 1917–1926.
25. Hu, C. *et al.* 2011. Modification of keap1 cysteine residues by sulforaphane. *Chem. Res. Toxicol.* **24:** 515–521.
26. Keum, Y.S. *et al.* 2006. Mechanism of action of sulforaphane: inhibition of p38 mitogen-activated protein kinase isoforms contributing to the induction of antioxidant response element-mediated heme oxygenase-1 in human hepatoma HepG2 cells. *Cancer Res.* **66:** 8804–8813.
27. Sun, Z., Z. Huang & D.D. Zhang. 2009. Phosphorylation of Nrf2 at multiple sites by MAP kinases has a limited contribution in modulating the Nrf2-dependent antioxidant response. *PLoS One* **4:** e6588.
28. Cheung, K.L. & A.N. Kong. 2010. Molecular targets of dietary phenethyl isothiocyanate and sulforaphane for cancer chemoprevention. *AAPS J.* **12:** 87–97.
29. Jain, A.K. & A.K. Jaiswal. 2006. Phosphorylation of tyrosine 568 controls nuclear export of Nrf2. *J. Biol. Chem.* **281:** 12132–12142.
30. Jain, A.K. & A.K. Jaiswal. 2007. GSK-3beta acts upstream of Fyn kinase in regulation of nuclear export and degradation of NF-E2 related factor 2. *J. Biol. Chem.* **282:** 16502–16510.

31. Rada, P. *et al.* 2011. SCF/{beta}-TrCP promotes glycogen synthase kinase 3-dependent degradation of the Nrf2 transcription factor in a Keap1-independent manner. *Mol. Cell Biol.* **31:** 1121–1133.

32. Rojo, A.I. *et al.* 2008. Functional interference between glycogen synthase kinase-3 beta and the transcription factor Nrf2 in protection against kainate-induced hippocampal cell death. *Mol. Cell Neurosci.* **39:** 125–132.